CBT WITH JUSTICE-INVOLVED CLIENTS

TREATMENT PLANS AND INTERVENTIONS FOR EVIDENCE-BASED PSYCHOTHERAPY

Robert L. Leahy, Series Editor

www.guilford.com/TPI

Each volume in this practical series synthesizes current information on a particular disorder or clinical population; shows practitioners how to develop specific, tailored treatment plans; and describes interventions proven to promote behavior change, reduce distress, and alleviate symptoms. Step-by-step guidelines for planning and implementing treatment are illustrated with rich case examples. User-friendly features include reproducible self-report forms, handouts, and symptom checklists, all in a convenient large-size format. Specific strategies for handling treatment roadblocks are also detailed. Emphasizing a collaborative approach to treatment, books in this series enable practitioners to offer their clients the very best in evidence-based practice.

TREATMENT PLANS AND INTERVENTIONS
FOR DEPRESSION AND ANXIETY DISORDERS, SECOND EDITION
Robert L. Leahy, Stephen J. F. Holland, and Lata K. McGinn

TREATMENT PLANS AND INTERVENTIONS
FOR BULIMIA AND BINGE-EATING DISORDER
Rene D. Zweig and Robert L. Leahy

TREATMENT PLANS AND INTERVENTIONS
FOR INSOMNIA: A CASE FORMULATION APPROACH
Rachel Manber and Colleen E. Carney

TREATMENT PLANS AND INTERVENTIONS
FOR OBSESSIVE–COMPULSIVE DISORDER
Simon A. Rego

CBT WITH JUSTICE-INVOLVED CLIENTS:
INTERVENTIONS FOR ANTISOCIAL AND SELF-DESTRUCTIVE BEHAVIORS
Raymond Chip Tafrate, Damon Mitchell, and David J. Simourd

CBT with Justice-Involved Clients

Interventions for Antisocial and Self-Destructive Behaviors

Raymond Chip Tafrate
Damon Mitchell
David J. Simourd

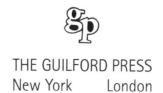

THE GUILFORD PRESS
New York   London

Copyright © 2018 The Guilford Press
A Division of Guilford Publications, Inc.
370 Seventh Avenue, Suite 1200, New York, NY 10001
www.guilford.com

Printed in the United States of America

This book is printed on acid-free paper.

Last digit is print number: 9 8 7 6 5 4 3 2 1

The authors have checked with sources believed to be reliable in their efforts to provide
information that is complete and generally in accord with the standards of practice that are
accepted at the time of publication. However, in view of the possibility of human error or
changes in behavioral, mental health, or medical sciences, neither the authors, nor the editor
and publisher, nor any other party who has been involved in the preparation or publication
of this work warrants that the information contained herein is in every respect accurate or
complete, and they are not responsible for any errors or omissions or the results obtained from
the use of such information. Readers are encouraged to confirm the information contained in
this book with other sources.

All case material is a composite of multiple individuals whose identities have been disguised and
fictionalized.

Library of Congress Cataloging-in-Publication Data

Names: Tafrate, Raymond Chip, author. | Mitchell, Damon, 1969– author. | Simourd, David J.,
   author.
Title: CBT with justice-involved clients : interventions for antisocial and self-destructive
   behaviors / Raymond Chip Tafrate, Damon Mitchell, and David J. Simourd.
Description: New York, NY : The Guilford Press, [2018] | Series: Treatment plans and
   interventions for evidence-based psychotherapy | Includes bibliographical references and
   index.
Identifiers: LCCN 2018011238| ISBN 9781462534920 (hardback) | ISBN 9781462534906
   (paperback)
Subjects: LCSH: Criminals—Mental health—Case studies. | Criminals—Rehabilitation—Case
   studies. | Forensic psychology—Case studies. | BISAC: PSYCHOLOGY / Forensic
   Psychology. | MEDICAL / Psychiatry / General. | SOCIAL SCIENCE / Social Work.
Classification: LCC RC451.4.P68 T34 2018 | DDC 616.89/142086927—dc23
LC record available at *https://lccn.loc.gov/2018011238*

To accuse others for one's own misfortunes is a sign of want of education. To accuse oneself shows that one's education has begun. To accuse neither oneself nor others shows that one's education is complete.

—ATTRIBUTED TO EPICTETUS (55–135 C.E.)

About the Authors

Raymond Chip Tafrate, PhD, a clinical psychologist, is Professor of Criminology and Criminal Justice at Central Connecticut State University. He co-chairs the Forensic Issues and Externalizing Behaviors special interest group for the Association for Behavioral and Cognitive Therapies, is a Fellow and Supervisor at the Albert Ellis Institute in New York City, and is a member of the Motivational Interviewing Network of Trainers. Dr. Tafrate frequently consults with criminal justice agencies regarding difficult-to-change problems such as anger dysregulation and criminal behavior. He has presented his research throughout North America, Europe, Asia, and Australia, and has published numerous journal articles, book chapters, and books.

Damon Mitchell, PhD, a clinical psychologist, is Professor of Criminology and Criminal Justice at Central Connecticut State University. As a criminal justice consultant, Dr. Mitchell has developed and delivered training workshops related to forensic assessment and treatment and has conducted evaluations of criminal justice programs. He has published numerous journal articles and book chapters as well as a coedited book.

David J. Simourd, PhD, CPsych, is in private practice in Kingston, Ontario, Canada, and has been involved in forensic psychological assessment and treatment since 1992. In addition to his clinical work, Dr. Simourd has published articles, delivered training workshops, and served as a consultant on offender assessment and treatment to a variety of correctional organizations throughout North America, Asia, and the Caribbean. He is on the editorial board of *Criminal Justice and Behavior* and is a member of the Ontario Review Board, the civil commitment board for mentally disordered offenders in Ontario.

Preface

This treatment planner is designed as a practical resource providing structure, guidance, and skills for working effectively with justice-involved clients (JICs). Since we recognize the immense variability within this clinical group, and the breadth of environments where treatment is delivered, a manualized session-by-session program seems unrealistic. Rather, this treatment planner is organized around broad phases of the treatment process that will be applicable to working with JICs across a wide range of forensic settings.

This is not the kind of book to read from cover to cover in one sitting. Also, just reading the material will not be enough for you to become proficient in working with this population. It is essential to try the skills described in this treatment planner in your clinical work and observe how JICs respond. Flexibility will also be important, as you will have to make decisions about which sections and chapters are most relevant for a particular case. We recommend that you review one chapter at a time while thoughtfully transferring the knowledge and skills to real-world sessions. The hope is that with practice and repetition, the material contained within this treatment planner will come alive in your day-to-day practice.

ORGANIZATION AND FEATURES OF THIS PLANNER

This treatment planner is organized into six parts. Part I, Forensic Basics (Chapters 1 and 2), provides an essential foundation of knowledge for applying the skills described throughout the subsequent sections of the planner. Part II, Engagement (Chapters 3 and 4), presents strategies for successfully engaging JICs in treatment and fostering their internal motivation for making changes in life domains most linked to criminal behavior. Part III, Assessment, Case Formulation, and Focus (Chapters 5, 6, and 7), offers guidelines for assessment, case formulation, and establishing collaborative treatment goals. The chapters in Part IV, Detailed Treatment Plans for Criminogenic Thinking and Antisocial Orientation (Chapters 8 and 9), describe specific interventions designed to restructure JICs' antisocial attitudes and improve their decision making. Part V, Detailed Treatment Plans for Harmful Lifestyle Patterns (Chapters 10, 11, and 12), emphasizes specific behavioral interventions for helping JICs alter their routines, relationships, and destructive habits (e.g., substance use and anger dysregulation). Finally, Part VI, Practice Management (Chapter 13), outlines a model for report writing and documenting treatment progress. The book concludes with a brief Postscript, two Appendices, and a References list.

In many chapters, you will find guidelines, scripts, and forms to help you utilize the specific skills presented and discussed. All scripts and forms are provided at the ends of their corresponding chapters. The scripts suggest specific wording for you to try when working with JICs. We have found in our own clinical work, and through research and consulting with practitioners across a variety of criminal justice agencies and programs, that a critical but often overlooked skill set is the ability to launch into productive conversations. The scripts help you introduce difficult-to-talk-about topics in a way that is beneficial to JICs. They also provide a structure for keeping conversations focused and efficient, which may be of particular concern if you are conducting brief supervision sessions in probation and parole contexts. You are more likely to experience immediate success with the proposed skills when sticking to the scripts. Finally, because you will go into interactions with a game plan for how to structure your discussions of treatment, you will have greater freedom to focus your attention on JICs' reactions.

A disadvantage of using scripts is that at first they can feel clunky and unnatural, because they are not your own words. It is important to try to deliver the scripted material in a way that is as natural as possible; just reading the words in a robotic fashion is unlikely to produce positive outcomes. Also, being too bound to the scripts can result in a loss of flexibility in conversations —flexibility that is often useful in real-world treatment. The scripts provided in this treatment planner are best viewed as starting points for conversations. In many cases, you will have to fill in the gaps in order to move conversations forward. Nonetheless, we recommend staying as close as possible to the wording as you begin to learn these scripts. With practice and repetition, the skills will begin to feel more natural. Of course, the goal is not to have you forever reading from scripts; rather, it is to allow you to become fluent enough with the skills that you develop a foundational competence. Once that competence is reached, you can feel free to put the scripts away, become more flexible with the material, and create variations of your own that work best for your JICs' needs. In that sense, scripts are a bit like training wheels on a bicycle.

At its heart, this is a "how-to" book about clinical assessment and treatment, with greater emphasis placed on treatment. A predominant theme of this book is the notion that treatment is driven by high-quality assessment. The guidelines for assessment and case formulation presented in this treatment planner are offered as clinical procedures for identifying the most relevant treatment targets for individual JICs. This is not a book about how to conduct *risk assessment* per se. The general topic of risk assessment is a specialty area with its own unique terminology and practices. A specific feature of risk assessment is the prediction of outcomes (e.g., reoffending) through using probability estimates. Our assessment guidelines are not recommended for making statistical estimates regarding probabilities of future criminal behavior. Nonetheless, we refer to materials to consider for conducting risk assessment, and we suggest ways to integrate information obtained from validated risk instruments into treatment planning.

LABELS AND LANGUAGE

There are too many terms commonly used to describe people receiving services in criminal justice settings: *offender, juvenile delinquent, probationer, parolee, prisoner, inmate, court-mandated client,* and *patient,* to name just a few. We have chosen to use the term *justice-involved client* (JIC) throughout this treatment planner. The abbreviation JIC is not intended to communicate any notion of inherent badness; instead, it is meant to convey the complexities and challenges associated with the larger context in which treatment is delivered. We believe that this term best captures the population this treatment planner addresses, while sidestepping the pitfalls of pejorative labels. The terms *traditional counseling client* and *psychotherapy client* are occasionally used to describe individuals seeking services for common mental health disorders, such as anxiety and depression.

Similarly, many terms are used to describe professionals who deliver services and care in criminal justice settings: *correctional counselor, therapist, clinician, case manager, probation officer, parole officer, social worker,* and so on. Often the terminology that emerges develops from the cultural norms and jargon of specific agencies, programs, and facilities. We have decided to use the term *practitioner* to describe the vast array of professionals who may work in forensic environments.

Finally, there is variation in how services are described across different environments; *intervention, programming,* and *supervision* are some examples. Since behavior change is at the heart of this treatment planner, we have decided to use the term *treatment* to describe the activities that are presented. Of course, such terminology sometimes falls short in accurately describing all people, roles, and circumstances. If you are more comfortable with other terms that depict your clients, job title, and work activities, please feel free to continue using them and to substitute them for our terms in the scripts.

Acknowledgments

We begin with thanks to Robert L. Leahy and Jim Nageotte for the opportunity to contribute this volume to the Treatment Plans and Interventions for Evidence-Based Psychotherapy series. We are most appreciative of their recognition of forensic treatment as an important area of clinical practice. Their enthusiasm, support, and ongoing editorial feedback helped to guide this project. We would also like to thank the production team at The Guilford Press for helping to shape this book into its final form; in particular, we thank Barbara Watkins for her feedback on an early version of the manuscript, Marie Sprayberry and Anna Brackett for their thoughtful editing, and Jane Keislar for organizing the many details inherent in bringing a project like this to completion.

There are many individuals and organizations who influenced our approach to this volume and to whom we owe many thanks. First and foremost, we are grateful to our friend and collaborator Tom Hogan, a retired probation officer who has worked with us for many years in the field perfecting the use of cognitive-behavioral therapy (CBT) principles in probation settings. Tom shares our passion for this work, and his ideas echo throughout this treatment planner. We are also indebted to the probation officer coaches in our Forensic CBT Program, which provided a kind of incubator for the development of some of the strategies and techniques discussed in this volume: Bethany LaPierre, Lisa Correa, Alex Dias, Margarita Gonzalez, Reginald Stanford, Sara Stone, Rick Sutterlin, and John Watts. The Forensic CBT Program was itself a product of the U.S. Bureau of Justice's SMART Probation grant 2012-SM-BX-0003, and we are thankful to that agency and all who worked on, and participated in, that project. On the juvenile probation side, we also thank Casey O'Neill, Meghan Korn, and Mark Irons for their creative ideas that emerged from the youth risk/need assessment project.

We are fortunate to have served as consultants to a number of state agencies and community organizations that have shaped our perspective on criminal justice practice, including the State of Connecticut Court Support Services Division, the State of Connecticut Department of Mental Health and Addiction Services, the State of Connecticut Department of Correction, Community Solutions Inc., the Connection Inc, and Wheeler Clinic. A special thanks to Ryan Quirk at King County Jails and Jon Venditti at Community Solutions, who made valuable suggestions that were incorporated into this treatment planner. As always, many thanks to long-time collaborator Howard Kassinove, whose ideas heavily influenced the material on managing anger.

We are grateful to work at an institution like Central Connecticut State University (CCSU), with great colleagues in the Department of Criminology and Criminal Justice, and with Dean Susan Pease, who fosters a culture of creative activity in the College of Liberal Arts and Social Sciences. CCSU has provided us with release time for research, financial support, and a sabbatical leave without which we could not have completed this project. We would also like to acknowledge our graduate assistants, Rebecca Bruey and Joseph Lupacchino, for their creative help with literature reviews and "office work" parts of the book.

Finally, special thanks to our families for their patience and support during the nights and weekends in which we prepared the book. We appreciate all you have done for us.

RAYMOND CHIP TAFRATE
DAMON MITCHELL

This book represents, for me, the expression of an ongoing professional journey of blending my understanding of the science of forensic psychology into assessment and treatment interactions with those in conflict with the law. I have been a clinician my entire professional career, and my influence in this book reflects what I have learned through clinical trial and error over the past 20+ years. The great enjoyment and success I have had as a psychologist during this time could not have been possible without the teaching, mentorship, and collegial relations of great people.

By sheer coincidence and great professional good luck, I began my forensic experience in Penetanguishene, Ontario, Canada, at the exact time the Violence Risk Appraisal Guide was being developed. My exposure to Vern Quinsey, Marnie Rice, Grant Harris, Terry Chaplin, and Catherine Cormier was professionally inspiring and socially enjoyable. Shortly thereafter, I began my doctoral studies in "the lab" at Carleton University in 1989; my time at Carleton coincided exactly, as it turned out, with the origins of the risk–need–responsivity (RNR) movement. The RNR philosophy produced a tectonic shift in corrections that is commonplace today. Being around Don Andrews, Jim Bonta, Steve Wormith, Paul Gendreau, and others, and participating in the infamous "lab meetings," provided the conceptual foundation that I have carried throughout my career. To top off all that, my supervisor, Bob Hoge, provided fantastic knowledge, support, encouragement, and mentorship—and along with his wife, Lynda, a lifetime of great social memories that I still cherish to this day.

My career and thinking have been blessed with influences from new relationships that have been equally inspiring to my professional and personal lives. My friends from Saskatchewan (Mark Olver, Kiera Stockdale, Ross Keele, and Steve Wong in the early days) easily come to mind. The professional discussions and debates with Tom Powell from Vermont have been insightful, and the socializing legendary. Bryan Brandenburg from Alaska has reinforced the idea that improving correctional operations can be easily achieved through commitment and a plan. There are also several people with whom I have had the pleasure of sharing occasional F-bombs about crazy correctional practices, and who are inspirations to "fighting the good fight" to ensure that correctional practice is done properly. In no particular order, they are Bree Derrick, Jason Stauffer, Rich Pudguski, Dan Lomardo, Jennifer Ferguson, Billie Grobe, and John Blette.

Professional careers, however, are nothing without family and friends. My lifelong "boys' weekend" buddies (my golfing and hunting friends) have always provided a basis in reality for my professional life and thinking. Nothing compares, however, to the joy and gratitude I feel toward my family. My daughters, Melanie and Lindsay, have been understanding and tolerant of my time commitments for this book and other professional obligations. (They have been even more accepting and tolerant of my humor, which they insist "isn't that funny.") Finally, my wife, Linda Simourd, has been with me every step of the way and has aided in my professional and personal growth over many years. There is no way I could have done what I have done without her.

DAVID J. SIMOURD

Contents

List of Figures, Tables, Scripts, and Forms   xvi

PART I. FORENSIC BASICS

CHAPTER 1.   **The Forensic Treatment Landscape**   3

What Is Working with JICs Like?   4
Community versus Custody: Different Settings and Challenges   5
Justice Involvement: The Scope of the Problem   7
What Works in Reducing Criminal Behavior?   8
Is Diagnosis Important?   9
A General Treatment Plan   10
What Do Sessions Look Like?   10
Realistic Expectations   12

CHAPTER 2.   **An Integrated Forensic Cognitive-Behavioral Therapy Approach**   14

Focusing on Criminal Risk Domains   15
Addressing Thinking Patterns That Promote Criminality   21
Enhancing Motivation for Change   24
Clarifying Values and Life Priorities   27

PART II. ENGAGEMENT

CHAPTER 3.   **Successfully Engaging Justice-Involved Clients**   31

Motivational Interviewing and OARS Skills   32
Engaging: Tips for the Initial Session   36
Putting It into Practice   37

CHAPTER 4.   **Clarifying Values and Life Priorities**   42

Why Work on Values with JICs?   42
Distinguishing Values from Goals   44

Identifying and Discussing Values 45
*Discussing Discrepancy versus Consistency between Values
and Decisions* 50

PART III. ASSESSMENT, CASE FORMULATION, AND FOCUS

CHAPTER 5. **Assessing Criminal Risk Domains** 65

Overview of Assessment and Case Formulation 65
*Assessing Criminal Risk Domains:
Guidelines for the Assessment Interview* 66

CHAPTER 6. **Case Formulation** 88

Formulating Judgments about Risk 89
Identifying Treatment Targets 91
Formulating a Treatment Plan 93
Avoiding Bias in Case Formulation 105

CHAPTER 7. **Establishing Collaborative Goals and Focusing Conversations** 115

Evoking Motivation for Change in Criminal Risk Domains 116
What Is Focusing? 121
Strategies for Establishing Goals and Focusing Conversations 121
What If I Can't Get Agreement on a Focus? 125

PART IV. DETAILED TREATMENT PLANS FOR CRIMINOGENIC THINKING AND ANTISOCIAL ORIENTATION

CHAPTER 8. **Connecting Criminogenic Thinking to Decision Making in Criminal Risk Domains** 135

Cognitive versus Behavioral Components of Criminal Risk Domains 135
Levels of Criminogenic Thinking 136
*Connecting Criminogenic Thoughts and Decisions within Criminal
Risk Domains* 140
*Connecting Criminogenic Thinking Patterns and Decisions across Criminal
Risk Domains* 144

CHAPTER 9. **Monitoring and Restructuring Criminogenic Thinking** 155

Monitoring 155
Restructuring 158

PART V. DETAILED TREATMENT PLANS FOR HARMFUL LIFESTYLE PATTERNS

CHAPTER 10. **Developing New Routines: Leisure Activities and Employment/Education** 173

Leisure Activities 174
Employment and Education 179

CHAPTER 11. **Restructuring Relationships: Friends and Family** 198

Altering Close Friendships 199
Changing Family Dynamics 204

CHAPTER 12. **Managing Destructive Habits: Substance Use and Anger Reactions** 215

Changing Substance Use Patterns 215
Managing Anger 226

PART VI. PRACTICE MANAGEMENT

CHAPTER 13. **Documentation and Report Writing** 249

Tips for Writing an Effective Assessment and Treatment Plan Report 250
A Template for an Assessment and Treatment Plan Report 251
Providing Feedback to JICs on Their Clinical Data 254
Monitoring and Documenting Clinical Progress within Sessions 262
A Template for a Treatment Summary Report 263

Postscript 281

APPENDIX A. **Standardized Test Recommendations** 283

APPENDIX B. **Resources for Practitioners** 287

Books 287
Professional Organizations 287

References 289

Index 297

List of Figures, Tables, Scripts, and Forms

FIGURES

FIGURE 2.1.   Criminal Risk Domains Quiz   16

FIGURE 4.1.   Hank's Completed Values Helpsheet   47

FIGURE 6.1.   Criminal Event Analysis: Hank's Most Recent Offense   94

FIGURE 6.2.   Criminal Event Analysis: Jackie's Most Recent Offense   95

FIGURE 6.3.   Hank's Criminal Risk Domains Worksheet   96

FIGURE 6.4.   Jackie's Criminal Risk Domains Worksheet   96

FIGURE 6.5.   Hank's Case Formulation Worksheet   97

FIGURE 6.6.   Jackie's Case Formulation Worksheet   101

FIGURE 7.1.   Recognizing Change Talk Exercise   118

FIGURE 8.1.   Relationship between Criminogenic Thinking Patterns and Thoughts   137

FIGURE 9.1.   Jackie's Completed Thinking Helpsheet   159

FIGURE 10.1.   Jackie's Completed My Typical Weekday Form   177

FIGURE 10.2.   Jackie's Completed Questions to Ask Myself   178
               about How I Spend My Time Form

FIGURE 10.3.   Jackie's Completed Questions to Ask Myself   181
               about Education and Employment Form

FIGURE 10.4.   Checklist of Practical Issues to Address Prior to Job Searching   183

FIGURE 11.1.   Jackie's Completed Looking at My Close Friends Form   201

FIGURE 11.2.   Jackie's Completed Questions to Ask Myself   203
about My Close Friends Form

FIGURE 11.3.   Jackie's Completed Looking at My Family   205
and Romantic Relationships Form

FIGURE 11.4.   Jackie's Completed Questions to Ask Myself about My Family   207
and Romantic Relationships Form

FIGURE 12.1.   Hank's Completed Looking at My Substance Use Form   220

FIGURE 12.2.   Hank's Completed Questions, Answers, and Next Steps   223
for My Substance Use Form

FIGURE 12.3.   Hank's Completed Announcing Change Form   225

FIGURE 12.4.   The Anger Episode Model   228

FIGURE 12.5.   Hank's Completed Anger Episode Record   231

FIGURE 13.1.   Assessment and Treatment Plan Report for Hank   255

FIGURE 13.2.   Assessment Profile for Hank   261

FIGURE 13.3.   Session Record: Initial Session with Hank   264

FIGURE 13.4.   Session Record: 10th Session with Hank   265

FIGURE 13.5.   Treatment Summary Report for Hank's Anger   267
Management Intervention

TABLES

TABLE 1.1.   General Plan of Treatment for JICs   10

TABLE 1.2.   General Session Structure   12

TABLE 2.1.   Criminal Risk Domains   18

TABLE 2.2.   Overview of Criminogenic Thinking Patterns   23

TABLE 3.1.   Converting Fact-Gathering, Closed Questions to Open Questions   33

TABLE 3.2.   Forming Affirmations   34

TABLE 3.3.   Forming Reflections   35

TABLE 3.4.   Forming Summaries   35

TABLE 3.5.   Responding to Challenging JIC Statements in the Initial Session   38

TABLE 5.1. Additional Questions for Eliciting Specific Criminogenic Thinking Patterns 71

TABLE 6.1. Secondary Domains to Consider in Case Formulation 92

TABLE 7.1. Questions Likely to Evoke Change Talk 119

TABLE 7.2. Focusing Questions 122

TABLE 7.3. JIC Reactions to Assessment Feedback and Practitioner Responses 125

TABLE 8.1. Criminogenic Thinking Patterns and Criminogenic Thoughts 138

TABLE 12.1. Examples of Cognitive Restructuring for Anger 234

TABLE A.1. Selected Instruments for Assessing Broad-Based Criminal Risk Domains 284

TABLE A.2. Specialized Tests for Assessing Criminogenic Thinking 284

TABLE A.3. Specialized Tests for Assessing Substance Use 285

TABLE A.4. Specialized Tests for Assessing Dysfunctional Anger 285

TABLE A.5. Specialized Tests for Assessing Response Bias 285

TABLE A.6. Specialized Tests for Assessing Readiness to Change 286

SCRIPTS

SCRIPT 3.1. Sample Opening Statements 40

SCRIPT 4.1. Instructions for Introducing the Values Helpsheet 55

SCRIPT 4.2. Following Up on Next Steps Connected to Values 57

SCRIPT 4.3. Discussing Discrepancy versus Consistency between Values and Decisions 58

SCRIPT 5.1. Introducing Assessment: Opening Statement 73

SCRIPT 5.2. Sample Questions for Assessing History of Criminal/Antisocial Behavior 74

SCRIPT 5.3. Sample Questions for Assessing Dysfunctional Family/Romantic Relationships 76

SCRIPT 5.4. Sample Questions for Assessing Lack of Connection to Work/School 78

SCRIPT 5.5. Sample Questions for Assessing Antisocial Companions 81

SCRIPT 5.6. Sample Questions for Assessing Maladaptive Leisure Time 83

SCRIPT 5.7. Sample Questions for Assessing Substance Abuse/Misuse 84

SCRIPT 5.8. Sample Questions for Assessing   86
            Criminogenic Thinking/Antisocial Orientation

SCRIPT 5.9. Sample Questions for Assessing Anger Dysregulation   87

SCRIPT 7.1. Examples of Focusing and Presenting Options   127

SCRIPT 7.2. Focusing on Criminal Risk Domains (to Be Used with Form 7.1)   128

SCRIPT 7.3. Focusing on Criminogenic Thinking Patterns (to Be Used with Script 7.4) 129

SCRIPT 7.4. Describing Criminogenic Thinking Patterns to JICs   130
            (to Be Used with Script 7.3)

SCRIPT 7.5. Providing Feedback on Standardized Assessments   131

SCRIPT 8.1. RTD–Companions Sequence   147

SCRIPT 8.2. RTD–Leisure Sequence   148

SCRIPT 8.3. RTD–Family/Romantic Sequence   149

SCRIPT 8.4. RTD–Substance Misuse Sequence   150

SCRIPT 8.5. RTD–Work/School Sequence   151

SCRIPT 8.6. RTD–Anger Sequence   152

SCRIPT 8.7. TPI Analysis   153

SCRIPT 9.1. Assigning the Thinking Helpsheet   164

SCRIPT 9.2. The Two Voices Role Play   166

SCRIPT 9.3. Guidelines for Other Restructuring Strategies   168

SCRIPT 10.1. Introducing Activity-Monitoring Forms   188
             (My Typical Weekday/My Typical Saturday)

SCRIPT 10.2. Script for Rating Activities   189

SCRIPT 10.3. Questions to Ask JICs about Work   190

SCRIPT 11.1. Discussing Close Friendships   209

SCRIPT 11.2. Discussing Family Relationships   210

SCRIPT 12.1. Assigning the Log of Weekly Substance Use   236

SCRIPT 12.2. Steps for Announcing Change   237

SCRIPT 12.3. Steps for Analyzing Anger Episodes   239

SCRIPT 13.1. Describing an Assessment Profile: The Example of Hank   269

FORMS

FORM 3.1.   Coding Sheet for the First Session   41

FORM 4.1.   Values Helpsheet   60

FORM 6.1.   Criminal Event Analysis   109

FORM 6.2.   Criminal Risk Domains Worksheet   110

FORM 6.3.   Case Formulation Worksheet   111

FORM 7.1.   Life Areas That Put Me at Risk   132

FORM 9.1.   Thinking Helpsheet   170

FORM 10.1.   My Typical Weekday   192

FORM 10.2.   My Typical Saturday   193

FORM 10.3.   Looking at My Life and Rating My Activities   194

FORM 10.4.   Questions to Ask Myself about How I Spend My Time   195

FORM 10.5.   Questions to Ask Myself about Education and Employment   196

FORM 10.6.   Education and Employment History Checklist   197

FORM 11.1.   Looking at My Close Friends   211

FORM 11.2.   Questions to Ask Myself about My Close Friends   212

FORM 11.3.   Looking at My Family and Romantic Relationships   213

FORM 11.4.   Questions to Ask Myself about My Family and Romantic Relationships   214

FORM 12.1.   Looking at My Substance Use   240

FORM 12.2.   Log of Weekly Substance Use   241

FORM 12.3.   Questions, Answers, and Next Steps for My Substance Use   242

FORM 12.4.   Announcing Change   243

FORM 12.5.   Anger Episode Record   244

FORM 12.6.   Questions to Ask Myself about My Anger   246

FORM 13.1.   Assessment and Treatment Plan Report Template   271

FORM 13.2.   Assessment Profile Template   277

FORM 13.3.   Session Record Template   278

FORM 13.4.   Treatment Summary Report Template   279

PART I

FORENSIC BASICS

CHAPTER 1

The Forensic Treatment Landscape

Brenda has a master's degree in counseling and has recently completed a clinical internship at a university counseling center, where she mainly works with college students experiencing adjustment, depressive, and anxiety disorders. Eager to broaden her clinical experiences, she begins an internship at a criminal justice day reporting center that provides case management, urine drug testing, individual and group counseling, and psychoeducational programs for clients in various stages of criminal justice involvement (e.g., pretrial, probation, and parole). Her first client is Hank, a 25-year-old male referred by the court for "evaluation/counseling" after an arrest for assaulting a female acquaintance. His case is awaiting trial/plea bargaining.

Before her first appointment with Hank, Brenda reviews the limited available information. The referral document from the court provides few details about the incident, except the list of charges and the bail amount. There is also a dearth of information on Hank's psychosocial history. He is noted to have prior convictions for possession/sale of drugs, larceny, and driving under the influence (DUI). To make matters even murkier, on the standard intake form where clients are asked to write the nature of their presenting problem, Hank has only written: "Court sent me here." When Brenda enters the waiting room to meet Hank, he looks up and makes minimal eye contact, scowling. He nonverbally communicates irritation and a sense of being unfairly put upon by the referral to the day reporting center.

In the face of such an unpromising beginning, Brenda senses that she is in a landscape quite unlike that of her prior clinical experiences. Among the questions she silently asks herself are these:

"What did I get myself into?"
"Are all the clients going to be like this?"
"What will it take to develop a therapeutic relationship?"
"What is effective with these types of clients?"
"Does the fact that Hank is court-involved change the clinical focus of treatment and intervention?"
"What risk does Hank pose to me and the community?"

This treatment planner provides a practical guide for working with justice-involved clients (JICs). It is designed for a diverse range of professionals who work with JICs, including psychologists, social workers, counselors, case managers, community program practitioners, probation officers, and parole officers. The plans and interventions discussed in this book are generally applicable to a wide array of JICs who may be seen in various forensic environments, such as prisons, jails, detention centers, probation and parole departments, day reporting centers, halfway houses, sober houses, and court-mandated community programs. The plans and interventions can also be integrated into different types of activities relevant to behavior change, such as treatment, case management, and supervision.

The initial chapters of this treatment planner address some of the questions raised by Brenda. They highlight key issues for working with JICs that are different from working with individuals in traditional counseling and psychotherapy. Subsequent chapters focus on matters of engagement, as well as assessment and case formulation; describe specific interventions to modify harmful thinking/orientation and lifestyle patterns; and offer templates for documentation and report writing. The present chapter provides an overview of the forensic treatment landscape and offers recommendations for getting the most out of this treatment planner.

WHAT IS WORKING WITH JICs LIKE?

If you have worked in traditional counseling or psychotherapy settings, it was probably quite natural for you to have sympathy, empathy, and a desire to help those seeking services. This may not be initially the case in conducting forensic treatment. By definition, a JIC has been arrested for some type of criminal act that may have caused harm and suffering to someone else, which makes forensic work a perpetrator-based enterprise. For example, JICs may readily acknowledge engaging in physical assault, sexual abuse, drug selling, conning, and theft. They may justify their actions, express no remorse for their behavior, minimize its consequences to others, or even blame those who have been victimized. It is not uncommon—indeed, it is quite typical—to experience automatic, and negative, emotional responses to such individuals. Displaying compassion toward some JICs may not feel natural. Compassion, generally defined as "sensitivity to the suffering of others and a desire to alleviate suffering" (Kolts & Chodron, 2013, p. 7), is foundational in most helping relationships. As with traditional mental health clients, genuine caring about JICs' lives is an essential ingredient for establishing productive working relationships, and thus a prerequisite for overall effectiveness. Burnout is a particular concern in settings where high-volume contact with JICs is the norm, and in some environments practitioners must continually monitor their capacity to approach treatment with a level of empathy and compassion for those with whom they work.

The ramifications of weak or unsuccessful treatment constitute another key issue. The costs of failing to effect change with JICs can be quite serious, resulting in a loss of their freedom that will negatively affect such individuals (and their families) for years to come. Suboptimal treatment with JICs can also result in unchanged criminal risk profiles, the consequences of which are future criminality and victimization that can ripple out and create suffering for others and the larger community.

The mechanisms through which JICs are referred for services are usually different from those in traditional counseling, where clients willingly seek out services in order to alleviate distressing symptoms or receive support for dealing with problems. In traditional counseling, even when clients are compelled to get help, the process is typically initiated by concerned others, such as family members (e.g., "I'm really concerned your depression is getting worse"), friends ("Go to counseling; your worrying is driving me crazy"), or employers ("You should attend a stress management program to help you manage the workload"). In contrast, the ubiquity and degree of the coercion that brings JICs into treatment ("Attend a treatment program as a condition of probation, or go to jail") are hallmarks of working in forensic settings.

In many ways, JICs can be strikingly similar to unmotivated psychotherapy clients. However, because of the external factors that usually compel JICs to participate in treatment, you will initially find yourself devoting more time and energy to engaging such clients and identifying appropriate goals. The development of a productive working alliance and agreement on a treatment focus is likely to be more labor-intensive with JICs. Even when JICs appear willing to try treatment, they may exhibit a lack of enthusiasm and eagerness to participate fully in the intervention process.

Understanding two basic assumptions underlying treatment with JICs will help you navigate criminal justice bureaucracies and more effectively focus assessments and interventions.

1. *Reductions in criminal behavior and recidivism are the overarching goals of treatment.* The primary aim of forensic treatment is to prevent future criminality. In contrast, mental health counselors and psychotherapists usually focus on diagnosable disorders, and the symptoms associated with those disorders are viewed as problems to be resolved. JICs are a diverse client group, and many individuals will not meet the diagnostic criteria for any specific disorder. For the benefit of both the clients and the community, success with JICs is best measured in terms of subsequent declines in criminal behavior and criminal justice involvement.

2. *The focus of treatment is on improved functioning in life domains statistically linked with criminal behavior.* It is not uncommon for JICs to attend treatment with minimal symptoms and not much subjective distress. Therefore, their functioning within specific criminal risk domains, and not their symptoms, is what will most often dictate the targets of treatment. These criminal risk domains are introduced later in this chapter and described in detail in Chapter 2. They become the clinical focal points of the interventions presented throughout this treatment planner.

COMMUNITY VERSUS CUSTODY: DIFFERENT SETTINGS AND CHALLENGES

Treatment and intervention with JICs occur in settings that vary in their degree of integration into the larger community—from correctional institutions far from clients' families and friends, to day reporting centers in the same communities where JICs live. You are probably reading this treatment planner because you work (or will be working) in a setting similar to one described below. Keep in mind that the strategies we present are designed to be flexible and easily adapted to the types of environments where JICs are most commonly seen.

Community Settings

The largest proportion of the JIC population is not physically confined in a jail or prison; it comprises the millions of individuals who are living in the community under some form of criminal justice supervision. JICs supervised in the community include *probationers* (who are typically serving their entire sentence in the community), *parolees* (who are released from prison early and serving the remainder of their sentence in the community), and *pretrial defendants* (who are permitted to reside in the community on bail bond while awaiting trial). Community settings that specialize in services for JICs include day reporting centers, drug courts, halfway houses, and transitional housing programs. Some facilities are operated directly by government agencies, while others are run by not-for-profit or private organizations. At day reporting centers, clients are typically mandated to report several days per week for periods as brief as 30 days or as long as several months or more. Day reporting centers often provide treatment, educational, and employment services, as well as drug and alcohol monitoring. Halfway houses and transitional housing programs typically provide similar services as well as housing and meals, and stays can be as long as a year. Some JICs end up in traditional outpatient settings where they pay for services or use insurance to reimburse treatment providers, although this arrangement is less common.

One common challenge about working in community settings is that services are most often court-mandated. The clients may not want to be there, present as uninterested in treatment, and be resentful of supervision and other mandated conditions such as drug testing. JICs' progress in community programs is typically monitored by the referring courts or criminal justice agencies. You may be required to submit regular written reports documenting clients' attendance, participation, and progress (Chapter 13 provides sample reports). Such documentation is typically more burdensome for practitioners in community settings than for those who work in custody settings (described below). Confidentiality is generally more limited than it is in traditional counseling and psychotherapy. You may be expected to be in regular telephone contact with a probation or parole officer, and provide information on JICs' verbal disclosures, employment status, violations of protective and no-contact orders, and drug test results. For this reason, working in the community with JICs involves a more complex practitioner role—a role that often blends the goals of behavior change, monitoring, and community safety in different proportions, depending on the job and setting.

Custody Settings

Custody settings include state and federal prisons, jails (which are distinct from prisons in that clients are awaiting trial or serving only short sentences), and juvenile detention centers. For JICs who are incarcerated, the treatment environment poses some unique challenges that are not commonly encountered in outpatient settings. In correctional institutions, the clients are, in principle, always available for their appointments. However, in actual practice, the needs of the custody staff—which are focused on the safe and orderly operation of the institution—take precedence over any therapeutic activities. There are periods allotted for "inmate movement," when clients may move from their cells or dormitory to other locations for work, school, or counseling. Within these confines, appointments may be canceled due to lockdowns, staffing shortages, or a host of other administrative concerns that are beyond a client's or practitioner's control.

Similarly, the termination of care may be dictated by reasons other than the successful attainment of treatment goals: No warning may be given about a JIC's transfer from one institution to another, leading to an abrupt and unplanned ending of an intervention protocol. Such premature terminations may exacerbate dysfunctional thinking and behavior patterns. To minimize harm and the potential loss of treatment gains in custody settings, you should occasionally discuss the possibility of unwanted termination and develop a plan to counter potential negative reactions.

Some correctional institutions may not have traditional professional office arrangements. Sessions are sometimes conducted at a JIC's cell door, in the "chow hall," in a visitation/interview area where JIC and practitioner are separated by glass, or in multipurpose rooms within the facility that afford limited privacy. In any of these settings, conversations can be overheard, and a JIC's status as a "mental health patient" is visible to staff and inmates. Even in institutions where professional space exists, practitioners may be surprised to find that offices are equipped with large windows so that staff–inmate interactions can be observed for safety purposes. This can be distracting and limit privacy, as other inmates, as well as custody staff, can see who is in treatment. Another consideration is that JICs who are assigned homework as part of treatment will typically be bringing their assignments back to a small cell shared with one or more other people; or they can be housed in a single large room with as many as 100 bunk beds, affording even less privacy and more distractions. In custody settings, you may need to be sensitive regarding the content of sessions and homework assignments, and to shift topics depending on the degree of privacy afforded to a particular case.

While treatment in correctional institutions is unlikely to be court-mandated, as it is in probation, parole, and some community program settings, it may not be free from other external pressures. JICs in custody may seek treatment to place themselves in a more positive light before the parole board or to obtain a placement in a less restrictive environment. As in working with JICs in the community, you will need to be savvy in understanding the external and internal motivations that go into inmates' decision to participate in treatment.

Finally, for JICs nearing release, the sheer passage of time in a prison environment can make former problems areas seem like historical factors that have been successfully resolved. For example, 3 years of incarceration-induced sobriety may lead a JIC to believe that his or her substance abuse problem has been resolved and treatment is therefore unnecessary, even though such treatment has been imposed as a condition for early release.

JUSTICE INVOLVEMENT: THE SCOPE OF THE PROBLEM

The U.S. Bureau of Justice Statistics has estimated the 2014 rate of incarceration for the country at 612 per 100,000 people (Carson, 2015), making it among the highest in the world. Over 1.5 million U.S. residents are incarcerated (Carson, 2015), and almost 5 million are supervised in the country's parole and probation systems (Kaeble, Maruschak, & Bonczar, 2015). In the United States, among the general population, justice involvement occurs at about the same rate as commonly treated psychological problems, such as panic disorder and generalized anxiety disorder (National Institute of Mental Health, n.d.). It is important to keep in mind that 90% of those incarcerated in the United States will be released and returned to the community.

Comparable statistics in other English-speaking nations with similar criminal justice systems are less dramatic but still indicate large numbers of prisoners and probationers. The estimated incarceration rate in England and Wales is 148 per 100,000 people (Walmsley, 2013), and there are about 88,000 people incarcerated and 225,000 on probation (U.K. Ministry of Justice, 2017). In Canada, which has an estimated incarceration rate of 118 per 100,000 people, there are approximately 37,000 federal and provincial inmates and another 102,000 individuals on probation (Correctional Services Program, 2015). The estimated incarceration rate of Australia is 201 per 100,000 people (Walmsley, 2013), with about 37,000 incarcerated and another 62,000 on probation (Australian Bureau of Statistics, 2015).

WHAT WORKS IN REDUCING CRIMINAL BEHAVIOR?

In an oft-cited review of the correctional treatment literature, titled "What Works?: Questions and Answers about Prison Reform," Martinson (1974) commented in the concluding section: "With few and isolated exceptions, the rehabilitation efforts that have been reported so far have had no appreciable effect on recidivism" (p. 25). Building off the title of the report, the phrase "nothing works" came to characterize beliefs about the ineffectiveness of treatment for justice-involved individuals for decades, and paved the way for punitive approaches as the principal means of attempting to reduce criminal behavior. However, with the expansion of cognitive-behavioral interventions to justice-involved populations and the advent of meta-analysis, improving researchers' ability to synthesize treatment outcome studies quantitatively, a body of literature has emerged to challenge the "nothing works" assumption.

Three key conclusions have emerged from this growing meta-analytic literature. First, criminal sanctions without treatment tend to be ineffective in reducing recidivism. In fact, incarceration with no treatment is associated with an increase in reoffending, and community supervision with no intervention is associated with small or no reductions in reoffending (Andrews, Zinger, et al., 1990; Lipsey & Cullen, 2007; Smith, Goggin, & Gendreau, 2002). Second, treatment and intervention focused on risk domains that are commonly intertwined with criminal behavior consistently produce the greatest reductions in recidivism (Andrews & Bonta, 2010a; Lipsey, Landenberger, & Wilson, 2007; Martin, Dorken, Wamboldt, & Wooten, 2012; Morgan et al., 2012; Skeem, Steadman, & Manchak, 2015). Third, across treatment modalities, interventions based on cognitive-behavioral therapy (CBT) have the greatest impact on reducing future criminality (Hoffman, Asnaani, Vonk, Sawyer, & Fang, 2012; Landenberger & Lipsey, 2005; Lipsey, Chapman, & Landenberger, 2001)—even among specialized JIC groups, such as women (Dowden & Andrews, 1999a), youth (Dowden & Andrews, 1999b), those convicted of sexual offenses (Hanson, Bourgon, Helmus, & Hodgson, 2009), and those convicted of domestic violence (Babcock, Green, & Robie, 2004).

The growing literature on the relative effectiveness of CBT with JICs has not gone unnoticed by criminal justice agencies (Bonta & Andrews, 2007; U.K. Ministry of Justice, 2013; National Institute of Corrections [NIC] & Crime and Justice Institute [CJI], 2004; Scott, 2008). Among the NIC and CJI's (2004) eight principles of effective intervention, CBT is specifically highlighted in Principle 4: "Provide evidence-based programming that emphasizes cognitive behavioral strategies and is delivered by well trained staff" (p. 5). The use of CBT-based interventions has more recently been extended into the field of probation and parole. Programs training supervision officers to use CBT skills in their sessions with JICs have shown promising results, such as measurable improvements in officers' skills and significant reductions in recidivism (Bonta et al., 2011; Rugge & Bonta, 2014).

IS DIAGNOSIS IMPORTANT?

A customary first step in implementing CBT interventions is to establish an accurate diagnosis. In work with JICs, however, diagnosis may be less important in guiding treatment decisions, because there is no acute clinical syndrome that adequately captures JICs experiences. The most popular diagnostic schemes for this client group are related to personality pathology: antisocial personality disorder (ASPD) as outlined in the *Diagnostic and Statistical Manual of Mental Disorders*, fifth edition (DSM-5; American Psychiatric Association, 2013); dissocial personality disorder (dissocial PD) as defined in the *International Classification of Diseases*, 10th revision (ICD-10; World Health Organization, 1992); and psychopathy as formalized by the Psychopathy Checklist—Revised (PCL-R; Hare, 2003). A conundrum for practitioners is that these conceptualizations are overlapping but not identical, emphasizing different symptom clusters.

ASPD in DSM-5 emphasizes overt conduct through criteria that includes criminal behavior, lying, reckless/impulsive behavior, aggression, and irresponsibility in the areas of work and finances. In contrast, the criteria set for dissocial PD is less focused on conduct; it includes a mixture of cognitive signs (e.g., a tendency to blame others, an attitude of irresponsibility), affective signs (e.g., callousness, inability to feel guilt, low frustration tolerance), and interpersonal signs (e.g., a tendency to form relationships but not maintain them). The signs and symptoms of psychopathy are more complex and blend in almost equal degrees conduct, interpersonal, and affective aspects of functioning. The two higher-order factors of the PCL-R reflect this blend. Factor 1, Interpersonal/Affective, includes signs such as superficial charm, pathological lying, manipulation, grandiosity, lack of remorse and empathy, and shallow affect. Factor 2, Lifestyle/Antisocial, includes thrill seeking, impulsivity, irresponsibility, varied criminal activity, and disinhibited behavior (Hare & Neumann, 2008; White, Olver, & Lilienfeld, 2016). Psychopathy can be regarded as the most severe of the three disorders. Patients with psychopathy would be expected to meet criteria for ASPD or dissocial PD as well, but not everyone diagnosed with ASPD or dissocial PD will meet criteria for psychopathy (Hare, 1996; Ogloff, 2006).

As noted by Ogloff (2006), the distinctions among the three antisocial conceptualizations are such that findings based on one diagnostic group are not necessarily applicable to the others and produce different prevalence rates in justice-involved populations. Adding a further layer of complexity is the fact that practitioners will encounter JICs who possess a mixture of features from all three diagnostic systems, rather than a prototypical presentation of any one disorder. In addition, we recommend caution in using labels such as *antisocial, sociopathic,* or *psychopathic* for JICs, because these labels are likely to trigger defensiveness that can undermine treatment engagement. In discussions with JICs, we sidestep specific personality labels altogether and emphasize the nature of problematic *lifestyle* patterns in areas related to thinking (Chapters 8 and 9) and to routines, relationships, and destructive habits (Chapters 10, 11, and 12). In referring to this family of diagnoses in this treatment planner, we use the umbrella terms *antisocial orientation* and *antisocial*, rather than any particular diagnostic label.

JICs rarely have just one problem, and their comorbidity patterns are often complex. Some common overlapping conditions are well captured by existing diagnostic categories, while other problems are not. For example, a JIC may meet DSM-5 criteria for a substance use disorder and borderline personality disorder, and may also have significant family dysfunction and vocational instability. We discuss the complexities of conceptualizing individual, social, and contextual factors, as well as mental health problems, in Chapter 6.

A GENERAL TREATMENT PLAN

We recommend that treatment be tailored to meet the unique needs of JICs. Nonetheless, Table 1.1 outlines a general treatment plan, to guide you as you become familiar with this approach to treatment. This outline is considered a template for the broad phases of the treatment process. How much time you will spend in each phase will depend on the characteristics of a particular case and the setting in which you work.

WHAT DO SESSIONS LOOK LIKE?

Effective treatment with JICs involves conducting sessions that are structured, organized, and active. Here we highlight five session characteristics that are emphasized throughout this treatment planner and are consistent with general CBT principles.

1. *Case formulation guides treatment.* Before launching into active change techniques, you will need to spend time assessing and considering the criminal risk domains that are most important in maintaining a JIC's criminal behavior. A common error among forensic practitioners is to adopt a superficial "check-in" style of interacting with JICs (e.g., "Are you staying out of trouble?"). Such check-ins rarely address the long-term patterns that contribute to risky and harmful behavior. Another common error is to become entirely crisis-focused. In this style, each session is about the latest upheaval in a JIC's life. Being flexible and responsive to crises is important; however,

TABLE 1.1. General Plan of Treatment for JICs

- Engaging
- Clarifying values and life priorities
- Assessing criminal risk domains
- Formulating each case and identifying relevant treatment targets
- Establishing collaborative goals and focusing conversations
- Addressing criminogenic thinking and antisocial orientation
- Restructuring routines, relationships, and destructive habits
- Documenting and reporting

there also needs to be *continuity* in terms of attention to risk domains and long-term patterns that are connected to criminality. The third error is to take on a "pass the buck" stance with JICs. In this style, practitioners refer JICs to all sorts of "other" programs and services in hopes that something will work. Such practitioners operate more like brokers, doing very little work themselves to change the patterns of their clients. Even if you typically conduct brief sessions (e.g., as community supervision officers do), your work will be more effective if it focuses on the criminal risk domains (listed in Table 1.2 and described in the next chapter) that are most relevant to a JIC's life. Case formulation means developing an individualized game plan for each JIC and having a clear rationale for which patterns and life areas will become the focal points across sessions.

2. *Sessions are structured and organized.* In addition to having an overall game plan for the course of treatment, you will need to approach sessions in an organized and structured manner, with an identified agenda, beginning, middle, and end. This means thinking ahead about the focus of a particular meeting and the strategy to be used in the session. Of course, not all sessions go according to plan. The ability to be flexible and adjust "on the fly" is often necessary. Table 1.2 provides a general session structure that can be adapted to most forensic settings. In using this structure, you will be providing the focus for the session, while also maintaining the necessary flexibility to address any significant developments that have occurred since the last contact. When homework is applicable, you will review progress on previous assignments. The centerpiece of the session, to which the majority of time is typically devoted, is a focus on a specific risk domain related to a JIC's criminal behavior. Administrative issues are dealt with toward the end of the meeting, and discussions in this area are kept relatively brief. The session ends with a summary highlighting what was most important and reinforcing any next steps to be taken. Finally, documentation related to session content and the JIC's progress is completed.

3. *A skills-building orientation is adopted.* The emphasis in sessions is on improving JICs' functioning (e.g., decision-making capacity, thinking, and behavior) in criminal risk domains. Although listening to and understanding JICs' perspectives are critical skills for successful engagement, discussions that end up as complaining sessions (about others, the system, etc.) will rarely be productive. Similarly, while JICs may develop awareness about how aspects of their personal histories have influenced their present life circumstances, insight in and of itself will not be enough to bring about change. Rather, you will be introducing new skills to alter a JIC's entrenched patterns of thinking and behavior, and thus to reduce criminal potential.

4. *Sessions are active.* JICs are not merely "along for the ride"; they are actively involved in coming up with their own reasons for change, ideas for improving their lives, and participating in repeated practice of new thoughts and behaviors. Your energy and creativity in utilizing activities and assignments to actively engage JICs in sessions will be vital for successful treatment.

5. *Treatment incorporates homework.* In forensic settings, homework is one of the main predictors of treatment success (Morgan et al., 2012), and it is an essential mechanism for transferring skills to JICs' day-to-day lives. The more homework completed, the greater the impact of the intervention (Kroner & Morgan, 2014). Assignments that work best are concrete and specific, easily understood by JICs, easy to implement, and have a real-world emphasis. We have found that when the issue is approached properly, the majority of JICs are willing to complete homework assignments. In fact, many are appreciative for the opportunity to take active steps to improve their lives.

TABLE 1.2. General Session Structure

1. *Set the agenda.* Take the lead in introducing the agenda and focus for the session.

2. *Inquire briefly about new developments.* Inquire about any significant developments since the last meeting (e.g., new police contacts, disciplinary tickets, eviction, a new job, end of a significant relationship).

3. *Review previous assignments.* Conduct a brief review of assignments from the previous meeting (e.g., follow up on referrals, homework, job search efforts).

4. *Focus on a relevant criminal risk domain.* These domains include a history of criminal/ antisocial behavior, criminogenic thinking/antisocial orientation, antisocial companions, dysfunctional family/romantic relationships, lack of connection to work/ school, maladaptive leisure time, substance abuse/misuse, and anger dysregulation.

5. *Address administrative issues.* Conduct a brief review of practical issues related to supervision or custody conditions that have not yet been addressed during the session (e.g., change of living situation, employment changes, restitution payments).

6. *Provide a summary.* Summarize what was accomplished and what the JIC should be doing (homework) between sessions.

7. *Complete documentation.* Document progress, put notes into record, file, etc.

REALISTIC EXPECTATIONS

Working with JICs has many challenges and rewards. No matter how high your skill level, you will not be successful with every case. Since behavior is determined by multiple influences, you are likely to do exemplary work with some individuals who will nonetheless make poor decisions and continue on the path of creating suffering for themselves and others. The flip side is that you will also have a significant effect in changing the life trajectories of some of the JICs you work with. We have witnessed such successes in our own clinical work, and we have heard many JICs describe caring practitioners whom they credit with influencing them over the longer term. We encourage you to embrace the opportunity to work with JICs, as it presents opportunities to provide services that contribute to the safety of our communities, reduce the human suffering caused by criminal victimization, and afford a chance for a more positive future for some of society's most marginalized members.

We end this chapter where it began. With Brenda's first session under her belt, she is getting ready for her next appointment. Once again, she finds herself with very little information to go on. All she knows is that her next case is a 24-year-old unemployed woman named Jackie, who has been referred to the day reporting center as part of her probation after an arrest for public intoxication, criminal mischief, and trespassing. In the chapters that follow, the cases of Hank and Jackie are used to illustrate the application of the concepts presented in this treatment planner.

KEY POINTS

- Justice involvement is common in the United States: Among the U.S. general population, it occurs at about the same rate as panic disorder and generalized anxiety disorder.

- The primary emphasis of forensic treatment is on the prevention of future criminality. Therefore, criminal behavior and reoffending—not symptom reduction—are the outcomes of most concern.

- Because referrals in forensic environments almost invariably involve some form of external coercion, a significant amount of time and clinical effort must often be devoted to engaging clients and fostering motivation to make changes.

- Compassion is foundational to most helping relationships. Caring and concern for JICs' lives are essential elements of successful treatment.

- The use of diagnostic labels is less helpful in guiding treatment with JICs than treatment with mental health clients, since many targets of intervention are not captured in existing diagnostic schemes.

- Optimism is warranted! Many JICs will benefit from high-quality treatment.

CHAPTER 2

An Integrated Forensic Cognitive-Behavioral Therapy Approach

Brenda's confidence is a bit shaken after her initial session with Hank. Her second client is Jackie, a 24-year-old woman on probation for criminal mischief and trespassing. The arrest occurred when Jackie and two older male coworkers were found trying the doors of cars at an auto dealership late at night, hoping to find one that was unlocked.

Jackie has a 4-year-old son who spends half of his time with her and half with his father, with whom she has a contentious relationship. In the year prior to Jackie's arrest, her mother became disabled after a car accident and struggled with her health. Jackie decided that she would work full-time in order to help with the family's expenses, and she obtained employment at a car wash. During this past year, Jackie's social network primarily consisted of the two friends with whom she was arrested. She met them when she started working at the car wash, which was adjacent to the auto dealership. The two men took Jackie "under their wing," and invited her to hang out after work, which often involved aimlessly driving around and occasionally selling small amounts of marijuana to acquaintances. Before she began working full-time, Jackie had several friendships with men and women close to her age who had more conventional lifestyles; however, she unintentionally allowed these friendships to drift away. As a result of her recent arrest, Jackie was fired from her job. Brenda is also aware that Jackie seems to suffer from a moderate level of depression, but she questions to what extent Jackie's mood symptoms are causes versus results of her criminal justice problems.

Brenda feels like a fish out of water. She is wondering to herself what part of her clinical training will be applicable to this new treatment environment and whether she has the right knowledge to be successful with this population. A recurring and nagging question pops into her mind:

"To what extent will my skills for treating anxiety and depression transfer to clients like Hank and Jackie who are justice-involved?"

In this chapter, we introduce four components that form the foundation of an integrated approach for decreasing criminal behavior: (1) focusing on criminally relevant risk domains, (2) addressing thinking patterns that promote criminality, (3) enhancing motivation for change, and (4) clarifying values and life priorities. Each component comes from a distinct theoretical model with its own unique history, philosophy, and clinical approach.

FOCUSING ON CRIMINAL RISK DOMAINS

A key principle for working effectively with JICs is designing interventions with an overall goal of *risk reduction* rather than mental health symptom reduction. The good news is that you are already familiar with the philosophy of a risk reduction approach as it applies to other areas, such as heart disease (for which risk factors include a family history of heart disease, high cholesterol, smoking, diabetes, hypertension, obesity, poor diet, increased age, and lack of physical activity; Centers for Disease Control and Prevention, 2015). A risk reduction approach to heart disease can be likened to going through life with a shopping cart: The more factors in the cart, the more risk. The goals for interventions are thus to remove those factors from the cart, fill it with healthier options, and avoid putting more risk factors into the cart in the future—all of which will reduce a person's risk profile as much as possible.

A risk reduction approach to criminal behavior is analogous, but the items in the shopping cart are different. Over the years, a theoretically sound and empirically supported risk reduction model of antisocial and criminal behavior has emerged and has become firmly ensconced in the field of forensic treatment. The *risk–need–responsivity* (RNR; Andrews, Bonta, & Hoge, 1990) model and its companion listing of the "Central Eight" risk domains for criminal behavior (Andrews, Bonta, & Wormith, 2006; Bonta & Andrews, 2017) now guide much of the assessment and rehabilitation work conducted with JICs around the world. The Criminal Risk Domains Quiz (Figure 2.1) contains 25 client characteristics. Take the quiz and try to identify the 8 domains that have been found to be most predictive of criminal behavior.

Reviewing the answers to the quiz (found at the end of this chapter), you may find that you have provided some answers you expected to be correct, but you may also have experienced a few surprises at which domains made the list, and some puzzlement at which ones did not. Several of the "Central Eight" (e.g., current alcohol/drug abuse, unemployment, and dysfunctional family relationships with spouse/partner and family) are often included in standard intake and assessment procedures that occur within generic therapeutic activities, whereas other factors (e.g., spending time with criminal friends and companions, low levels of involvement in prosocial hobbies and activities, criminal thinking) are not typically identified in traditional counseling and psychotherapy. In previous conceptualizations, these risk factors were grouped into two tiers: the "Big Four," or those risk factors most strongly linked with reoffending (history of antisocial behavior, antisocial associates, antisocial cognition, and antisocial personality patterns and the "Moderate Four" (school/work, family/marital circumstances, leisure/recreation, and substance abuse). However, the "Big" versus "Moderate" distinction has fallen out of favor to some extent, as the relative strength of these factors seems to vary across different JIC groups (Bonta, Blais, & Wilson, 2014).

Circle the eight items that are most predictive of reoffending.	
Low self-esteem	Criminal thinking
Antisocial personality	Living in a high-crime neighborhood
Depression	Currently prescribed psychotropic medication
Lack of opportunity to express one's creativity	Record of prior criminal behavior
Having an enlarged forehead	Unemployment
Current alcohol/drug abuse	History of childhood physical abuse
History of opiate addiction	Low-income family
Low levels of involvement in prosocial hobbies and activities	Dysfunctional relationships with spouse/partner and family
More than 10 hours a week playing violent video games	Lack of transportation
Spending time with criminal friends and companions	Lack of basic identification documents
	Anxiety
Schizophrenia	Being adopted
Bipolar disorder	History of a learning disability

FIGURE 2.1. Criminal Risk Domains Quiz.

What about Girls and Women?

Although the risk domains that predict recidivism are the same for men as they are for women, there are some gender-related differences that should be considered in treatment. Compared to male JICs, female JICs are more likely to have histories of childhood abuse, mental health symptoms, and at least one dependent child, among other psychosocial stressors (Salisbury & Van Voorhis, 2009). The extent to which these factors loom large in female JICs' lives will influence their abilities to improve functioning within relevant criminal risk domains. Rates of girls and women entering the juvenile and criminal justice system have dramatically increased over the past decade (Garcia, 2015). In work with women such as Jackie, it will be beneficial to help female JICs enhance their existing strengths and develop new resources, to address the complex social needs of this marginalized and growing population (Van Dieten & King, 2014).

Mental Health Symptoms and Criminal Behavior

Noticeably absent from the "Central Eight" are traditional mental health disorders (with the exception of substance use and antisocial personality, which are included as criminal risk domains rather than disorders). Diagnosable mental disorders (e.g., mood and anxiety disorders, schizophrenia spectrum problems) are common in forensic populations, with prevalence rates exceeding those found in the community (Steadman, Osher, Robbins, Case, & Samuels, 2009). This observation has fostered the belief among practitioners (and the public) that mental health treatment is the best means of reducing JICs' risk for future criminal behavior. In fact, the empirical literature indicates that the relationship between mental illness and criminal behavior is contrary to this common wisdom. An emerging body of research indicates that mental health symptoms, even those of psychosis, rarely precede criminal or violent activity (Peterson, Skeem, Kennealy, Bray, & Zvonkovic, 2014; Skeem, Kennealy, Monahan, Peterson, & Appelbaum, 2016). Indeed, a meta-analysis comparing predictors of recidivism among JICs with and without mental health disorders found that the same set of criminal risk factors predicted general and violent recidivism for both groups (Bonta, Law, & Hanson, 1998). More strikingly, mental health symptoms did *not* predict recidivism. A more recent meta-analysis by Bonta and colleagues exploring the predictors of recidivism in JICs with mental health disorders supported these conclusions: Criminal risk domains predicted general and violent recidivism, whereas mental health symptoms, including diagnoses of psychosis or mood disorders, were unrelated to recidivism (Bonta et al., 2014). Although there are certainly individual cases in which JICs' mental health symptoms relate directly to their offending behavior, it appears to be a general guideline that criminal risk domains, rather than mental health symptoms, drive criminal behavior.

In order to appreciate the relevance of the above-described research findings to practical clinical challenges, let's consider Jackie. Targeting only her depression may help her feel better, but it will not reduce her likelihood to reoffend (and could possibly increase it, since she may have more energy to hang out with the guys from the car wash, drink alcohol, and sell drugs). Addressing her connection with antisocial companions and assisting her in obtaining meaningful employment will reduce her likelihood of reoffending. However, such an approach will be difficult to implement if she is too depressed to engage in activities designed to break ties with existing friends, develop prosocial connections, and take steps to build a career path. In this sense, mental health symptoms (her depression) may interfere with forensic treatment. JICs with mental illness may thus require interventions that target symptoms of mental illness, so that they can later work productively on improving the risk-relevant domains of their lives. Therefore, addressing mental health symptoms is regarded in this book as an adjunct to treatment for JICs, not as a replacement for focusing on criminal risk domains.

Criminal Risk Domains Addressed in This Treatment Planner

This treatment planner focuses on a constellation of criminal risk domains that are similar to the "Central Eight." One modification is that we blend the concepts of criminal thinking and antisocial personality (we use the term *antisocial orientation* for the latter). *Criminal thinking* reflects issues of cognition related to criminal behavior (i.e., thoughts, attitudes/beliefs, and maladaptive thinking styles), whereas *antisocial orientation* reflects a broad range of personal tendencies (e.g., feelings, behaviors, ways of interacting with others) related to criminality. We emphasize the thinking component in our combined term, *criminogenic thinking/antisocial orientation,* because entrenched criminal thinking patterns often underlie an antisocial orientation. We have included *anger dysregulation* as an additional criminal risk domain to be considered in treatment, because anger regulation difficulties appear to be common among forensic populations, and anger is the emotional excess most likely to be connected to criminal behavior (Novaco, 1994, 2011a, 2011b;

Skeem et al., 2006). Descriptions of the criminal risk domains that form the foundation for this treatment planner are provided in Table 2.1.

Implications of a Risk Reduction Model

Below are several implicit principles of a risk reduction approach that will be helpful in understanding this perspective as it applies to the treatment of JICs.

An Optimistic Outlook

A risk reduction perspective views JICs as having the potential for change. The criminal risk domains represent broad areas of life functioning that are changeable (dynamic), rather than the factors that are unchangeable (static). Seven of the eight domains have dynamic components (the one exception is history of criminal/antisocial behavior). Moreover, we have found that even this lone (but certainly not least important) static factor can be addressed in treatment. When approached with the right spirit and tone, discussions with JICs about their criminal/antisocial history and its impact on their lives can be useful in enhancing motivation to change thinking and

TABLE 2.1. Criminal Risk Domains

Risk domain	Description
History of criminal/ antisocial behavior	A history of criminal/antisocial behavior that persists over time
Criminogenic thinking/ antisocial orientation	Thoughts and beliefs that facilitate criminal, antisocial, and maladaptive behavior; personal disposition of an antisocial nature
Antisocial companions	Connection with people involved in, or oriented toward, criminality; absence of prosocial friends
Dysfunctional family/ romantic relationships	Family or marital/couple relationships that are emotionally detached and/or ignore, reinforce, or model antisocial behavior
Lack of connection to work/school	Lack of success/negative attitudes/low levels of performance and satisfaction related to work/school
Maladaptive leisure time	Aimless use of leisure time/lack of structure to daily routines; low levels of involvement in positive prosocial pursuits; enjoyment of antisocial and risky activities
Substance abuse/misuse	Misuse of alcohol and/or other drugs (including prescription medications)
Anger dysregulation	Inability to modulate anger (e.g., frequency, intensity, and/or expression); anger reactions that create social, vocational, or interpersonal difficulties

behavior within other risk domains. Rather than beginning treatment with a pessimistic outlook, Brenda can view Hank and Jackie as JICs whose criminal trajectories can be altered if treatment can improve their functioning within the unique constellation of risk domains relevant to each of their lives.

A Preventive Orientation

To return to the example of heart disease, it is possible for people to be at high risk for heart disease and have few noticeable symptoms; to remain relatively unaware of how their current lifestyles undermine their long-term well-being; and not to consider change until they suffer a cardiac event. Similarly, chronic criminality has been described as a *lifestyle disorder* that develops over time and that affects judgment and behavior (Mitchell, Tafrate, & Freeman, 2015). JICs can remain relatively unaware of their problematic patterns until they have suffered serious losses (e.g., incarceration, reincarceration, financial instability, damaged relationships). When a risk reduction perspective is applied to criminal behavior, the orientation is preventive; the aim is to reduce risk before the person suffers more serious losses and consequences. The goal of treatment is to reduce a JIC's risk profile as much as possible before damage gets worse.

Individually Tailored Treatment

Embedded in the RNR model are three core principles intended to inform assessment and treatment considerations. One of these is referred to as the *need principle* (Andrews & Bonta, 2010b); the other two principles are discussed later. According to the need principle, the interventions provided to any given JIC should address the risk domains pertinent to the client's particular case. As a practitioner, you should take care to avoid the cookie-cutter approach that often creeps into forensic programming, in which every JIC is provided with the same program, regardless of the program components' applicability to the person's risk profile. Second, you should consider individual differences in how a given risk domain translates into criminal behavior. For example, two JICs may both have problems with antisocial companions, but *how* their companions influence criminal behavior may be different. One JIC's friends may present opportunities for impulsive criminal activities that the person might not have sought out or initiated independently. For another JIC, the desire to obtain the respect of friends may lead the client to initiate criminal behavior that he or she believes will meet their approval.

The Synergistic Nature of Risk Domains

Although Table 2.1 presents the criminal risk domains as a list of discrete factors, it is important to appreciate the interrelationships between them and the unique ways they may be manifested across individuals. Given the multidetermined nature of human behavior, risk domains are often connected in ways that can be complex in how they amplify or reduce each other. Let's consider Hank as an example. Prior to his most recent arrest, his lifestyle might be characterized as impulsive, unstable, and self-destructive (criminogenic thinking/antisocial orientation). He did not have steady full-time employment, because he was reluctant to work in the low-wage positions for which he was qualified and did not spend enough time in one position to work his way to better opportunities (lack of connection to work). He spent the better part of his considerable amount of free time (maladaptive leisure time) with friends who drank heavily and used marijuana (antisocial companions, substance abuse/misuse). His friends reinforced his unproductive beliefs about work; his drug use eliminated any hope of his passing preemployment drug screens; and his alcohol use increased his poor behavioral control, leading to altercations with acquaintances (anger dysregulation). Thus the various risk domains relevant to Hank's case influenced each other in an interrelated destructive system. Clearly, due to such synergistic effects, the influence of risk domains can be multiplicative rather than simply additive.

On the optimistic side, because the domains are interconnected, a positive change in one of these areas can facilitate positive changes in the others. In Hank's case, if his treatment could successfully address his negative attitudes toward work, he might be willing to stop smoking marijuana and drinking temporarily and obtain full-time employment. Full-time employment would result in less time with his antisocial friends, less time to engage in substance use, and exposure to new peers who express prosocial thoughts and who model more productive lifestyles. A strategic focus on one or two risk domains can thus create a positive ripple effect in a JIC's life.

Other Treatment Elements: Risk and Responsivity

As noted above, the RNR model has emerged as a core competency for working with JICs, and several other elements of the model are worth noting. Another core principle of the RNR model is the *risk principle* (Andrews & Bonta, 2010b). The risk principle concerns the importance of matching the intensity of an intervention with a JIC's overall risk. More intensive interventions should be reserved for higher-risk JICs (those for whom more risk domains are applicable), while lower-intensity interventions should be reserved for lower-risk JICs. The literature surrounding the risk principle has found that providing high-risk JICs with low-intensity interventions will have only a minimal effect on reducing criminal behavior (Lipsey & Cullen, 2007; Lipsey et al., 2007). Startlingly, providing low-risk JICs with high-intensity interventions not only will fail to reduce criminal behavior, but may even increase recidivism rates (Andrews & Bonta, 2010b). This latter finding may seem counterintuitive, but consider what happens when an employed low-risk JIC, with few criminal companions and limited criminal thinking, is referred to an intensive residential program by a well-intentioned judge or prosecutor. This JIC may lose his or her job, make a large network of new criminal companions, be exposed to their criminal thinking patterns, and have excessive leisure time once the program is completed. Moreover, he or she may develop an antagonistic attitude toward treatment and/or the "system," increasing the "pissed-off = turned-off" dynamic. Thus the client's risk level has been raised, and responsivity to future treatment has been degraded, as the unintended results of a misguided attempt to help the JIC.

In practical terms, decisions will need to be made about how frequently, and for how long, to meet with a particular JIC (e.g., periodic contacts, consistent ongoing meetings, intensive treatment and supervision). With this client group, it is important to think beyond the traditional 50-minute counseling session once a week. Decisions about treatment dosage must be based on assessment (Chapter 5) and case formulation (Chapter 6), with more intensive services going to higher-risk JICs.

The third core principle of the RNR model is the *responsivity principle* (Andrews & Bonta, 2010b). This principle concerns the orientation of the intervention and the factors that influence a JIC's reaction to treatment. Two points related to the responsivity principle are highlighted here. First, as noted in Chapter 1, CBT interventions produce greater reductions in reoffending, compared to the psychodynamic and nondirective therapies that have historically prevailed in forensic settings. Second, the JIC's characteristics can influence receptivity to an intervention. Consider two JICs who are referred to a substance abuse program for similar alcohol-related offenses. One is a 50-year-old white male; the other is a 22-year-old black female. They attend the same program, which is populated overwhelmingly with middle-aged white men. Their reactions to this intervention may be quite different: One client may respond positively; the other may be uncomfortable, due to factors related to gender, age, and ethnicity rather than to any particular quality of the program itself. A variety of individual responsivity factors (e.g., mental health symptoms, motivation to change, cognitive ability, and maturity) should be considered in treatment delivery. These are discussed further in connection with case formulation in Chapter 6.

ADDRESSING THINKING PATTERNS THAT PROMOTE CRIMINALITY

A curious finding emerged from a doctoral dissertation that focused on the irrational beliefs of convicted felons: On two separate self-report paper-and-pencil measures of irrational beliefs, the felon group (at pretest) reported fewer such beliefs than other populations, including college students who had previously completed the same measures (Swanston, 1987). Were the felons to be considered the standard for accurate, rational, and healthy thinking? Were they simply less than honest in completing the questionnaires? Or were the cognitive targets measured in the instruments not entirely relevant to their criminality?

If you are unaccustomed to working in the forensic area, the beliefs and cognitions of JICs may seem somewhat bewildering. In some cases, the cognitive profiles of JICs are mirror images of the profiles of clients suffering from anxiety and depression (Kroner & Morgan, 2014; Mitchell et al., 2015; Seeler, Freeman, DiGiuseppe, & Mitchell, 2014; Walters, 2014). For example, anxious and depressed individuals often overestimate and exaggerate potential dangers, are overly concerned about others' opinions, and harshly blame and judge themselves when things do not go well. JICs, on the other hand, tend to present with a tendency to underestimate danger, challenges, or difficulties in favor of overly optimistic and self-serving predictions, and often display a lack of concern for the opinions of others and for how their actions affect others.

At about the same time as the CBT models of Albert Ellis (1957, 1962) and Aaron T. Beck (1963, 1967) were being developed, a cognitive literature focused on the thinking patterns of JICs began to emerge in the field of criminology. In one of the seminal works in this area, Sykes and Matza (1957) proposed that offenders "neutralize" the wrongfulness of their criminal actions by embracing specific cognitions that free themselves of guilt, self-blame, or disapproval from others. These neutralizations exculpate the JICs from their past actions and facilitate future antisocial behavior. Subsequent empirical work has identified an array of cognitive patterns that facilitate antisocial and self-destructive behavior. If you are comfortable with conceptualizing clients' thinking in terms of established CBT models (e.g., schemas, intermediate beliefs, automatic thoughts), you will find that these constructs can be applied to JICs, but that the contents of thinking patterns within those constructs will be noticeably different.

Levels of Cognition

Cognitive therapy takes into account several levels of cognitive processes. At the most basic level are *core beliefs* (or *schemas*), which tend to be global and overgeneralized conceptions about the self, other people, and the world. These beliefs are formed in early childhood and often remain below the level of conscious awareness. Core beliefs influence the next level of thinking, *intermediate beliefs* (*attitudes, rules,* and *assumptions*), which form the basis for how an individual thinks, feels, and behaves across different situations. Lastly, *automatic thoughts* are quick evaluative thoughts that spring up in response to different stimuli and form the stream of consciousness that people can learn to identify with minimal effort (J. S. Beck, 2011).

The thinking patterns at the heart of this treatment planner operate at the level of intermediate beliefs and automatic thoughts. Our focus on these two cognitive levels in treatment is not intended to negate the importance of schemas in personality pathology. We focus on intermediate beliefs and automatic thoughts because such thinking patterns are instrumental in guiding JICs' decision making and behaviors. Also, these cognitive levels are the most practical to address in the brief interactions and time-limited treatment common in forensic settings. Efforts to address schemas are better pursued in those environments where longer-term individual treatment is an option. If you are interested in schema-focused therapy for JICs, see Keulen-de Vos, Bernstein, and Arntz (2014) and Sun (2014).

Intermediate Beliefs: Criminogenic Thinking Patterns

Intermediate beliefs that are relevant for JICs can be conceptualized effectively by taking into consideration the empirical literature that has developed around the assessment of criminal thinking patterns. We use the term *criminogenic* to highlight the role of these patterns in facilitating criminal, antisocial, and destructive behavior. At the core of this literature are seven instruments that have been developed for assessing criminal/criminogenic thinking in adult JICs: the Psychological Inventory of Criminal Thinking Styles (Walters, 1995); the Criminal Sentiments Scale—Modified (Simourd, 1997); the Measures of Criminal Attitudes and Associates (Mills, Kroner, & Forth, 2002); the Texas Christian University Criminal Thinking Scales (Knight, Garner, Simpson, Morey, & Flynn, 2006); the Measure of Offender Thinking Styles (Mandracchia, Morgan, Garos, & Garland, 2007); the Criminogenic Thinking Profile (Mitchell & Tafrate, 2012); and the Criminal Cognitions Scale (Tangney et al., 2012).

Each instrument measures multiple thinking patterns (ranging from 3 to 8). The total number of thinking patterns measured across all the instruments is an unmanageable 32; however, taking into account overlapping content reduces the number to a more clinically practical 13. These 13 criminogenic thinking patterns are introduced in Table 2.2. The patterns in the first column represent beliefs about the self and others, and those in the second column are related to interactions with the environment. Detailed descriptions of these criminogenic thinking patterns are presented in Chapters 5 and 8 of this treatment planner.

We provide one caution with regard to interpreting this literature. The terms *criminogenic thinking* and *criminal thinking* may inadvertently reinforce the idea that JICs are somehow qualitatively different from other people and perhaps inherently resistant to change. Our overall point of view places criminality and JICs on a continuous spectrum rather than at one end of a dichoto-

TABLE 2.2. Overview of Criminogenic Thinking Patterns

Beliefs related to self and others	Beliefs related to interacting with the environment
Identifying with antisocial companions	Demand for excitement
Disregard for others	Exploit
Emotionally disengaged	Hostility for law and order
Hostility for criminal justice personnel	Justifying and minimizing
Grandiosity and entitlement	Path of least resistance
Power and control	Inability to cope
	Underestimating

mous spectrum. Therefore, criminogenic thinking patterns (at the level of intermediate beliefs) represent a somewhat normative, but maladaptive, cognitive coping style that becomes ingrained over time. In the face of life's challenges and struggles, everyone has the potential to crave excitement, to believe that certain problems cannot be resolved, or to fail to consider the impact of one's actions on the suffering of others. For JICs, such patterns may become pervasive, setting the stage for choices (reflected in the automatic thoughts described below) that lead to problems with the criminal justice system as well as problems in other risk domain areas. In that sense, criminogenic thinking patterns such as those listed in Table 2.2 are simply beliefs that guide day-to-day choices that will ultimately influence one's life trajectory.

Interplay of Criminogenic Thinking Patterns across Life Areas

The case of Jackie provides an example of how criminogenic thinking patterns manifest themselves in criminal justice involvement. Her perspective on her recent offense reflects her belief that the trespassing incident was a way to create excitement after a boring shift at the car wash: "We were just looking for something fun to do" (demand for excitement). She also mentions the influence of her male companions on her decision to break into cars: "I felt that if I didn't go along with them, they would be disappointed in me" (identifying with antisocial companions). She adds: "Not sure why everyone is making such a big deal about this; we didn't steal the car" (justifying and minimizing).

Jackie's criminogenic thinking is also apparent in several other criminal risk domains that are relevant to her case. First, she doesn't see any urgency in taking steps to develop a career path: "I'll just find another job somewhere" (path of least resistance). Second, she has a tendency to give up easily in the face of challenges: "School was hard, so I gave up on it" (inability to cope). As a general rule, a handful of such thinking patterns will become targets for intervention.

Automatic Thoughts: Criminogenic Thoughts and Decision Making

At the level of automatic thoughts, the thinking that precedes JICs' risky decision making becomes another focal point of treatment. This emphasis on decision making is slightly different from traditional cognitive therapy, which usually seeks to uncover thinking that precedes episodes of excessive emotional upset. Depending on the therapeutic circumstances, JICs are often very willing to discuss their history of poor decisions in relevant criminal risk domains (e.g., friendships, family relationships, substance use). With skill and effort, you can elicit what JICs typically think when they make poor decisions, and determine what the thinking looks like when choices are made that lead to more positive outcomes.

To understand the role of automatic thoughts and decision making, try this experiment: Focus on a recent time where you made an unhealthy choice, and try to recall the fleeting moment where you gave yourself permission to go in that direction (e.g., "I worked hard today and deserve to [have a drink, go shopping, stay out late]"). See if you can identify this type of "green light" moment—when you gave yourself permission to do something self-defeating. It may be difficult, because such thoughts become more automatic and harder to detect with repetition. Developing awareness of the thinking that occurs in these decision-making moments is an important first step in changing automatic reactions. Helping JICs become less automatic and more deliberate in their thinking and decision making is a prerequisite to enhancing longer-term positive life outcomes.

ENHANCING MOTIVATION FOR CHANGE

Motivation for change varies both within and among all client groups, and JICs are no different. However, some dynamics related to motivation are more likely to occur with JICs. For example, whereas traditional psychotherapy clients often seek help voluntarily, are able to identify and acknowledge their symptoms, and want those symptoms reduced or removed with the hope of improved functioning and well-being, JICs may be unaware of any symptoms and therefore quite naturally see no urgent need to engage in treatment.

As noted in Chapter 1, individuals formally connected to the justice system commonly come to treatment either through coercion by the court or through an incentive presented by a correctional institution. For example, JICs in pretrial status may seek counseling as part of a court program that dismisses charges once they have completed a period of intervention (this is the situation for Hank). JICs who have already been convicted and on probation may have evaluation and intervention as conditions of their probation, and face incarceration if they drop out or refuse to participate (this is Jackie's situation). Those who are incarcerated may attend treatment because they have been informed that doing so is essential in successfully securing parole or another form of early release. Although such mechanisms do not technically force the persons into treatment (even probationers, after all, can refuse treatment and serve their sentences in prison rather than in the community), the clients may well believe that they are "forced to come here."

In regard to personal insight, JICs like Hank and Jackie may initially be unable to identify or acknowledge areas in need of change. The internal distress that typically motivates behavior change among traditional psychotherapy clients is often lacking. In some cases, JICs find their current destructive patterns enjoyable, largely harmless to themselves, and worth continuing (e.g., "If I don't sell drugs in my neighborhood, somebody else will get rich, so it might as well be me"). Even when awareness of negative consequences exists, some JICs see the cause of their difficulties as other people or external circumstances, rather than their own behavior (e.g., "There were five other people dealing in that park, so why did the cops pick on me? That's not fair"). They may also see themselves as victims rather than perpetrators, and may argue that any change ought to lie in other people and institutions, rather than themselves (e.g., "Weed is legal in lots of places now. The state should leave me alone. I'm just trying to make a living").

Since few people react well to being pressured into getting help, it is not surprising that under such circumstances JICs present with a lack of interest in making changes, if not outright hostility toward intervention programs and practitioners. A recent meta-analysis examining forensic treatment reached the stark conclusion that mandated programs were generally ineffective, whereas voluntary treatment in both institutional and community settings was associated with positive effects (Parhar, Wormith, Derkzen, & Beauregard, 2008). An important implication of this finding is that in order for treatment to be effective, coerced clients must develop an interest in treatment and change akin to that of their voluntary counterparts. In essence, you will need to create an atmosphere in which JICs who say they are "forced to be here" become willing to look at themselves and are eventually able to say that they "want to make changes anyway."

Motivational Interviewing: A Core Competency for Working with JICs

Motivational interviewing (MI) has immediate practical advantages in the early stages of treatment: moving JICs toward greater engagement and collaboration, and moving practitioners away from confrontation, advice giving, and practical steps for which the clients are not yet ready. The main objectives of using MI in forensic practice are to promote engagement in the treatment process, and to explore and elicit JICs' inner motivation to change behaviors related to criminal risk domains, with the aim of preventing future criminality. Instead of relying on the practitioner–client power differential that exists in most justice settings, which often results in practitioners' telling clients what to do, JICs and practitioners collaboratively discuss reasons *why* change would be important, as well as *how* the clients might go about achieving it. MI is a complex communication style built on a platform of four core counseling skills (known as OARS: *open questions, affirmations, reflections, summarizations*) that are used across four broad and dynamic processes: *engaging, focusing, evoking intrinsic motivation,* and *change planning* (Miller & Rollnick, 2013).

The Four Processes of MI

There is often a strong temptation to jump straight into identifying solutions and offering suggestions intended to help JICs solve their problems. In this type of prescriptive interaction style, a practitioner determines what a client needs to change and what steps the client needs to take in order to be successful. Because of the motivational challenges noted above, this approach rarely succeeds with JICs; it most often leads to a lack of movement, or to treatment plans that a JIC cannot or will not follow.

The four processes of MI provide a more useful guide, serving as a road map in helping you navigate treatment. The first process, *engaging,* is about connecting and establishing a productive working relationship. In MI-based work with JICs, this means using a person-centered style that is caring, curious, and patient. This may at first seem difficult, given the perpetrator-based nature of some JICs' behavior. With time, however, approaching treatment with compassion and a willingness to understand JICs' perspectives becomes easier. The second process, *focusing,* occurs when a practitioner and a JIC come to agreement in clarifying a general direction and establishing change goals. At the strategic heart of MI is the third process, *evoking intrinsic motivation*—in other words, eliciting and encouraging JICs' own motivations for making changes. When this is done skillfully, the JICs are the ones who talk themselves into making life changes. The final process, *change planning*, has to do with establishing realistic and manageable steps for reaching agreed-upon change goals. By often asking yourself the question "Where am I with this client?" (developing a connection, establishing a direction, eliciting reasons for change, or working on practical steps toward a goal), you can become more strategic in your treatment efforts.

In thinking about the four processes of MI, it is important to be flexible, as the amount of time spent in each process will vary across different clients. Also, the processes are best thought of as fluid and overlapping, rather than as discrete stages. For example, even when JICs make progress, skilled practitioners will shift back and forth between processes as challenges arise. In that sense, there is no precise beginning or end to each process (Miller & Rollnick, 2013). In MI, the OARS skills are used throughout each process. Specific strategies for the first process (making the initial approach and enhancing JIC engagement) are outlined in Chapter 3, and the other processes (focusing, evoking intrinsic motivation, and change planning) are discussed in Chapter 7 and integrated into the later Chapters.

A Personal Experiment: Launching into Productive Conversations about Change

To better understand the dynamics of MI, try this experiment. The list below contains four common health-related behaviors that many people struggle with. Pick the one that is most relevant to your life.

1. Eating less fatty food
2. Smoking less
3. Reducing alcohol use
4. Exercising more frequently

Now imagine that you have to undergo a health and wellness exam as part of a new health insurance program initiative. In the waiting room, you complete a lengthy health behavior questionnaire that includes many questions on lifestyle, diet, exercise, and so forth. When you are called back to meet with the nurse to review the results of your questionnaire, the nurse suggests that you make a lifestyle change in the health behavior you have identified from the list above. He or she then provides several reasons why you should make this change and recommends a bold course of action. If your health behavior is eating less fatty food, the nurse recommends cutting out fats and following a low-fat, plant-based diet; supplies a fact sheet with foods to target; and provides a referral to a nutritionist. If your health behavior is smoking less, the nurse proposes a smoking cessation medication and provides a referral to a smoking cessation clinic. If your health behavior is reducing alcohol use, the nurse suggests attending Alcoholics Anonymous meetings once a week. If your health behavior is exercising more frequently, the nurse recommends 45 minutes of exercise three times a week, membership in a gym, and an appointment with a personal trainer.

During this process, the nurse never asks you about your perspective on the issue or your level of interest in following this course of action. He or she seems most concerned about documenting the recommendation and making sure you sign an acknowledgment that you have received the proper counsel.

What would your reaction to this interaction be? For many people, their natural reaction would be to become defensive and noncompliant. It would not be uncommon for you to do one or more of the following: minimize the seriousness of the health behavior ("My grandmother smoked for 70 years, and she lived to be 90"); justify your current unhealthier ways ("I need to do something to relax, and wine is a fairly healthy option"); argue why the recommended change is not practical, given your lifestyle ("I can't get to the gym regularly; who has that kind of free time?"); or scowl, sigh deeply, roll your eyes, and sign the form, while telling yourself you will ignore the nurse's advice. Of course, if you reacted in any of these ways, the nurse would probably view you as unmotivated and uncooperative.

Unfortunately, since few people react well to being pressured to change, the dynamics represented above are very similar to the types of unproductive conversations that happen countless times per day in forensic settings around the world. JICs are told that they have a problem (confrontation) and that they must get treatment (coercion). The JIC becomes defensive and counters with minimizations of, or justifications for, his or her self-defeating and risky behaviors (resistance); the practitioner argues with logic and counterevidence (more confrontation). The client feels frustrated, becomes self-protective, and resists a plan for change. The practitioner feels frustrated in turn and concludes that the JIC is noncompliant.

In contrast, productive conversations can be held with clients like Hank and Jackie if you listen to their perspectives (engaging), explore what they see as important in terms of change within relevant risk domains (focusing), elicit reasons for making changes (evoking), and collaboratively develop ideas for how change might happen (planning). In this sense, the four processes of MI provide a practical structure for moving forward with JICs who feel coerced into treatment.

CLARIFYING VALUES AND LIFE PRIORITIES

The positive psychology movement, with its emphasis on character strengths, virtues, and fundamental values that make life meaningful and fulfilling, may seem better suited to individuals in positions of corporate leadership than to those incarcerated, living in halfway houses, or attending day reporting centers. Nonetheless, in recent years, positive psychology's impact has influenced treatment with JICs, and strength-based models of offender rehabilitation such as the *good lives model* (GLM) are being integrated into forensic practice (Dumas & Ward, 2016; Fortune & Ward, 2014; Ward, 2010).

A guiding principle of the GLM is that working with JICs to help them avoid high-risk behaviors (*avoidance goals*) is only part of the change process; helping them develop behavioral paths to a life worth living (*approach goals*) is an equally important component. Although the importance of reducing risk for future criminal behavior is not ignored, the emphasis is placed on identifying JICs' aspirations and enhancing competencies that will help them to achieve their life goals through prosocial means. In the GLM, the exploration of values helps to identify the types of resources JICs will need in order to live according to their values in a constructive rather than an antisocial manner.

A similar concept from *acceptance and commitment therapy* (ACT) has also been applied to JICs (Amrod & Hayes, 2014). In ACT, the clarification of values is used to establish anchor points to guide future behavioral choices; these anchor points aid in minimizing behaviors that will interfere with core values and developing behavioral activation plans likely to lead to a more prosocial and meaningful life. Specific guidelines for having discussions with JICs about clarifying personal values are provided in Chapter 4.

As you continue reading this book, you will recognize the risk-based, motivational, cognitive, and values components intertwined in many of the "how-to" chapters that follow. In the next chapter, we discuss strategies for the initial approach to JICs and ways to successfully engage them.

KEY POINTS

- We recommend an integrated approach that incorporates focusing on criminal risk domains, addressing criminogenic thinking patterns, enhancing motivation for change, and clarifying JICs' values and life priorities.

- Criminal risk domains are the primary drivers of criminal behavior. Targeting these domains in treatment is the best path to reducing recidivism and increasing public safety.

- The relationship between criminal risk domains and mental health symptoms is complex. Mental health symptoms most commonly emerge as responsivity factors that will interfere with forensic treatment (e.g., a JIC may be too anxious to make new prosocial companions). In some cases, mental health symptoms will need to be addressed before JICs can successfully work on the risk-relevant areas of their lives. Addressing mental health symptoms is seen as an adjunct to forensic treatment, not as a replacement for focusing on criminal risk domains.

- Mandated and coerced treatment appears to be ineffective, whereas voluntary treatment shows positive results. Therefore, assisting JICs in developing their own inner motivation to change those behaviors most related to the criminally relevant areas of their lives is a critical part of the treatment process.

- Criminogenic thinking patterns guide day-to-day choices that will ultimately influence JICs' life trajectories. To prevent future criminality, practitioners will need to focus on a constellation of thinking patterns that are different from those commonly found among people suffering with anxiety and depression.

- A sole focus on avoidance goals (e.g., avoiding high-risk behaviors) will not be sufficient. Helping JICs create a life worth living (approach goals) is an equally important component of effective treatment.

Answers to Criminal Risk Domains Quiz (Figure 2.1): Record of prior criminal behavior; antisocial personality; current alcohol/drug abuse; spending time with criminal friends and companions; criminal thinking; dysfunctional relationships with spouse/partner and family; low levels of involvement in prosocial hobbies and activities; and unemployment.

PART II

ENGAGEMENT

CHAPTER 3

Successfully Engaging Justice-Involved Clients

Hank's demeanor remains relatively unchanged during his second session with Brenda. After attempting the usual pleasantries and small talk, Brenda is able to establish some semblance of rapport, but making headway on assessment and a case plan is a slower process than she is used to. Hank provides only brief answers to her questions, and conveys a sense that the session is something being done *to* him rather than something being done *for* or *with* him. Brenda finds it difficult to pinpoint any symptoms of subjective distress; Hank's biggest complaint is that his arrest, and subsequent referral to the day reporting center, are unfair and taking up his time. As Brenda works through the interview, she finds Hank's way of thinking about himself and relating to others to be highly self-destructive. Also, Hank's reluctance to engage in the session shapes how Brenda interacts with him. In an attempt to gather relevant information, she finds herself asking mostly closed-ended, fact-gathering questions. This unintentionally produces an interrogative quality to the session, a rushed pace, and a lack of depth, rather than a collaborative conversation. Toward the end of the session, Brenda finds herself trying to convince Hank that he needs to change and offering several suggestions for steps he can take. Her advice is met with a list of reasons why these suggestions are unnecessary or impossible to implement. The session ends at a standstill. In thinking about her two sessions with Hank, Brenda wonders what she could have done in these sessions, or can do in subsequent sessions, in order to get treatment off to a more productive start.

The reality of working with JICs is that tremendous variability exists regarding issues of insight, honesty, and motivation. Therefore, you should resist the temptation to paint this client group with a broad brush. Remember that to a large extent, successful engagement is a matter of how such clients are initially approached.

Contrary to what is portrayed on popular reality television shows, a "get tough," "get real," or "confrontational" approach to work with JICs is likely to increase resistance and undermine the foundation of a productive working relationship; it is thus not often advocated by forensic experts (Tafrate, Mitchell, & Novaco, 2014). Instead, you will need to take time to establish a good working relationship, elicit from JICs their own motivations for making changes within criminal risk domains, explore the impact of antisocial patterns on broader life goals, investigate potential strengths, and delve into what JICs value most. Being warm, being collaborative, providing intelligent direction, being rewarding, and showing that you can quickly understand a client's perspective are critical with this population. We have met many practitioners whose hearts are in the right place in wanting healthy change for their JICs—but in the absence of proper skills, confrontation becomes their default option, providing the illusion that the practitioners are doing something productive.

There is certainly no "single solution" or "one right way" to engage JICs, so several options are described. Our experiences with these engagement strategies have been overwhelmingly positive. We have been consistently surprised at the extent to which, if they are approached skillfully, JICs will verbalize a desire for help and work constructively toward making meaningful life changes.

MOTIVATIONAL INTERVIEWING AND OARS SKILLS

If you are new to the concepts of motivational interviewing (MI; introduced in Chapter 2), the good news is that the OARS skills (open questions, affirmations, reflections, and summarizations) are not exotic and are commonly taught across many models of counseling. However, within an MI framework, they are used with a certain precision, fluency, and rhythm. Since these skills are foundational, a quick review of how each is utilized in a forensic context is provided.

Open Questions

Thoughtful open questions promote in-depth responses and provide JICs with the latitude to reveal what is of most concern to them. Although most practitioners intellectually grasp the difference between open and closed questions (closed questions can be answered with minimal information; open questions require more elaboration), emphasizing open questions in practice is more challenging than it seems.

In the initial sessions, it is important to deliver open questions from an exploratory and curious stance ("What are your biggest concerns about work?"), rather than attempting to fix problems or find solutions ("What can you do to make things better at work?"). Also keep in mind that a barrage of fact-gathering, closed questions in the first session with a JIC will have the effect of narrowing the conversational focus and shutting the JIC down. Several examples contrasting closed and open questions are provided in Table 3.1. Notice how fewer questions can be used to gather the same information in an initial session, with the added benefit of allowing the JIC more space to reveal important details about his or her life.

Affirmations

Negative feedback from others is a common experience for JICs, and over time such individuals develop cognitive mechanisms that allow them to quickly dismiss or ignore criticism. Because of this tendency, you will need to show at the outset of treatment that you can quickly grasp the problem areas, but at the same time can recognize those things that are going well and acknowledge specific competencies that might help a JIC move forward. Keying into things that are positive will

TABLE 3.1. Converting Fact-Gathering, Closed Questions to Open Questions

Closed questions	Open questions
Family life	
"Are you married?"	"Tell me about your family relationships and *how* they are going right now?"
"How many kids do you have?"	
"Do you have stepchildren?"	
Employment	
"Are you working?"	"What have been your biggest successes and challenges regarding work?"
"Have you ever been fired from a job?"	
"How many times have you changed jobs in the past year?"	
Criminal history	
"Have you ever been incarcerated?"	"In what ways have you been involved with the criminal justice system?"
"Are you on probation?"	
"What is your current charge?"	

reduce defensiveness and enhance engagement. In addition, affirming provides the opportunity to verbally reinforce specific behaviors.

Affirmations are statements of appreciation for the client's accomplishments or strengths, formulated according to a specific structure. These guidelines for forming affirmations are offered by Miller and Rollnick (2013) and Rosengren (2018): (1) organizing each statement around the word *you*, and resisting the temptation to start with the word *I*; (2) affirming specific behaviors and descriptions of those behaviors; (3) attending to strengths rather than deficits; and (4) being genuine by keying into legitimate strengths and avoiding compliments that might seem superficial or insincere. Examples of affirmations that might be delivered in an initial session are provided in Table 3.2.

Reflections

The purpose of reflections is to convey an understanding of a JIC's perspective. Practitioners trained in various counseling modalities may have different conceptions of what reflections actually look like in practice. Skillful reflections involve more than parroting back what a client has just said. A reflection is a reasonable guess—delivered in the form of a statement—that emphasizes the meaning behind what a person has communicated (Miller & Rollnick, 2013). Reflecting is like holding up a mirror so that the person can see him- or herself clearly.

Forming reflections can feel clunky and artificial when practitioners first learn to do it. Becoming proficient with this skill takes time, and you can learn quickly by paying attention to JICs' reactions after reflections are delivered. Reflections that are on target produce nodding, continued talking, or sometimes enthusiastic agreement ("Yes, that's often the way I feel, and . . .").

TABLE 3.2. Forming Affirmations

"It is obvious that being a good parent is something you take very seriously."

"In spite of the fact that you are being pressured into coming here, you show a great openness in talking about your struggles."

"For someone who has faced so much hardship in finding full-time employment, you continue to get part-time work and resist the temptation to go back to selling drugs."

"You have worked hard to avoid the people who have negatively influenced you in the past, and you've been successful in making new friends."

"You have shown great determination in taking steps to slow down your drinking."

Reflections that miss the mark are followed by a facial expression of disagreement or by the JIC's correcting the statement and possibly providing additional information (e.g., "No, it's more than just the money; I crave the rush of excitement"). Once you know what to look for, you can perfect this skill with practice.

The skill of reflecting becomes incredibly valuable once a level of fluency in it is reached, because it allows smooth responses to all sorts of difficult statements by JICs. Although there are many ways to reflect, we recommend using certain sentence stems when you are learning to launch into reflections ("It sounds like . . . ," "You're feeling . . . ," "It seems . . . ," "So you . . . ," and "You . . ."). Examples of reflections in response to increasingly challenging JIC statements are presented in Table 3.3. Keep in mind that in the initial sessions, reflections are designed to clarify meaning, express understanding, reduce defensiveness, and move the interaction forward. For information about additional complex subtypes of reflections, see Rosengren (2018); for video demonstrations, see Miller, Moyers, and Rollnick (2013).

Summarizations

Summarizations are common endings in MI conversations. The key distinction between a summary and a reflection is that in reflecting, practitioners convey a moment-by-moment understanding of what the JIC means. In contrast, summaries reach back further and encapsulate larger amounts of information that help JICs organize their experiences. It is best to launch into summaries with sentences like these: "Let's pull together what we have been talking about," "Let me see if I understand what you have told me so far," or "We're running low on time, so let's pull together what is most important."

Summaries may be strategically inserted at various points in a conversation and serve different purposes. For example, a *collecting summary* highlights what is most important for the JIC; it pulls together relevant information into a well-structured and coherent package. Another type of summary is a *transitional summary*, which guides the conversation in a specific direction by ending with an open question. Examples of both types of summaries are presented in Table 3.4. The art of developing effective summaries is related to decisions about brevity and selectivity, since it is the practitioner who strategically decides what to include (Rosengren, 2018).

TABLE 3.3. Forming Reflections

JIC statements	Practitioner reflections
"Glad to be starting this program. Things have gotten really bad, and I'm hoping you can help me do something so that Child Services won't take my kids."	"*It sounds like* keeping your kids with you is your highest priority."
"I've never been to any type of counseling before. I'm not sure what is supposed to happen."	"*You're feeling* a little apprehensive, because this is new for you."
"I don't see how talking about my past abuse will change anything. It just makes me feel worse."	"*It sounds like* facing some of the things in your past is difficult, and you're not sure it's worth it."
"This drug testing is new. I don't really see the big deal. I use a little, but never on the job, and I always get my work done."	"*You think* that your drug use isn't really anyone else's business, because it doesn't get in the way of you performing your job."
"The system is unfair to men. She should be here and not me. She's the one who starts things. I'm just defending myself."	"*It seems* unfair that everyone is focused on you and not recognizing her role in what has been happening."
"I'm only here because my attorney thinks it would be a good idea; it's not because I want to do any of this crap."	"*You* are not here because you think you have a problem. You're here because your attorney thinks it will help with your legal problems. That's the only reason you're here."

TABLE 3.4. Forming Summaries

Collecting summary

"Let's pull together what we have been talking about. You are really trying to get your life back on track. Part of that involves finding other ways of coping with your problems besides using drugs. Finding consistent work is also a priority, and you are considering getting training to become an electrician. Finally, you want to improve things with your family, but recognize that it will take time to rebuild trust in your relationships."

Transitional summary

"You're not happy about having to come here as a condition of your parole, but you are willing to do whatever it takes not to go back to prison. In talking about things that put you at risk for ending up back in prison, you have identified one relationship that is a concern. It is clear to you that Matt's drug use and temper make him a risky friend to be around. And now that you are going to be a mother, you want to avoid situations that might lead to more legal problems. What do you see as the next step in dealing with this relationship?"

ENGAGING: TIPS FOR THE INITIAL SESSION

In some cases, engagement may happen quickly; in other cases, it may take considerable time or may never fully emerge. Without a foundation of engagement, it will be difficult to advance to the CBT strategies described in subsequent chapters. Of course, it is worth noting that even with the highest level of skill, you cannot expect to be effective with every JIC.

We recommend that in the first session, you position yourself as a good listener and strive to maintain a respectful, curious, supportive, empathic, and compassionate stance. Throughout the engagement process, a client-centered style is usually preferred over an active–directive approach. The initial session is relaxed and unrushed, and you should give up your own agenda in favor of meeting the JIC where he or she is. It is also important to maintain a moment-to-moment focus, without getting too far ahead of the JIC. Steering the interaction is subtle and somewhat akin to internet surfing: "clicking" (by using reflections and open questions) on what has been said that seems most important in the moment, carefully following what is next communicated by the JIC, and then "clicking" again on what seems most useful (Tafrate & Luther, 2014). This is stylistically different from traditional CBT, where practitioners operate like chess players—thinking several moves ahead, conceptualizing how their clients' beliefs are linked to behaviors, and pursuing strategies for altering dysfunctional patterns. Shifting to a more client-centered and present-moment focus requires you to take a leap of faith that the interaction will go somewhere useful. It usually does, and in a way that is more efficient than if you attempt to be overly directive.

We also recommend that you pull back from lengthy assessment activities in the initial session. Assessment of JICs will be more valid once a level of engagement is established. One possible strategy is to break apart engagement and comprehensive assessment by having separate meetings for these (engagement first and assessment second). Guidelines for assessment are discussed in detail in Chapter 5. Other practitioner behaviors to minimize in the first session (and beyond) include confrontation; judgmental statements; fact-gathering, closed questions; providing advice and solutions; and lecturing, moralizing, threatening, shaming, or arguing.

It is best to keep goals for the initial session modest. Although expectations about what is to be accomplished in a first meeting may vary across treatment settings, here is a sample checklist of reasonable goals for the first session:

- Understanding the circumstances that brought the JIC into treatment
- Exploring how the JIC views the situation
- Inviting the JIC to share his or her concerns
- Eliciting from the JIC how treatment might be beneficial
- Ending the session in a way making it likely that the person will continue to participate in treatment

Opening Statements and OARS Skills

In the first 60 seconds of the initial meeting, the stage is often set for successful (or unsuccessful) engagement. You can expect that a JIC who has been mandated or otherwise coerced into attending the appointment will be looking to you for cues about what to expect from treatment.

Therefore, the way you introduce yourself, describe your role, and explain the treatment process will be particularly influential in how the JIC responds. For this reason, it is important to develop an effective opening statement. Successful "openers" for working with JICs usually include four components: (1) introducing yourself and clarifying your role; (2) providing a general statement about the purpose of treatment; (3) conveying a sense of collaboration; and (4) ending with an open question that invites a response from the JIC. Once an opening statement is delivered and the JIC responds, you will shift into a curious, supportive, and empathic stance—utilizing OARS skills to keep the conversation moving. It is also helpful to get into the habit of ending the first session with a collecting summary.

Scripted examples of opening statements from diverse treatment settings (e.g., outpatient counseling, probation/parole, case management, and prison) are presented at the end of this chapter (Script 3.1). These examples can be used as a general guide in constructing your own opening statement that will fit best for your work environment.

Responding to Challenging JIC Statements in the Initial Session

While this style of engagement works well with the majority of JICs, provocative and antagonistic statements can, and do, emerge in the first meeting. A good rule of thumb is to expect the unexpected when working with this population. It also important to keep in mind that antagonistic JIC statements in the first session are not necessarily predictive of treatment failure, especially if they are responded to skillfully. We recommend that you strive to be patient, steer away from confrontation, and resist the urge to convince a JIC of the benefits of treatment. Instead, reflections and open questions that elicit more information about the JIC's concerns usually work best. With practice, you can learn to sidestep arguments and smoothly move the interaction in a productive direction. Table 3.5 provides some examples of how to respond constructively to difficult scenarios.

PUTTING IT INTO PRACTICE

As a practical first step to becoming proficient in engaging JICs, we recommend that you thoughtfully craft an opening statement—one that fits well with your specific work environment and adheres to the guidelines presented earlier. Opening statements are often works in progress, in that several variations can be pilot-tested to determine which version works best.

Developing fluency with OARS skills is another important element for successful engagement. Practice increasing reflections, emphasizing open questions, weaving occasional affirmations into the conversation, and ending sessions with summaries that highlight the most important things discussed. Even though these skills may seem basic, sustaining the OARS communication style throughout a conversation is not necessarily easy.

One procedure to help you quickly improve your skills is to record several sessions and code them afterward. Form 3.1 (located at the end of this chapter) provides a basic coding sheet for an initial session. Section 1 of the form is a checklist for evaluating the quality of the opening statement. Section 2 is structured to provide a running count of what *you* actually verbalize during the interaction, contrasting OARS skills with less desirable forms of communication. Several bench-

TABLE 3.5. Responding to Challenging JIC Statements in the Initial Session

JIC statements	Practitioner responses
"I don't belong here. It was just an argument that got out of hand. I'm not an abuser. "	"This incident was unusual, and it doesn't represent who you are." [Reflection]
"I've been to a lot of treatment programs, and nothing has ever worked."	"Tell me more about what you have tried." [Open question]
"What's the point in developing job skills? No one is going to hire me with my record."	"You don't think the effort is worth it, because it seems like no one is going to overlook your past and give you a chance." [Reflection]
"This is bullshit! I like drinking, and I'm not hurting anyone. Nobody is going to tell me to stop."	"What do you like about drinking?" [Open question]
"There is no way I'm going to tell you anything. You're not here to help me. You're gonna rat me out to my probation officer."	"You think this whole thing is about trying to keep you stuck in the system, and no one is really here to help you." [Reflection]
"My parole officer sent me. I'll be honest, I don't want to do this. I'm just here so I don't go back to prison. How many sessions can I miss and still get credit for completing this program?"	"You want to figure out the easiest way to get through this, and you also want to make sure you don't have any problems with parole and end up back in prison." [Reflection]

marks to strive for include the following: (1) using more open than closed questions, (2) having at least as many reflections as questions, and (3) pulling back from offering advice or solutions. Section 3 provides a checklist of the overall objectives accomplished in the first meeting.

The advantage of the coding and counting approach is that you can quickly see what you are doing well, what is missing, and what types of verbalizations should be minimized or increased as you move forward. By increasing your awareness and consistently practicing, you will improve your OARS skills and decrease unproductive communications. Even coding 5 or 10 minutes of a session will often provide clarity about what is going well and highlight areas for improvement. Keep in mind, however, that becoming too rigid in tracking your own in-session statements can be counterproductive, because you can end up focusing too much on yourself and not enough on the JIC. Also, relevant closed questions will not derail the session and can often be useful. It is the overall pattern that is most important. This coding exercise is meant as a way to take a "snapshot" of your natural style, in order to determine where to make adjustments.

In agencies and programs with large numbers of practitioners, the coding form (Form 3.1) can be incorporated into supervision, coaching, or quality assurance activities to promote consistency in how JICs are engaged. For interested readers, more advanced coding instruments for assessing MI proficiency are available (Miller, Moyers, Ernst, & Amrhein, 2008; Moyers, Martin, Manuel, Miller, & Ernst, 2010; Rosengren, Baer, Hartzler, Dunn, Wells, & Ogle, 2009).

KEY POINTS

- In the initial session, first and foremost, position yourself as a good listener and maintain a curious and exploratory stance.

- Try to minimize fact-gathering, closed questions, and to shift toward open questions that broaden the focus and allow JICs to reveal important details about their lives.

- Develop a well-prepared and structured statement for opening the first session. Effective opening statements set the stage for engagement in the first few seconds of the meeting.

- Even though most practitioners already have some familiarity with the OARS skills, it takes a good deal of practice to become proficient in using them to engage challenging clients.

- Remember that engagement is the primary goal of the first session. Assessment follows engagement and will be more valid once JICs feel they have been listened to.

SCRIPT 3.1. Sample Opening Statements

OUTPATIENT COUNSELING

"Hello, [JIC's name]. My name is Mark, and I'm a clinical psychologist. I work with people who are struggling to make changes in their lives. I'd like to spend a bit of time talking about what brought you here, the problems you have been having, and the history of those problems. Tell me, what brought you here?"

PROBATION/PAROLE

"Hello, [JIC's name]. Thanks for coming in on time today. My name is Meghan. I'll be your probation [parole] officer. Part of my job is to uphold the expectations of the court and the conditions of probation [parole]. Another part of my job is to provide support and information about community resources, and to help you gain skills and knowledge to successfully complete your probation [parole] and keep you from returning to the court [prison] in the future. We will work together on identifying some of your strengths and some of the things you've struggled with. We will also focus on those things you think might put you at risk for having future problems. Before we directly discuss those things, I'd like to know how you think being on probation might be helpful to you."

CASE MANAGEMENT

"Hello, [JIC's name]. My name is Denise, and I'm the clinical social worker at this program. People usually get referred here by the court as a condition of probation [parole]. I've read over your file and have an understanding of the conditions of your probation [parole], and my job is to help you get through this period successfully. During our meetings, we will work on identifying those factors in your life that might put you at risk for having future problems with the law. We will also talk about resources and skills to help you make changes that you think might be important. What are some things you might want to get out of this program?"

PRISON

"Hello, [JIC's name]. My name is Ryan. I am the counselor on this unit, and also your primary therapist. On this unit, you will have the opportunity to participate in a variety of individual and group mental health services, in addition to other out-of-cell activities. I heard that you just arrived on the unit, and I would like to learn more about you, so we can decide together what would be most helpful. Tell me about some of the things you have been struggling with."

FORM 3.1. Coding Sheet for the First Session

SECTION 1: OPENING STATEMENT

Session began with a structured opening statement: ☐ Yes   ☐ No

If yes: In the opening statement, the practitioner:

☐ Introduced him- or herself

☐ Briefly clarified his or her role

☐ Provided a general statement about the purpose of treatment

☐ Conveyed a sense of collaboration

☐ Ended with an open question that invited a response from the client

SECTION 2: COUNT OF PRACTITIONER VERBALIZATIONS

OARS skills	Verbalizations to minimize	Verbalizations to avoid
No. of open questions _____	No. of closed questions _____	No. of confrontational statements _____
No. of affirmations _____	No. of unsolicited pieces of advice/solutions offered _____	No. of judgmental statements _____
No. of reflections _____	No. of mini-lectures (don't count the opening statement) _____	No. of threatening statements _____
No. of summarizations _____		

SECTION 3: SESSION OBJECTIVES

Practitioner accomplished the following objectives:

☐ Understood the circumstances that brought the JIC into treatment

☐ Explored the JIC's view of the situation

☐ Invited the JIC to express his or her concerns

☐ Elicited the JIC's reasons why treatment might be beneficial

☐ Ended the session in a way making it likely that the JIC will continue to participate in treatment

CHAPTER 4

Clarifying Values and Life Priorities

It is obvious to Brenda after the first two sessions with Hank that his life would improve considerably, and his chances of involving himself in the criminal justice system would lessen, if he could better manage certain life areas—for instance, if he could decrease his use of alcohol, stop using and selling drugs, change his circle of friends, and better control his anger when things don't go his way. What is less clear to her (and probably to Hank) is this: What would Hank's life look like if he weren't doing those things? What would he do with his time instead? Who would he do it with? This relates to a larger question: What kind of life does Hank want for *himself*?

WHY WORK ON VALUES WITH JICs?

We place clarifying values and life priorities in the initial phase of treatment, because such discussions tend to sidestep resistance and enhance engagement. This strategy also provides a different, but important, piece of baseline information that is not obtained in the formal assessment procedures outlined in the next chapter: Learning what JICs value will help you understand what motivates them at a basic level. Although it will be necessary to address the criminogenic treatment targets discussed in the following chapters, values can serve as a useful anchor point in treatment and are something you can always come back to if you get lost or off track.

On the surface, discussions about values may seem tangential, or at best ancillary, to work with JICs. For the most part, the focus in forensic treatment is on reducing behaviors such as stealing cars, lying, skipping school, quitting jobs, hanging out with certain friends, arguing with family members, staying out until 3:00 A.M., using heroin, and so on. With so many treatment goals that are based on behaviors we want to stop, where does a discussion of values fit into treatment planning?

The presence of the words *reduce* and *stop* in the description of treatment goals above is key to one of the main reasons to include a discussion of values and life priorities early in treatment. For JICs, reducing and stopping behaviors such as the ones noted above mean pursuing a series of avoidance goals. However, helping JICs develop behavioral paths to a life worth living (approach goals) is an equally important treatment component. As noted in Chapter 2, there are at least two intervention models—the GLM (Dumas & Ward, 2016; Fortune & Ward, 2014; Ward, 2010) and ACT (Amrod & Hayes, 2014) —that emphasize approach goals as part of the change process in forensic treatment. A few questions are worth considering: What do we want JICs to be starting, not just stopping? What do we want them to do instead of their risky activities? And, at a larger level, what do they themselves want out of life? Understanding JICs' underlying values helps answer these questions.

We see treatment planning related to values as productive for two primary reasons: When approached properly, working on values (1) results in JICs' pursuing prosocial goals that often reduce maladaptive behaviors within criminal risk domains; and (2) raises JICs' awareness of areas where they are falling short of their own expectations for themselves and their lives, thereby providing a powerful motivator for behavior change. The remainder of this chapter addresses these points in more depth and provides practical guidelines for having powerful discussions of what matters most to JICs.

Values Can Help Establish Prosocial Goals that Reduce Risk

Let's return to the case of Jackie. The high-risk nature of Jackie's friendships with the older men from the car wash makes "distancing" from them a logical (avoidance) goal. The reestablishment of former friendships with women her age is a good example of an approach goal that not only enhances the richness of Jackie's life, but also reduces her risk for recidivism. Reestablishing some of her old healthy relationships increases her connection to positive social influences, diminishes the importance of her car wash friends, and allows her to see—in a new light—the impact these men have recently been having on her life.

Values Can Help Build Motivation for Change

Clarifying values helps create discrepancy between JICs' current destructive behavior patterns and their underlying values and aspirations. In a general sense for all of us, being aware of the discrepancy between how we are living and how we want to live can act as a powerful catalyst for change.

In discussing values, you may discover a potentially powerful motivator for behavior change that can be harnessed throughout the treatment process. Using the MI skills reviewed in Chapter 3, and the more advanced skills presented in Chapter 7 (it is OK to peek ahead to the Chapter 7 discussion of evoking motivation), you can help JICs become aware of how specific thinking and behavior patterns are undermining their own underlying values. You can also assist JICs in developing their own arguments for change so that they can live more harmonious lives—ones that are consistent with what they view as their most important life priorities.

Let's again consider the case of Jackie. One of her priorities is taking care of her mother, who has been disabled by a car accident. Once Jackie begins to explore the relationship between her current lifestyle and her underlying values, it becomes obvious to her that she has been living in a way inconsistent with "Staying involved with family members" and "Being a supportive daughter." Little things like checking in on her mom regularly, playing cards with her, and having dinner with her—as well as bigger things like taking her mother to doctor's appointments and making sure she has her medications—have been wholly taken over by her siblings. As Jackie looks back on times when she acts according to this core value, she notes that she feels closer to her mother, feels better about herself, and has a sense of satisfaction in doing something for her family that is highly rewarding.

Another of Jackie's identified values is "Doing work that I find rewarding or important." As Jackie discusses the connection (or lack thereof) between her job at the car wash and what she values, she realizes again that she has been living in a way inconsistent with what she views as a very important value in her life. She has found her job at the car wash neither rewarding nor challenging. As Brenda soon learns, Jackie didn't even seek out the position, but only took the job because a friend who was quitting recommended her to the manager. She did not intend to stay long, but after a few months became complacent and set aside other aspirations such as pursuing her education. Helping Jackie gain an awareness of how she has gradually drifted from a life based on her core values becomes a compelling source of motivation for doing things differently and making changes in her lifestyle. Pursuing goals consistent with her values also puts Jackie on a path toward addressing the relevant criminal risk domains of her life.

DISTINGUISHING VALUES FROM GOALS

It is not uncommon for values and goals to be confused by both practitioners and JICs. Clarity on these issues is necessary before you initiate discussions of values. Although the strategies presented in this chapter touch upon both values and goals, the difference between the two is more than a semantic one, and it has implications for treatment planning.

A *value* is a direction or overarching aspiration in a particular life area. Ideally, values guide the choices that lead to a meaningful life or a "life worth living." In this regard, values can never be achieved in a tangible sense; they are directions that can be followed over the long term. *Goals*, on the other hand, are tangible objectives. Although energy related to goals may ebb and flow, goals are essentially finite in duration, and their success can be measured (e.g., fully achieved, partially achieved, or not achieved). Goals in major life areas can be consistent or inconsistent with our values. If we set goals that are consistent with our values, we keep ourselves moving in a direction or path that is meaningful. Once a goal is achieved, the underlying value remains and will be expressed through new goals and the related behaviors we engage in to achieve those goals.

As a concrete example of these concepts, a mother may question her teenage daughter (e.g., "How will you spend the afternoon hours after school? Who will you spend time with? Where will you be?"). This simple behavior pattern of parental monitoring is probably annoying to the adolescent, but if you were to ask the mother why she does it, she might say that the goal is "Making sure my kid stays out of trouble." This behavior and goal will likely end (or lessen) with high school graduation, but the underlying value "Being a concerned and involved parent" will remain after high school graduation and manifest itself in new goals (and, ideally, behaviors that are more appreciated by the daughter as she grows older).

Once more, Jackie's case can be used as an illustration of these concepts. As part of her probation supervision, Jackie is referred to an employment skills program. Successful completion of the program, and adherence to other probation conditions, will allow Jackie to avoid incarceration. The program assists clients with the development of résumés, job search strategies, and job interviewing skills. In Jackie's case, completing the program becomes a goal consistent with her underlying value of "Doing work that is rewarding or important." Although the goal ends with the completion of the program, the underlying value provides direction for her to pursue both part-time work and admission to a technical program at a community college. This path thus continues long after her probation period has ended.

IDENTIFYING AND DISCUSSING VALUES

The Values Helpsheet (Form 4.1, provided at the end of this chapter) helps JICs identify their values and set goals that will allow them to live in a manner consistent with those values. While these objectives can be accomplished through less structured discussions, having a stimulus like the Values Helpsheet will be useful because, although JICs certainly have values, they may have never articulated them and therefore remain relatively unaware of what they are. Generic lists of values for use in clinical practice can be found in several places in the public domain (simply enter the online search terms *core values* or *personal values*). The Values Helpsheet is by no means exhaustive. It contains 16 values across four major life areas relevant to JICs. If you are already familiar with existing lists of values, you may be surprised to see that we do not include those that consist of highly abstract nouns (e.g., *creativity, wisdom, perseverance*); instead, we present values in the form of life directions related to criminal risk domains. This is a strategic attempt to get JICs working in those specific areas of functioning that are directly connected with future criminal behavior. As an example, a completed Values Helpsheet for Hank is provided in Figure 4.1.

We recommend that you start by working through the Values Helpsheet with a JIC in a structured manner. A complete script for using the Values Helpsheet can be found at the end of this chapter (Script 4.1). Start by explaining the nature and purpose of the helpsheet, and then provide a copy to the JIC, directing his or her attention to the values in the left-hand column. Ask the JIC to read over the list and circle 2 values (of the 16) that are most important. If a JIC has strong values that are not on the helpsheet, there is an option in each life area where the client can write in his or her own. Ask the JIC to rank-order the 2 values he or she has circled in terms of their importance, and explore why these values are priorities for the person (see the sample dialogue below). Make sure the values that JICs circle are the ones that actually matter to the clients, not the ones they think they should have. For example, not every JIC who has children strongly values being a concerned and involved parent, and not every JIC who has a significant other values being a nurturing and committed partner. Sometimes JICs may choose certain values to avoid negative judgments from others.

You want to use the Values Helpsheet to clarify what JICs value most, because that's where you will have the greatest likelihood of establishing meaningful goals that the clients will potentially work toward, and that will reduce their risk of reoffending. Let's return to the case of Hank. Brenda introduces the Values Helpsheet as follows:

> "I'd like to spend some time today talking about the things that are important to you, the things that make life worth living. Let's call these *values*. We all have values, but we may not always know exactly what they are because we don't take the time to tell them to ourselves and to clarify them. When people aren't making decisions in line with their values, they tend to lead less satisfying lives. So figuring out our underlying values gives us more chances to make decisions in life that are in line with our values. This helpsheet lists values in some

What's most important to you?

Life Area (My values)	Goal (What I want to see happen in the next 6–12 months)	Next Step (What I need to do next to move toward the goal)
Intimate and Family Relationships		
(Being a nurturing and committed partner)	Have a good relationship. Go on dates with positive women.	Text or call Denise.
Staying involved with family members		
Being a nurturing and involved parent		
Being a good role model for my child		
Other _____		
Friends and Community		
Being a supportive and trusted friend		
Having friendships that are close/accepting		
Being actively involved in community service or organizations (e.g., school board, PTO, town council)		
Other _____		

46

Career and Learning	Become a commercial driver.	Get information on three schools that offer classes for the commercial driver's license (CDL).
Being excellent in my line of work		
(Doing work that I find rewarding or important)		
Learning new skills		
Keeping my mind active through education		
Other _____		
Lifestyle		
Maximizing my physical health		
Being of service to others		
Being involved in sports		
Maintaining my sobriety		
Developing my spirituality		
Other _____		

FIGURE 4.1. Hank's completed Values Helpsheet.

major life areas. Take a look at the left-hand column, and read through the different values in the life areas. Circle the two from the list that are most important to you right now. It is OK if the two that you select appear across different life areas. Try to circle two things that you really value, and not what other people expect you to value. Not everyone strongly values parenting or career, for instance. This helpsheet is meant to get you in touch with what you really value right now. There are also spaces where you can write down a value if the ones on the sheet don't really match yours."

Brenda and Hank then engage in this dialogue:

> BRENDA: I'd like to learn more about what these mean to you. You circled "Doing work that I find rewarding or important." What makes that one stand out for you?
>
> HANK: Pretty much that I've just had jobs here and there. Nothing real.
>
> BRENDA: So nothing in the work area has meant much to you so far.
>
> HANK: You wouldn't think it from my history, but work is important to me. I want to get up and go to work. When I'm working, I'm there early. I'll stay late. But if I don't like what I'm doing while I'm there, I don't stay.
>
> BRENDA: So work that is meaningful is important, and that's something that has been missing for you.
>
> HANK: Right. I've just done stuff that I fell into or found. I was glad to have the work, have money coming in, but there was nothing to it beyond that.
>
> BRENDA: And you're looking for more. (*Moves on to the next core value that Hank has circled.*)

Setting Goals Consistent with Values

Once the JIC's core values have been identified and discussed, help the JIC pick one to focus on for the Goal and Next Steps columns of the Values Helpsheet. Don't try to address more than one core value at a time. Start with one value, and wait until you think sufficient progress has been made before going back to the helpsheet and starting on the next one. Working on values will become an ongoing activity—something that you and the JIC revisit with new goals and homework assignments as the course of treatment progresses.

Getting started on one value begins with setting a goal for the JIC to work toward that is consistent with this value, and then identifying the next step to be taken that moves the person in the direction of achieving this goal. Ideally, the next step is concrete and specific—one that can be achieved before your next appointment, and that you are confident does not exceed the JIC's current skills and resources. This next step then becomes a homework assignment and a starting point for the next appointment. Again, Brenda and Hank provide an example:

> BRENDA: Now that we've talked about specific values, I'd like you to take a look at the Goal column of the helpsheet and write down a goal you want to work toward in the next 6 to 12 months. Your goal needs to fit with the value "Doing work that I find rewarding or important."
>
> HANK: (*Writes on sheet.*)

BRENDA: (*Reading from sheet*) "Become a commercial driver."

HANK: I've had one job I liked—working for a trucking company. Other than that, there hasn't been anything that I looked forward to, or even liked. I did odd jobs for people around the neighborhood, such as painting and yard work. Also odd jobs for my uncle, who's a contractor. I've worked in a few restaurants, washing dishes and cleaning. I worked in a factory, also cleaning. I just did them because I had to.

BRENDA: So most of what you've done hasn't really been for you. But the trucking company was different?

HANK: I got that job through my uncle. He knows the owner of a trucking company. I didn't have a commercial license, so I wasn't a driver. I just worked moving the trucks on the lot and helping him out.

BRENDA: How did moving the trucks on the lot connect with something meaningful?

HANK: I like cars and trucks. I like working on them. I like driving them. I'd really like to be a driver. I've wanted that for a long time.

BRENDA: Great! Now that we've got a goal for the next few months, the next step is to set up a very short-term action that moves you toward completing this goal—something you think is actually worth doing but that is also realistic, even if it won't be easy. Try to think of what that would be, and write it down in the Next Steps column on the helpsheet.

HANK: Well, if I want to become a driver, I need to get my CDL [commercial driver's license]. That's something I've thought about over the years.

BRENDA: That doesn't sound like something that happens overnight.

HANK: No. You have to go to a licensed school, take a course, and then take a test.

BRENDA: What's one thing you can do between now and our next appointment that will get you a little closer to the goal?

HANK: I could look into some CDL schools.

BRENDA: That sounds good. How would you do that, and what information would you be looking for?

HANK: I'd be looking at the cost, when classes start, and location. I think I can find information over the internet. I've thought about doing it in the past.

BRENDA: How many different schools do you think it makes sense to look at?

HANK: I don't know. I guess at least three.

BRENDA: So how about for a next step, you bring in the information you find on three different schools? Bring that information to our next appointment, and we'll look at it together and then figure out another next step—and think about how to keep moving forward from there.

Following Up on Next Steps and Goals

We recommend the use of specific behavioral homework assignments for next steps that are connected to larger goals and underlying values. This gets JICs working toward their goals in a structured manner. It also provides an opportunity for them to receive positive reinforcement for engaging in newer, more productive behaviors; this gives them a sense of accomplishment and self-efficacy. It is important to provide affirmations for effort and for homework that is successfully completed.

When you are developing homework assignments for next steps, we recommend taking an active role in making sure that these steps are well within the range of a JIC's capabilities. For example, we have seen cases in which JICs who have not applied for a job in over a year suggest a next step of applying for a dozen or more jobs in the span of 1 week. Although that would certainly be a productive use of time, there seems a high likelihood of failure, given the clients' history and context. In such situations, adjusting the assignment to one or two job applications is preferable, because it's more likely to be successfully completed. In the early stages of treatment, you want to establish a pattern in which homework gets completed and to set up success experiences related to between-session assignments.

Once the Values Helpsheet has been introduced, working on values becomes an ongoing component of treatment, with new next steps being set as the JIC moves forward, new goals being established as the client fulfills existing goals, and new values being targeted. Whenever new next steps are assigned, time should be allocated for their review in the following appointment. Failing to review homework can be deflating to a JIC who has made the effort to complete it; even worse, this failure will communicate that any homework you assign is unimportant.

A step-by-step outline and sample script for following up on the Values Helpsheet is provided at the end of this chapter (Script 4.2). Begin by encouraging the JIC to discuss his or her progress on the next step. If the JIC was successful in completing it, take advantage of the opportunity to offer an affirmation. If relevant, allow the JIC to talk about what it was like to work toward the goal, and what he or she has learned. This helps raise the JIC's awareness of, and highlight the reward of, acting consistently with values. After reviewing the progress on the next step, build on the JIC's success by working with him or her to identify a new next step that moves the client further toward the goal, and discuss homework for the next appointment.

If the next step has not been successfully completed, do not simply reassign it without first discussing the nature of the difficulty that came up. If the barrier appears to have been motivational, consider taking a step back and developing a different goal or next step about which the JIC seems more enthusiastic or energized. If the barrier is related to a lack of skills or resources, help the JIC troubleshoot the difficulty. JICs may have limited experience advocating for themselves, successfully navigating organizations, or engaging others cooperatively. Your assistance as a resource can sometimes be valuable and necessary. Once you feel confident that barriers have been resolved and the JIC is in a position to succeed, go ahead and reassign the next step.

DISCUSSING DISCREPANCY VERSUS CONSISTENCY BETWEEN VALUES AND DECISIONS

We have noted earlier that one of the benefits of completing the Values Helpsheet is the opportunity to make JICs aware of their values in the first place. Although they have values, these may have never been articulated—and, by extension, the opportunity to consciously set goals according to their values and live in a manner consistent with them may never have materialized. The Values Helpsheet discussion can set the stage for conversations focused on making JICs aware of the discrepancy between their underlying values and any recent antisocial or self-defeating decision making. This awareness can then become a powerful motivator for making better decisions as the clients move forward.

A structured follow-up script for discussing discrepancy versus consistency between values and decisions is provided at the end of this chapter (Script 4.3). To begin, select one of the JIC's values, and elicit an example of a specific decision the client recently made that was contrary to this value. If the JIC offers an example from the distant past, probe for a more recent example (the more recent, the better). Once the situation and decision have been described, prompt the JIC to verbalize how he or she considers the decision to be inconsistent with the selected value. Use the MI skills discussed in Chapter 3 to explore the discrepancy more fully, and to elicit from the JIC his or her view regarding how such decisions might create risk for further involvement with the criminal justice system. You want JICs to increase their own awareness of how making decisions that are contrary to their values can put them at risk for more problems. We recommend that you avoid explaining or directly telling JICs about these connections. The discussion will have more impact if JICs make such connections themselves.

The second part of the discussion is essentially the inverse of the first part. Elicit an example of a specific decision that was consistent with the selected value. Again, probe for a recent example. Once you have an understanding of the situation and decision, explore with the JIC how he or she sees the decision as consistent with the selected value. Encourage the JIC to look for connections between this type of decision and a more positive lifestyle, which includes steering clear of criminal involvement in the future. The aim is to increase awareness of how living in accordance with values can reduce overall risk and lead to more satisfying life outcomes. To conclude the discussion, provide a summary that contrasts the nature and outcomes of both types of decisions. In the case of Hank, the following dialogue illustrates a brief discussion about the second value he has selected: "Being a nurturing and committed partner."

BRENDA: I want to follow up on some of the values we touched upon last time, and explore some decisions you've made that were in line with your values and those that were not. Tell me about a decision you made since I last saw you that maybe wasn't consistent or wasn't in line with your value of having a healthy dating relationship.

HANK: I went out with one of my sister's friends. She'd said she liked me, and I liked her. It didn't go well. I fucked it up.

BRENDA: What about this date didn't fit with your value of having a healthy relationship?

HANK: The date ended in an argument. I was telling her about how money is kind of tight right now. She said, "So why do you spend your money on alcohol and pot?" That made me kind of mad, and I got loud and blew it out of proportion.

BRENDA: I think I'm getting the picture. Tell me a little more about what happened.

HANK: It's not like I am spending all this money on pot and booze. She was saying this, and I'd just bought her a margarita. She should be supportive. When I got loud, she got really pissed. My blow-up ended the relationship, and it was just getting started.

BRENDA: So, for you, reacting with anger pushed her away. And you wanted to go in the other direction with this relationship.

HANK: Yeah. She has a good head on her shoulders. I overreacted and messed it up.

BRENDA: Tell me how reacting with anger could potentially lead to problems with the criminal justice system.

HANK: It's kind of like my last arrest. When I get angry, I sometimes put my hands on people. Even when I don't get physical, I get loud, and people get afraid, and sometimes the cops get called.

BRENDA: It sounds like that's happened in the past.

HANK: It has, and not just with my last arrest.

BRENDA: So not managing your anger doesn't help you get close to women. It also puts you at risk for more problems with the police. Now tell me about a decision you made recently that was in line with your value of having a healthy dating relationship.

HANK: I guess just calling her in the first place was a good step, because she is a stable person. I don't always make the right choices with people I get involved with.

BRENDA: Tell me more about making better choices.

HANK: Usually the person I would be with would never bring up my drinking and smoking, because they would be right there doing it with me. She recognized that what I was doing wasn't a good thing, given my situation.

BRENDA: What's the best thing for you about making better relationship choices?

HANK: If I want to have a healthy relationship, I have to pick more stable women. I probably have to change the way I act, too.

BRENDA: If you make decisions more in line with this value, how can that help you avoid problems with the criminal justice system?

HANK: I will be with people who are doing the right thing and who are a better influence on me—less alcohol and drugs, less conflict, and less drama all around.

BRENDA: That sounds like the type of relationship you want. It seems like when you act impulsively with anger, it moves you further away from your goal of having a healthy relationship, and it puts you more at risk for getting arrested. In the past, you have chosen to get involved with people who don't bring out the best in you. You recognize that getting a handle on who you spend time with and how you deal with your anger will be important in moving toward this value.

Concerns about JICs with Destructive Values

We have noticed that some practitioners avoid discussing values with JICs, because they assume JICs will express values that are highly antisocial and/or self-destructive (e.g., "My dream is to be the biggest drug dealer in the state," or "I want to be the most feared gang member in my neighborhood"). It is, of course, possible that you will encounter JICs whose core values are focused on harm and destruction to both themselves and others. Fortunately, expressions of outright antisocial values seem to be extremely rare, and in our experience, these concerns should not dissuade you from discussing values. Although we have repeatedly pointed out areas of differences in clinical work between JICs and traditional mental health clients, discussions of values with JICs reveals that most of them have the same core values as those suffering from mental health problems do: being a good provider for the family, having meaningful relationships, experiencing fun and enjoyment in life, and being successful at work.

The difference between JICs and traditional mental health clients may not be in the nature of the core values they hold, but in the degree to which they make choices that are inconsistent with their values and the strategies that they adopt in pursuit of their values. The cases of both Jackie and Hank provide examples. Jackie has made a lot of recent choices inconsistent with her values of "Staying involved with family members," "Being a supportive daughter," and "Doing work that I find rewarding or important." Similarly, Hank has made many choices inconsistent with his values of "Doing work that I find rewarding or important" and "Being a nurturing and committed partner." The discrepancy–consistency discussion is intended to make this pattern evident to JICs.

How a person goes about pursuing a value may be another difference between JICs and traditional mental health clients. For example, consider two fathers who share the same value of "Being a good role model for my child." Each father takes his son to a baseball game, where the child accidentally spills a drink on the person in the seat in front of him. A volatile situation quickly develops with the drink-drenched, angry patron. Both fathers know that their sons are keenly observing them. One father may seek to defuse the situation and placate the angry patron, because he believes that by defusing tense situations, he is serving as a good role model. The other father shouts and shoves the angry patron, threatening to do further harm if he doesn't sit down and shut up, because he believes that showing toughness will help his son to grow up strong. It is not hard to see how antisocial and self-destructive actions can often be made in pursuit of an ordinary and prosocial value.

Clarifying values provides anchor points that can be useful in guiding future behavioral choices by decreasing choices that interfere with personal values and that put JICs at risk for future criminal justice involvement. Clarifying values also assists JICs in developing more prosocial and meaningful lives.

KEY POINTS

- Discussions that clarify values and life priorities are useful in the initial stages of treatment, because they enhance engagement and provide critical information regarding what JICs want out of life.

- Once identified, values can serve as beneficial anchor points throughout the treatment process, help to establish prosocial goals that offset risk, and foster motivation for change.

- *Values* are big life directions that require ongoing attention across a lifetime. *Goals* are tangible objectives that can be completed and have a clear end point. *Next steps* are concrete and specific actions JICs can take to move them toward their desired goals and values.

- Decisions that are contrary to JICs' values can lead to more risk for future criminal justice problems, whereas decisions in harmony with underlying values tend to reduce risk. Thus aligning everyday decision making with values is an important treatment objective.

- When asked—at a basic level—what they ultimately value in life, the overwhelming majority of JICs will verbalize values similar to those of most other people. The expression of psychopathic and sadistic values is quite rare.

- Living in accordance with values and life priorities sets the stage for JICs to develop a more positive lifestyle and live more meaningful lives.

SCRIPT 4.1. Instructions for Introducing the Values Helpsheet

Step 1: Briefly review the nature and importance of values.

Sample explanation: "I'd like to spend some time today talking about the things that are important to you, the things that make life worth living. Let's call these *values*. We all have values, but we may not always know exactly what they are, because we don't take the time to tell them to ourselves and to clarify them. When people aren't making decisions in line with their values, they tend to lead less satisfying lives. So figuring out our underlying values gives us more chances to make decisions in life that are in line with our values."

Step 2: Introduce the Values Helpsheet and have the JIC identify values.

Sample introduction: "This helpsheet lists some values in some major life areas. Take a look at the left-hand column, and read through the different values in the life areas. Circle the two values that are most important to you right now. It is OK if the two that you select appear across different life areas. Try to circle only the things that you really value, and not what other people expect you to value. For example, not everyone strongly values parenting or career; these may be important, but not core values. This helpsheet is meant to get you in touch with what you really value right now. There are also spaces where you can write down a value if the ones on the sheet don't really match yours."

Step 3: Clarify the chosen values, using open questions, and have the JIC choose one value to work on first.

Sample prompt: "I'd like to learn more about what these mean to you. You circled [name of value]. What makes that value important for you?"

Step 4: Reflect back what is most important to the JIC.

Step 5: Have the JIC identify a goal related to the chosen value. Use open questions to clarify the goal.

Sample prompt: "Now that we've talked about specific values, I'd like you to take a look at the Goal column of the Values Helpsheet, and write down a goal you want to work toward or achieve in the next 6 months to a year that fits with [name of value]."

Step 6: Develop and identify a *next step* (an assignment the client can do that will move him or her closer to achieving the chosen goal). Assign it for the next session. Again, use open questions to clarify as necessary.

Sample prompt: "From here, we want to set up a very short-term action that moves you toward completing this goal—something you think is actually worth doing in your life, but that is also realistic, even if it won't be easy. The key to accomplishing goals is getting started. Even a small step in the

(continued)

direction you think is important is a step worth taking. So in the Next Step column of the Values Helpsheet, jot down something you can do between now and the next time we meet that will get you started."

Step 7: Recap the connection among thinking, actions, and values.

Sample closing: "To sum up, we've talked about how knowing our own personal values can help guide us to make better decisions. And when we set goals about the things that matter most to us, it can become clearer how to start the journey. You've set [name of value] as one of the life areas that is important to you; you've set [name of goal] as a goal you want to work on in relation to that value; and you've said that [name of next step] is the next step for you toward achieving that goal. When we meet next time, I'd like to hear how the next step went."

SCRIPT 4.2. Following Up on Next Steps Connected to Values

Step 1: Review progress on the next step that was assigned in the previous session.

"Last time we met, we discussed one of the values in life that is most important to you, which was [name of value]. We also discussed a longer-term goal related to that value, which was [name of goal], and we talked about a next step you could take that would move you in a valued direction. That step was [name of next step]. Tell me how working on that step went." [Explore progress as necessary. If the JIC did reasonably well, move to Steps 2a and 3a. If the JIC did not succeed, move to Step 2b and 3b.]

Step 2a (if the JIC has moved forward): Affirm the positive step, and elicit the JIC's motivation for moving forward.

"What did you learn from doing [name of next step]?"

"What are your thoughts about your ability to keep moving forward?"

Step 3a (if the JIC has moved forward): Work with the JIC to assign a new next step in line with the value, and/or establish a next step for a different value.

"So what can you do between now and the next time we meet that will keep you moving in this direction?"

"What is something you can do between now and the next time we meet that will get you started on your other value, [name of other value the JIC has previously identified]?"

Step 2b (if the JIC has not moved forward): If the JIC has not been successful, explore the nature of the barrier to achieving the next step. Troubleshoot ways to move forward.

"What got in the way?"

"What would help you to succeed the next time?"

Step 3b (if the JIC has not moved forward): Depending upon the outcome of Step 2b, reassign the previous next step, or develop a new assignment in line with the value, or assign a next step related to a different value.

Step 4: Close the discussion by expressing confidence in the JIC's ability to move forward, and remind the person that this topic will be on the agenda for the next session.

"I'm sure if you decide to make a change here, you will do it. Thanks for your willingness to talk about this issue. We will check in on how you are doing with this the next time we meet."

SCRIPT 4.3. Discussing Discrepancy versus Consistency between Values and Decisions

PART 1: EXPLORING DISCREPANCY

Step 1: Identify a recent decision by the JIC that was inconsistent with an identified value.

"Take a look at the Values Helpsheet that we completed together, and tell me about a decision you made recently that wasn't in line with [name of value the JIC has identified in the previous session]."

Step 2: Explore the discrepancy between the decision and the value.

"What makes the decision inconsistent with the value?"

"What's the worst thing for you about making decisions that aren't in line with what you value most?"

Step 3: Reflect back what is most important to the JIC.

Step 4 (if appropriate): Explore the potential relationship between the decision and future criminal justice involvement.

"How could this decision have led to further problems with the criminal justice system?"

"In the past, how have decisions like this gotten you in trouble?"

Step 5: Again, reflect back what is most important to the JIC.

PART 2: EXPLORING CONSISTENCY

Step 1: Identify a recent decision by the JIC that was consistent with the identified value.

"Now tell me about a decision you made recently that was in line with [name of value the JIC has identified in the previous session]."

Step 2: Explore the consistency between this decision and the value.

"What makes the decision seem consistent with the value?"

"What's the best thing for you about making decisions that are in line with what you value most?"

Step 3: Reflect back what is most important to the JIC.

(continued)

Step 4 (if appropriate): Explore the potential relationship between the decision and avoiding future criminal justice involvement.

> "If you keep making decisions more in line with this value, how can that help you avoid problems with the criminal justice system and lead to a better life?"

> "How do you think your life can be different if you keep making decisions that are consistent with this value?"

Step 5: Again, reflect back what is most important to the JIC.

PART 3: SUMMARIZING DISCREPANCY–CONSISTENCY

"So when you make decisions such as [name of inconsistent decision] that are not in line with what you value, you set yourself up for more problems. On the other hand, when you make decisions in line with your values, such as [name of consistent decision], you are more likely to create a better life for yourself."

FORM 4.1. Values Helpsheet

What's most important to you?

Life Area (My values)	Goal (What I want to see happen in the next 6–12 months)	Next Step (What I need to do next to move toward the goal)
Intimate and Family Relationships Being a nurturing and committed partner Staying involved with family members Being a nurturing and involved parent Being a good role model for my child Other _____		
Friends and Community Being a supportive and trusted friend Having friendships that are close/accepting Being actively involved in community service or organizations (e.g., school board, PTO, town council) Other _____		

(continued)

FORM 4.1. Values Helpsheet (page 2 of 2)

Life Area (My values)	Goal (What I want to see happen in the next 6–12 months)	Next Step (What I need to do next to move toward the goal)
Career and Learning		
Being excellent in my line of work		
Doing work that I find rewarding or important		
Learning new skills		
Keeping my mind active through education		
Other _____		
Lifestyle		
Maximizing my physical health		
Being of service to others		
Being involved in sports		
Maintaining my sobriety		
Developing my spirituality		
Other _____		

ASSESSMENT, CASE FORMULATION, AND FOCUS

CHAPTER 5

Assessing Criminal Risk Domains

Brenda knows that effective treatment is based on assessment and case formulation, because an understanding of what makes a client "tick" allows for the development of clear treatment targets and for appropriate planning. In order for Brenda to establish sound case formulations for Hank and Jackie, she must collect information about both clients by way of assessment. Brenda has spent some time trying to understand the literature regarding "what works" with JICs, and has acquired a conceptual knowledge base regarding relevant criminal risk domains pertinent to this client group. Unfortunately, her limited clinical exposure to JICs makes her unsure how to transfer this conceptual knowledge into actual practice. She wonders:

"What changes do I need to make to my standard assessment interview?"
"How do I assess areas that I'm not overly familiar with or comfortable discussing?"
"What kinds of questions do I ask clients about these aspects of their lives?"

As noted in Chapter 1, casual perusal of the scientific literature related to JICs shows that an enormous volume of scholarly activity has occurred during the past three decades related to assessment and treatment. However, the clinical practice literature contains few descriptions of how to put this scientific knowledge into actual practice. Gendreau and his colleagues (see Gendreau, Goggin, & Paparozzi, 1996; Gendreau & Smith, 2007) have commented about the importance of bridging the science–practice gap, so that JICs are offered treatment that has the greatest opportunity for promoting clinical improvement. This chapter describes a practical approach to assessing the most important criminal risk domains for JICs.

OVERVIEW OF ASSESSMENT AND CASE FORMULATION

In the construction industry, a vital component of the building process is some type of schematic drawing or blueprint. Building plans are important because they provide some detail about what is to be accomplished, the relationship between important pieces, and the order in which they are to be completed. This same concept can apply to forensic treatment planning. Your goal is to assist JICs in altering their criminal behavior, and this will require determining which specific criminal risk domains are most instrumental for a particular JIC, understanding the manner in which the relevant risk domains interact with each other, and strategically prioritizing treatment targets. Identifying and understanding the specific factors influencing criminality are the goals of *assessment* (discussed in this chapter), and synthesizing relevant assessment information to create a tailored treatment plan is called *case formulation* (discussed in Chapter 6).

The assessment and case formulation process with JICs often involves the same procedures that occur with traditional mental health clients: an interview with the client to gather socio-developmental and background information; perhaps an interview with a collateral source, such as a family member; a review of available file records; administration of psychometric tests; and thoughtful integration of the information into a case formulation. The difference with JICs is largely one of focus, with assessment directed toward the criminal risk domains discussed in Chapter 2: history of criminal/antisocial behavior; criminogenic thinking/antisocial orientation; antisocial companions; dysfunctional family/romantic relationships; lack of connection to work/school; maladaptive leisure time; substance abuse/misuse; and anger dysregulation. Some of the criminal risk domains encompass specialized areas of practice (e.g., substance abuse/misuse, criminogenic thinking/antisocial orientation, anger dysregulation), for which standardized assessment instruments exist that can be incorporated into your assessment (see Appendix A for recommendations). Understanding JICs' status or functioning in these domains aids in prioritizing treatment targets and tailoring interventions to specific cases.

Ideally, by adhering to the practices outlined in Chapters 3 and 4, you will have been able to attend to and improve (or at least understand) responsivity factors such as motivation and excessive defensiveness, prior to formal assessment. Guidelines for evaluating general psychopathology are beyond the scope of this treatment planner. If you are interested in further assessment resources, we recommend Morrison (2014) as a general guide; Leahy, Holland, and McGinn (2012) for assessment of depression and anxiety disorders; and A. T. Beck, Davis, and Freeman (2015) for assessment strategies for the full range of personality disorders.

ASSESSING CRIMINAL RISK DOMAINS: GUIDELINES FOR THE ASSESSMENT INTERVIEW

For practitioners unfamiliar with working with JICs, obtaining information about criminal risk domains may require adjustments to their existing assessment interview protocols. These adjustments are likely to include (1) more extended exploration of JICs' criminal history; (2) probes for antisocial lifestyle elements (e.g., routines, relationships, and destructive habits); and (3) expansion of their typical interviewing questions to include areas not typically assessed (e.g., social connections, leisure activities, criminogenic thinking). A template for beginning the interview is provided at the end of this chapter (Script 5.1).

Detailed questions to assist you in exploring each of the criminal risk domains are also provided at the end of this chapter (Scripts 5.2–5.9). Questions are organized within each area to allow for the exploration of specific facets within each domain. In regard to the order of the interview, we recommend beginning with criminal history, because it is perhaps the only area where reasonable corroborating information (i.e., legal files) exists that can serve as a modest check on a JIC's honesty and openness, and establish a baseline of self-report reliability. The degree to which there is similarity between self-report information and data from other sources provides an approximate gauge of the JIC's "truthfulness" in other areas that are more challenging to corroborate (e.g., substance use patterns, aimless use of leisure time).

After criminal history, we recommend discussing topics that follow a natural order, such as family, employment/education, social connections, substance use, and so on. Of course, the order of the interview can be changed, depending on time constraints and other considerations. We generally recommend gathering assessment information during a single session, rather than spreading this process over multiple sessions. The initial assessment is designed as a point-in-time snapshot and summary of the JIC, rather than an ongoing collection of information. Conducting the initial assessment over multiple sessions introduces confounds in which JICs may alter their style of responding or change the type of information revealed altogether. Keep in mind that as treatment progresses, assessment activities will be ongoing, because you will be tracking the JIC's improvement across relevant criminal risk domains (see Chapter 13).

History of Criminal/Antisocial Behavior

For JICs who have been previously involved with the criminal justice system, criminal history may occupy a disproportionate amount of time in the interview relative to other criminal risk domains, although information gathering in this area can be done efficiently. In some ways, history of criminal/antisocial behavior can be likened to the "chief complaint" or "history of presenting problem" in a traditional mental health assessment, which means that it is a useful starting point for discussion. The referring offense, prior arrests, and possible other undetected criminal and antisocial behavior should be examined in sufficient depth that an understanding of the type and style of the JIC's criminal behavior patterns will emerge. The nature of the client's prior criminal involvements should be explored; it is not enough simply to obtain a list of charges and convictions. You should try to elicit the JIC's narrative about how previous arrests occurred, as well as his or her thought processes at the time, situational factors that facilitated prior offenses, and general attitude toward this criminal behavior now.

Early involvement in a variety of antisocial behaviors across situations suggests a higher level of criminal risk. Also, as a general rule, the greater the dissonance the JIC exhibits about past criminal behavior, the greater the JIC's likelihood for criminal desistance moving forward. Keep in mind that it is common for people to downplay their involvement in all sorts of antisocial behaviors, so it can be expected that JICs will offer some distortion in describing their criminal histories. Sample questions for assessing history of criminal/antisocial behavior are provided in Script 5.2.

Dysfunctional Family/Romantic Relationships

Assessing the family and marital/romantic domain includes exploration of family-of-origin relationships, current romantic attachments, and parenting. Past family circumstances (composition and dynamics) are important for several reasons, such as social attachments, development and maintenance of life habits/attitudes, and social support. Equally important is exploring the nature of the JIC's current relationships with family members. Identify which relationships are prosocial and which are antisocial, and how these relationships contribute to, or lower risk for, criminal behavior. Also, gauge the JIC's awareness of the links between high-risk family relationships and potential continued criminal justice involvement. Inquire about prosocial family members with whom the JIC once had a bond but no longer maintains a close relationship. In a similar manner, for a JIC currently involved in a romantic relationship, probe for stability, nurturance, and the degree to which the romantic partner is involved in antisocial activities. You are seeking information about family/romantic relationships that either directly or subtly reinforce criminal activity. General questions for assessing dysfunctional family/romantic relationships are provided in Script 5.3. Additional materials for exploring the relative influence of specific family members are provided in Chapter 11.

Lack of Connection to Work/School

Being involved in employment or education is important when it comes to reducing criminal risk, for several reasons—such as occupying time, providing a means for economic survival, affording opportunities for prosocial interactions, and supporting a general sense of accomplishment. You will want to expand the typical assessment of career and educational achievement to include negative or unrealistic attitudes and expectations toward employment or school; difficulties with supervisors and coworkers or with teachers and fellow students; behavioral problems at work or school; and low levels of satisfaction related to work or school. Consider the degree to which JICs' current or former employment difficulties may relate to their criminal and antisocial behavior. Ask about interests in furthering employment and education, if you have not already done so in your exploration of values. To get an initial overview of the employment/education area, sample questions are provided in Script 5.4. Additional questions about this area (e.g., perceived value of employment, conflicts with supervisors and coworkers, work absences, and terminations) can be found in Chapter 10.

Antisocial Companions

Being socially connected provides opportunities to learn from others and to receive feedback, by way of encouragement and disapproval from others. Generally speaking, antisocial companions tend to encourage antisocial behaviors and may directly or subtly disapprove of prosocial actions, whereas prosocial companions encourage prosocial behaviors and disapprove of and subtly punish antisocial actions. As with the assessment of family and marital/romantic relationships, the assessment of antisocial companions should involve gathering information about the full range of a JIC's current social relationships, both antisocial and prosocial. As a general rule, current friendships are more important than those in the past. The goal is to explore the extent (i.e., size of social circle), relative risk (i.e., prosocial vs. antisocial), and degree of exposure (i.e., proportion of time spent with prosocial vs. antisocial influences) related to various friends and companions. Also, gauge the JIC's susceptibility to companion influence. This can range from highly influenced (the JIC is a "follower") to unaffected (he or she is a "leader"). Also, ask about prosocial friendships that have lapsed. Prosocial friendships reduce risk by increasing feelings of belongingness (i.e., reduce isolation), provide opportunities for expressing and practicing social skills, and are sources of feedback to guide decision making (social learning). General questions for assessing antisocial companions are provided in Script 5.5. Chapter 11 includes additional materials for exploring the influence of companions.

Maladaptive Leisure Time

Leisure activities are often underappreciated, but they represent an important practical issue. That is, leisure activities require planning and intention, which means that they serve to some extent as proxies for general life management. Excessive free time, or an aimless use of free time, also increases the likelihood of criminal behavior related to other risk domains. Start by gathering information related to a JIC's perspective on, and involvement in, leisure pursuits. Probe for high levels of involvement in risky and antisocial activities. Ask for a description of a typical weekday and a typical weekend. Also, attempt to distinguish activities that are solitary from those that take place with other people. One way to operationalize what counts as leisure time is to define it as the time remaining once essential obligations (e.g., work or school, family responsibilities) have been managed. Sample questions for assessing maladaptive leisure time are provided in Script 5.6. These questions are provided to obtain a general understanding of this domain. If leisure time becomes a target for intervention, then additional materials related to activity planning should be incorporated into treatment (see Chapter 10).

Substance Abuse/Misuse

As with any client, assessing substance use involves determining the types of substances being used (i.e., alcohol, drugs [including prescription medications], or both) and its impact on functioning. As a general guideline, current use is more important than prior use. You should explore the degree to which substance use is part of a JIC's lifestyle, and, more importantly, determine the precise role substances have played in past offending behaviors (for this section of the interview, substance use itself is not considered a criminal behavior). That is, did it drive the JIC's criminal actions (e.g., was a crime committed to get money for substances, did substance use influence poor decisions, did use prompt aggressive or out-of-control behavior)? Or was it more an outcome of an offense (e.g., celebration after a "successful" crime)? Determine the JIC's perspective of the effects of substance use on his or her life, particularly criminal behavior. This may indicate insight and motivation related to modifying future use of substances. Sample questions for assessing this domain are provided in Script 5.7, and further guidance is provided in Chapter 12.

Criminogenic Thinking/Antisocial Orientation

As noted in Chapter 2, criminogenic thinking reflects two conceptual levels of beliefs (intermediate beliefs and automatic thoughts), and the intermediate beliefs are often what underlie an antisocial orientation. There are both formal and informal methods of assessing criminogenic thinking patterns and thoughts. Formal methods include the administration of standardized tests (several recommendations are found in Appendix A) and interview questions designed to elicit criminogenic cognitions. The informal method generally involves attending to JICs' verbalizations during clinical interactions—spontaneous descriptions of their thought processes related to other criminal risk domains, such as criminal history, lack of connection to work/school, antisocial companions, substance abuse/misuse, and so on. It is important to pay close attention to criminogenic thoughts that are verbalized in different risk domains, and it can be helpful to record specific phrases when they emerge. In addition to criminogenic thinking, it is equally important to recognize the degree to which prosocial attitudes may also be present. These types of thoughts will often emerge during discussions of values and life priorities (see Chapter 4).

Standard interview questions for assessing criminogenic thinking patterns are provided in Script 5.8. Since practitioners sometimes struggle with finding the right questions for accessing JICs' internal thought processes, Table 5.1 presents additional questions that can be used to assess the 13 criminogenic thinking patterns first introduced in Chapter 2. These questions should be used sparingly, as they are intended to get more detailed information when you believe that a certain thinking pattern reflects a JIC's general antisocial orientation. We do not recommend that you ask all possible questions for every thinking pattern.

Anger Dysregulation

An inability to regulate emotions makes it difficult to control behavior. Anger dysregulation contributes to a range of related problems, such as impulsiveness, verbal outbursts, aggressive behaviors, deficient problem solving, and poor decision making. The so-called "crime of passion" is an example in which unregulated emotion (usually anger) contributes directly to a criminal event, most likely an impulsive and aggressive act. Enhancing JICs' ability to regulate anger and slow down decision making can offset risk and increase interpersonal effectiveness. The first step, however, is to determine the extent to which anger dysregulation difficulties exist, and how such problems may influence a JIC's general functioning and his or her criminal potential.

As noted in Chapter 2, we focus on anger as a risk domain because it is the emotion most likely to be connected to criminal behavior, and treatment may be necessary for JICs who report problematic anger reactions. Other emotions may be important as well. For some JICs, anxiety and depressive symptoms can trigger substance use; in other words, drugs and alcohol become mechanisms of self-medication to relieve distressing symptoms. Anxiety and depression can also interfere with work and school performance, pursuit of enjoyable leisure activities, and healthy social functioning across family and peer relationships. For practical steps for treating anxiety and depression, see Leahy et al. (2012).

Sample questions for assessing anger dysregulation are provided in Script 5.9. These questions will provide a general understanding of whether or not anger is problematic. Chapter 12 offers additional information on assessing individual episodes of anger, as well as practical treatment steps for JICs who struggle with anger difficulties.

KEY POINTS

- *Assessment* is the process of gathering relevant information. Synthesizing that information into a coherent treatment plan is called *case formulation*.

- Assessment and case formulation help to identify relevant treatment targets and tailor interventions to the unique characteristics of a particular JIC.

- Assessment and case formulation are the cornerstones of effective treatment.

- Assessment activities revolve around developing an in-depth understanding of the specific criminal risk domains most relevant for a particular JIC, and of how those risk domains interact with one another to influence criminal behavior.

- You are encouraged to integrate the scripted material presented in this chapter into your assessment procedures, and to do so in a manner consistent with your own personal style.

TABLE 5.1. Additional Questions for Eliciting Specific Criminogenic Thinking Patterns

Criminogenic thinking pattern	Description of pattern	Sample questions to elicit pattern
Thinking patterns related to self and others		
Identifying with antisocial companions	Viewing self as similar to, and relating best to, antisocial peers; seeing relationships with prosocial peers as unimportant	"How important is it for you to get along with your friends, even if it might get you, or them in trouble? What do you think about people who live pretty normal lives—you know, like working regularly, taking care of their kids, maintaining a decent place to live?"
Disregard for others	Belief that the needs/rights of others are unimportant; antipathy/hostility to others; lack of empathy and remorse for hurting others	"Give me a recent example where you may have intentionally or unintentionally taken advantage of another person. [Once an example is identified, ask the following questions.] How was the other person affected? Did that person get hurt in any way? How do you think the other person felt or thought about the situation? How much do you care about what the other person felt or thought? Why?"
Emotionally disengaged	Belief that avoiding intimacy and vulnerability is good; lack of trust; fears about being taken advantage of	"What, if anything, makes it difficult for you to share your problems and feelings with other people? What do you think about letting yourself get close to others?"
Hostility for criminal justice personnel	Adversarial and suspicious attitude toward police, lawyers, judges, and so forth	"What do you think about people who work in law enforcement or corrections, such as police officers, lawyers, judges, or probation/parole officers?"
Grandiosity and entitlement	Inflated beliefs about oneself; belief that one is deserving of special treatment	"To what extent do you see yourself as smarter and more creative than others? Do you think sometimes different rules should apply to you compared to other people?"
Power and control	Seeking dominance over others; seeking to control the behavior of others	"Would you describe yourself as a leader or a follower? How often do you get your own way with other people? How important is it for other people to do what you say? Why is this so important?"
Thinking patterns related to interacting with the environment		
Demand for excitement	Belief that life should be focused on thrill seeking and risk taking; lack of tolerance for boredom	"Would you describe yourself as a thrill-seeking type of person? In the past year, what kinds of things have you done just for the rush of excitement or the thrill of it? Could these risky types of things have gotten you in trouble? What goes through your mind right before you do these types of things? How well do you handle boredom? What do you tell yourself when you are bored?"

(continued)

TABLE 5.1.   *(continued)*

Criminogenic thinking pattern	Description of pattern	Sample questions to elicit pattern
Exploit	General intent to manipulate situations or relationships for personal gain when given the opportunity	"To what extent do you use people for your own agenda, even when it is not in their best interests? What are your reasons for dealing with people in this way?"
Hostility for law and order	Animosity toward rules, regulations, and laws	"How important is it for you to follow rules on a scale of 0 to 10, where 0 is 'not at all important' and 10 is 'very important'? Why? What are some reasons why the rules should not apply to you?"
Justifying and minimizing	Rationalization and underestimation of harmful behaviors	"What do you see as the causes of your criminal behavior? Tell me about times where you know something was illegal or harmful, but a little voice inside told you it was OK to do it anyway. What did that voice say?"
Path of least resistance	"Easiest way" approach to problem solving; a "no worries," "no plan needed," and "in the moment" style of life	"When it comes to taking care of responsibilities, do you tend to put things off, or do you get to them right away? At those times when you put things off, what do you say to yourself?"
Inability to cope	Giving up in the face of adversity; low frustration tolerance	"How do you handle difficult situations? When you are faced with a new challenge or an obstacle, are you the kind of person who gives up or the kind who tries to figure out a solution? Tell me about the last few disappointments you experienced and how you coped with them. What do you usually say to yourself right before you give up on things?"
Underestimating	Underrating the negative consequences of risky behaviors; overconfidence in decision-making skills	"Tell me about situations where you did not think things through and you were surprised later by a bad outcome. What stops you from thinking things through? What do you tell yourself that blinds you to the risks in some situations?"

SCRIPT 5.1. Introducing Assessment: Opening Statement

"Hi, [JIC's name]. I want to talk to you about certain areas of your life, so I can better understand how you got involved with the criminal justice system. We are going to talk about several different topics, such as your history of problems with the law, your family background, social connections such as family and friends, substance use, and other things in general. I am going to start with some questions about your criminal justice involvement and then move on to other areas. Do you understand what we are trying to do today? What questions might you have before we begin?"

SCRIPT 5.2. Sample Questions for Assessing History of Criminal/Antisocial Behavior

I. CURRENT OFFENSE(S)

Introduction: "I'd like to find out what was going on in your life that led you into getting into trouble with the law. I have reviewed some information about your background, but I always like to hear it directly from the person. I'd like to start by discussing your current arrest(s). What I know is _____." [Provide a snapshot of the offense, such as "I understand you were indicted for burglary, and it was a residence. . . ."]

"So tell me, what were the circumstances of this event? How did all this happen?"

"What were you doing immediately beforehand?"

"Were you alone or with someone else?"

"Whose idea was it?"

"At the time it occurred, what were you telling yourself? In other words, what thoughts were in your head either just before or during this situation?"

"What do you think about it now?"

"Was there anything that could have happened differently so things turned out better?"

II. PRIOR OFFENSE(S)

"OK, thank you for your openness. I'd like to talk now about other offenses you may have been involved with. Tell me about the history of involvement with the criminal justice system in your life. Start with the first time you got in trouble, and walk me through what has happened since."

"How old were you when your first arrest occurred?"

"What was the outcome of the case?" [Repeat the first group of questions from the Current Offense(s) section above for each identified offense. If there is an extensive arrest history, you can ask about the most serious charges. If there is an array of different charges, you can ask one or two questions from each offense type.]

"Overall, do you see any patterns or connections between your prior offense(s) and your current one?"

"Tell me about any other situations in which the police could have been involved but were *not* called for some reason."

(continued)

Sample Questions for Assessing History of Criminal/Antisocial Behavior

III. INCARCERATION AND SUPERVISION

If relevant: "Have you ever spent time in a detention center, prison, psychiatric hospital, or group home?"

[If yes:] "Tell me, how long were you detained, and what setting were you in?"

"What was that like for you?"

"What kinds of tickets did you receive? Tell me about those incidents."

"Have you ever tried to escape or run away from [type of custodial placement]?"

[If yes:] "What happened?

"Did you participate in any treatment programs, and if so, what did you learn from them?" "Overall, how much time have you served? And how many different times?"

If relevant: "Have you ever had a probation or parole officer before?"

[If yes:] "Tell me about your experiences being on probation and parole. What was that like for you?"

"What have been some of the positives about being on community supervision?"

"What have been some of the negatives about supervision?"

"What programs did you participate in while on probation or parole?"

"Tell me what was helpful about those programs."

"Have you ever had an unsuccessful period of probation or parole?"

[If yes:] "Tell me about that; what happened?

"Overall, how much time have you served on community supervision? And how many different times?"

SCRIPT 5.3. Sample Questions for Assessing Dysfunctional Family/Romantic Relationships

Introduction: "Now I'd like to talk with you about your family situation. I'll start by asking about the circumstances in which you were raised. In talking about your family, I'd like to get a sense of the type of household you grew up in and what type of family relationships you have now. We learn a lot of our life habits from our family upbringing, so maybe we can understand some of the ways in which your family has influenced your life. Then I would like to ask you about any current romantic relationships you may be involved in, and, if you have children, what your relationships are like with them."

I. FAMILY OF ORIGIN

"Tell me about your family situation when you were growing up."

"Were you raised by your biological parents or someone else?"

"Tell me about any times in your life growing up where you were separated from your family."

"Tell me about any brothers or sisters that you grew up with. Did anybody in your family have any significant problems, such as mental health issues, problems with alcohol or drugs, or involvement with the law?"

[If yes:] "What influence did these events have on you?"

"What was your family life like when you were growing up? I mean, were there house rules and expectations, and if so, did people follow those?"

"How would you describe the relationships with people in your family as you were growing up?"

"How did the members of your family generally get along?"

"When disagreements occurred, how bad did arguments or fights get in your family?"

"How are your relationships with your family now?"

"How often do you talk to people in your family?" and "What types of things do you talk about?"

"How interested is your family in your life?"

"How supportive is your family toward you now?"

"Who in your family do you spend the most time with?"

"What are their lifestyles like?"

"What kinds of concerns do you have about them getting involved with the criminal justice system?"

"What connections exist between the way you were raised and the problems you have in your life now?"

"What connections exist between your current family relationships and your current problems?"

"What do you see as a possible solution to any issues you have with your family?"

(continued)

II. ROMANTIC PARTNERS/CURRENT FAMILY

If relevant: "I'd like to switch and now talk about your own family—I mean, a romantic partner and any children you may have. Tell me about your current romantic partner situation."

"Are you married or involved with someone?"

[If yes:] "What type of person is he [she]?"

"What does [partner's name] do for work?"

"What does [name of partner] like to do with free time?"

"To what extent does [partner's name] have life problems, such as mental health issues, problems with drugs or alcohol, or troubles with the law?"

"How would you describe your romantic relationship? I mean, how are things going?"

"Do you consider your most recent relationship as positive?"

"Have you ever had major disagreements or problems?"

[If yes:] "What are some of those problems, and how did they get resolved?"

"What type of connection exists between your romantic relationship and your criminal involvements, either current or past? In what ways have they been related?

If relevant: "Describe your relationship(s) with any children that you have"

"How often do you see them?"

"What types of things do you do together?"

"What do you like about having children?"

"What are the biggest challenges you have with your kids?"

SCRIPT 5.4. Sample Questions for Assessing Lack of Connection to Work/School

Introduction: "I'd like to talk with you about employment [school, for those solely involved in educational pursuits]. There are many benefits to working, such as giving us something to do, providing us with money, and feeling a sense of accomplishment. Of course, there are some downsides as well, such as having to show up at certain times, sometimes doing things that aren't enjoyable, and being told what to do. People have different opportunities for work due to their own circumstances, and there are many different types of jobs people can do over the course of their lives. I'm going to ask you about your current employment situation and some jobs you have done in the past. I'm interested in understanding your work patterns and history. I'm also interested in your educational history and have a few questions related to your experiences with school."

I. EMPLOYMENT

"Are you currently working?

[If yes:] "Tell me about your job and what you do."

"How long have you been at this job?"

"Are you employed full-time or part-time?"

"Approximately how much money do you make in a year?"

For a JIC who is unemployed: Determine if there is any reasonable explanation for not working (e.g., the JIC is in a period of transition from school to work force, is between jobs, was recently laid off due to legitimate work shortage). Find out the JIC's perspective on not working and how motivated the client is to find employment.

"What are the reasons why you are not working?"

"How long have you been unemployed?"

"What do you think about this situation?"

"Has this situation happened in the past?"

"Are you looking for another job or expect to get one soon?"

"Tell me about your career goals."

"What skills, training, or talents do you have?"

"Sometimes people work at jobs in which they don't pay taxes. These are often called 'under-the-table' jobs. Is your current job one in which you pay taxes, or is it an under-the-table job?"

For under-the-table employment: Determine reason for not paying taxes. This may range from the type of work (e.g., —drug dealing, etc.) in which easy money and an exciting lifestyle may be the motivating factor. Alternatively, the under-the-table job may be related to other circumstances (e.g., an honest business such as construction, landscaping, or hospitality, where tax avoidance may be related to issues such as immigration status).

(continued)

"How long have you been working under the table?"

"Can you tell me what a typical work week is like and the approximate number of hours you work?"

"Why don't you do a job that is 'above-board'?"

For all employed JICs:

"What do you like about your job?"

"What do you not like?"

"Is there a connection between your work situation and your criminal involvements, either current or past? What is the possible connection?"

II. EDUCATION

"How far did you go in school?

"What was school like for you?"

"What kind of effort did you put into it?"

"What were your favorite classes?"

"What were your grades like during your last year in school?"

Explore special education experiences, disciplinary problems, and social adjustment: "Did you ever struggle in school because of learning problems?"

"What subject areas did you struggle with?"

"Did you miss any substantial time at school?"

"How much school did you miss on average?"

"What were your reasons for missing school?"

"What kinds of things did you do when you were not at school?"

"Did you ever get suspended or expelled from school?"

[If yes:] "How many times?"

"What kinds of things led to your suspensions or expulsions?"

"What was school like for you socially?"

"How well did you get along with kids at school?"

"What kinds of problems or fights, if any, did you have with other students?"

"What types of organized after-school activities were you involved with?"

"What were your relationships like with teachers and staff members in high school?"

"How well did you get along with teachers and other staff members?"

"Who were your favorite teachers or staff members?"

"What teachers or school staff members did you have the most problems with? Tell me about those problems."

(continued)

Explore college or technical training and future educational pursuits:

"What kind of educational experiences have you had since you left regular school?"

"Tell me about your educational goals now."

"What interest do you have in furthering your education or training?"

If high school has not been completed:

"How important is it for you to complete high school?"

[If not important:] "Tell me why school is not important to you."

SCRIPT 5.5. Sample Questions for Assessing Antisocial Companions

Introduction: "Now I'd like to talk about the people you spend time with outside of your family. Being connected with people is important in life, because it can make us feel good and we can learn things from others. I'd like to start by saying that we often have close friends and acquaintances. *Close friends* are those people we spend more time with and have stronger connections to. These are people we often trust and share things with. *Acquaintances* are people we may know and see from time to time, but we really don't spend much time with them. At this point, my questions are related to your close friends. I'd also like to mention that people have different social networks; some have many friends, and others have very few. It doesn't matter how many you have. I'm interested in understanding your social connections and how your close friends fit into your life."

- "I'd like to begin by asking about how many people you consider to be your close friends. You don't have to tell me names, just the approximate number."
- For JICs who claim to have "many friends," ask about the closest five. It may also be important to clarify that you are asking about face-to-face friends and not relationships that occur exclusively online (e.g., Facebook, Instagram).
- For JICs who claim to have "no friends," determine if they are true "loners" (i.e., people with a preference to be solitary), or if they are social people who have temporarily limited their social connections for some reason (e.g., they are prevented due to their criminal justice circumstances), or if they desire social contact but are not successful due to various reasons (e.g., they are anxious or socially awkward).

For JICs with "no friends":

"You said that you don't have many friends and prefer to be by yourself most of the time. Can I ask why?"

"Is it related to circumstances such as being limited to certain locations, or because you are prevented for some reason or another?"

"Do you actually prefer to be by yourself?"

"If you are mostly by yourself, to what extent are you around other people at work or with family?"

For JICs with friends:

"I'd like to ask about the type of people your close friends are. Tell me something about each of them. For instance, what do they do?"

"How does each spend their spare time?"

"How many of your close friends use drugs or alcohol?"

"Sometimes we can describe people as 'positive people' because they live pretty normal lives and don't get into trouble or have a lot of problems. There are also 'negative people' who seem to get into trouble or have many serious problems. Approximately how many of your close friends are 'positive' and how many are 'negative'?"

(continued)

"In your mind, how do you view your close friends: Mostly positive or negative?"

"Tell me approximately how much time you spend with each of your close friends."

"Do you see them every day, once a week, or something else?"

"If you have both 'positive' and 'negative' people in your life, how much time do you spend with each?"

"With your close friends, what type of things do you do or talk about?"

"If you have both 'positive' and 'negative' friends, do you notice a difference in what you talk about or how you act when you are with each type?"

"Which of your close friends do you most admire and want to be like?"

"How much of a connection is there between contact with your friends, and your current or past criminal justice problems?"

What do you see as the connection, if there is one?"

"Changing friends can be difficult. Have you ever tried to change your friends or the amount of time you spend with them?"

[If yes]: "How did that work out? What happened?"

SCRIPT 5.6. Sample Questions for Assessing Maladaptive Leisure Time

Introduction: "I'd like to talk with you about your use of *free time,* which is the time after you deal with basic things in life, such as working, going to school, and family responsibilities. How people spend this time is important, because it creates enjoyment so that life doesn't get boring."

"Tell me what you do in a typical weekday. For example, what do your work, school, and family responsibilities look like?"

"Approximately how much time is left each day after you deal with these obligations?"

"How do you normally spend that time?"

"Now tell me about a typical weekend day, like a Saturday."

"What types of organized activities have you been involved with in the past year? You know, like clubs, sports, religious activities, or classes. How many times per week do you go?"

"Tell me about any interests or hobbies you have."

"How long have you been interested in these activities?"

"How often do you actually involve yourself in them now?"

If activities exist: "Is it a regular event that has set days and times, or is it more 'now and then'?"

"Do your interests or hobbies involve other people? If so, what people?"

"How are they involved and how do you all get along?"

"What types of risky activities have you engaged in during your free time in the past year?"

"Do you see any connection between how you spend your free time and having criminal justice problems?"

"What possible connection is there between having a lack of meaningful activities and your criminal involvements, either current or past?"

SCRIPT 5.7. Sample Questions for Assessing Substance Abuse/Misuse

Introduction: "I'd like to talk about substances, and in particular your use of them. We both know that a lot of people use substances—either alcohol, or street drugs, or prescription medications. What I'd like to figure out is the extent to which substances play a role in your life and to what degree substances are related to your criminal justice problems."

I. TYPES OF SUBSTANCES

"First of all, tell me about your use of substances. Let's start with alcohol. How often do you drink?"

"How much do you normally drink at a time?"

"How does this amount of drinking affect your life?"

[If relevant:]"Have you ever tried to stop using alcohol?"

[If so:] What was that like?"

"What worked? What didn't?"

"How difficult would it be for you to stop using now?"

"Now let's talk about other drugs that are not alcohol. What type of other drugs have you tried?"

[Follow the same pattern of questions of the other substances such as marijuana and other drugs (including prescription medications) that the client has identified.]

II. IMPACT ON LIFE AREAS

[Next, ask about the impact of the most frequently used substances on **work, school, sports, family, social activities, and health.**]

"How much time do you spend thinking about [normally used specific substance(s) of interest]?"

"How much energy do you spend trying to get [specific substance(s) of interest]?"

"When you think about [specific substance(s) of interest], what areas of your life have been most affected by your using it [them]?"

"Give me an example of how using [specific substance(s) of interest] has affected [relevant life areas]."

"How bad have things gotten with [relevant life areas] because of your use of [specific substance(s) of interest]?"

(continued)

III. CONNECTION BETWEEN SUBSTANCES AND CRIMINAL BEHAVIOR

"What connections do you see between your use of either alcohol or drugs and your current offence or an offense(s) in the past?"

[If relevant:] "Tell me how your current offense(s) would be different if there was no substance use."

"In the past year, have there been times when you could have gotten, or did get, in trouble when you were intoxicated or high because you were out of control?"

[If yes:] "About how many times?"

"What does it look like when you are out of control because you are using [specific substance(s) of interest]?"

"In the past year, have there been times when you could have gotten, or did get, in trouble for trying to get money to buy [specific substance(s) of interest]?"

[If yes:] About how many times?"

"How do you typically get money to buy [specific substance(s) of interest]?"

SCRIPT 5.8. Sample Questions for Assessing Criminogenic Thinking/Antisocial Orientation

Introduction: "I'd like to talk to you about what you may have been thinking at the time of your offense(s) and how you see things in general. This is important, because there is a general connection between how we think and how we act. You have already mentioned a few of your thoughts related to your criminal justice problems, so I'd like to talk a bit more about those."

"First of all, what do you generally think about crime?" [This neutral question often stimulates a rationalization of some sort, such as "It's OK to do X crime if you have a good reason."] and "Why do you think people commit crimes?"

"Now I want to ask you a couple of questions about laws and rules. What do you generally think about laws and the justice system? Why are laws important?"

"How about the people who work in the justice system—the police, lawyers, judges, and parole and probation officers? What do you generally think about them? Do you see them as regular people doing a job, or is it different from that?"

"What do you think about your own criminal offenses when you look at them now?"

"Tell me about the thoughts you had just before or during your most recent offense(s). You know, what you were thinking when you did [most recent criminal offense(s)]."

"What do you think about the sentence you got, or possibly could get, for your current offense(s)? Do you think it's fair?"

"Let's talk about some of your friends who may have had trouble with the law. Do you notice anything special about the way they think when making decisions in their lives?"

"What are some examples of the way your friends think that might encourage decisions to commit criminal acts, or at least make such decisions OK?"

"Now let's talk about people who live pretty normal lives, such as working, socializing with friends or family, and doing 'regular Joe' type of stuff. What do you think about those types of people? In what ways do you think they get excitement out of life?"

"One last area I want to talk about is how our minds can play tricks on us. Sometimes we do things we know we shouldn't, but then we later give an excuse or reason why we did it to make it seem OK. This is called a *rationalization*. We can also simply downplay how serious something is, which is called a *minimization*. Have you ever had these types of thoughts either before, during, or after doing a crime?"

[If yes:] "How do you see it as a rationalization or minimization?"

[See Table 5.1 for additional questions for assessing specific criminogenic thinking patterns.]

SCRIPT 5.9. Sample Questions for Assessing Anger Dysregulation

Introduction: "So far, we have talked about some of your thoughts and behaviors in certain areas of your life as these relate to trouble with the law. I want to talk with you now about emotions, particularly anger. Emotions such as anger are a normal part of life. For example, anger can sometimes be a useful signal about how we're feeling about things in our lives. Anger can also energize us to take action, fix problems, or change relationships that are not working. The downside of anger is that it can sometimes get out of control and make us say or do things we later regret. Also, over time, anger reactions can become automatic and lead to problems with relationships, work, or even the criminal justice system."

"How often would you say you get angry? More than once a day, about once a week, about once a month?"

"When you do get angry, where would you say you normally are on a scale of 0 to 10, where 0 is 'no anger' and 10 is 'the most anger you have ever experienced'?"

"Think about a time where you were a 9 or a 10; what did that look like? How did you act? How is that different from how you normally act when you are angry?"

"When you get angry about a situation, how long does your anger usually last? Days, weeks, or months?"

"Is there a situation or group of people such as friends, family, coworkers, or people at school, where you show your anger more?"

[If yes:] "What does that typically look like?"

"Have you ever thought about getting even with someone who has angered you?"

[If yes:] "Tell me about times where you have thought about getting even or times when you acted on these thoughts?

[If yes:] What did you do?"

"Overall, what effect would you say your anger has had on your relationships?"

"Tell me about times when your angry feelings have led you to the use drugs or alcohol."

"Give me an example of a recent experience, from the last 2 weeks, when you felt angry." [Explore with the JIC a recent anger episode; ask about what triggered the anger, thoughts, overall intensity of angry feelings, actions, and what happened afterward.]

CHAPTER 6

Case Formulation

ase formulation is the process of integrating assessment information and forming opinions about the causes and maintenance of a JIC's behavior. A well-developed formulation can provide a rich perspective on the JIC's functioning—one that will allow you to develop a treatment plan and form realistic expectations about potential improvement. Formulations can be simple and rudimentary, or complex and intricate. Any case formulation will be of benefit in treatment; however, the scientific notion of *Occam's razor* (the principle that parsimonious interpretations are as accurate as, if not more accurate than, complex interpretations) suggests that simple and broad explanations of JICs' criminal tendencies may be the preferred approach.

The case formulation process in forensic contexts typically has three components: (1) estimating the risk level for future criminal behavior (this often involves statistical probability estimates for reoffending); (2) identifying the relevant criminal risk domains to target in treatment; and (3) formulating a plan for improving a JIC's functioning within criminal risk domains. Depending on the setting where you work and on your role, the relative emphasis given to these three activities may differ. For example, community corrections officers (e.g., probation and parole officers) are often interested in establishing risk levels of new cases, in order to guide decisions about frequency of contacts during supervision. Social workers and psychologists may be less concerned about risk estimates and more interested in establishing goals and game plans for intervention. In many settings, these two objectives are often linked, as the assessment related to criminal risk domains provides baseline information for determining both risk level *and* treatment targets. In this chapter, we emphasize the treatment-planning aspects of case formulation.

To return to our two case examples, Brenda's goals in developing case formulations for Jackie and Hank are to understand why they have gotten into trouble with the law; to develop a general impression of their risk for continuing criminal behavior; and to formulate treatment directions that may improve their functioning within the criminal risk domains most closely related to their criminality. The case formulation model we present is generic, in that it can be applied to JICs across many offense types (violence, property crime, drug selling, etc.) as well as to complex cases (e.g., comorbid criminality and mental health concerns). In this chapter, after making a few general comments about risk, we focus on identifying relevant treatment targets. A template for recording and organizing information for the purpose of treatment planning is also provided.

Finally, we discuss types of human judgment biases that can interfere with interpretation of assessment data and the development of an accurate case formulation.

FORMULATING JUDGMENTS ABOUT RISK

The first step in case formulation is to establish an estimate for risk of future criminal behavior. The well-established *risk principle* (introduced in Chapter 2) suggests that your treatment efforts and resources should correspond with the magnitude of a JIC's risk for reoffending. Essentially, a higher dosage of treatment and programming (and more frequent sessions) should go to the highest-risk JICs, and the least amount of treatment to those with the lowest risk. Implicit in the risk principle is the assumption that you will be able to distinguish higher-risk from lower-risk JICs.

A whole cottage industry has been built around the assessment and prediction of recidivism. Numerous risk assessment tools have been developed on the basis of established risk factors, such as the "Central Eight" discussed in Chapter 2. Incorporating one of the widely used standardized risk instruments into your assessment will reduce uncertainty and biases that can affect case formulation (see Appendix A for several examples). If you are not using a standardized assessment instrument, the interview guidelines and questions for assessing the criminal risk domains, outlined in Chapter 5, can serve as a useful foundation for clinical case formulation. However, they should not be used to make statistical estimates regarding probabilities of future criminal behavior.

Estimating Risk Levels

Risk assessment instruments usually offer a categorical determination of criminal risk potential, described by terms such as *low, medium,* and *high.* When validated risk tools are used, statistical probability estimates based on actuarial data are attached to these categorical statements (e.g., "Of 100 individuals with the same score, approximately 90 will be convicted of committing a new criminal offense within 2 years"). Although we advocate the use of validated risk assessment tools in determining JICs' base criminal risk levels, we recognize that this may not always be possible for any number of reasons (e.g., lack of suitable instruments, scarcity of resources for training staff, and unique circumstances of individual JICs). In these cases, a general guide can be applied to establish some semblance of risk level. JICs with fewer problems within criminal risk domains, and/or with problems that are characterized as mild (creating only minimal interference in functioning) or transitory, are considered *low-risk.* At the *high-risk* end of the continuum are JICs with multiple and chronic patterns embedded within the criminal risk domains that have wide-ranging and long-standing negative effects on their lives.

The process by which a person engages in criminal behavior is complex and dependent on the convergence of several factors and circumstances. Therefore, risk prediction can be an inexact science, and the prognosis regarding a JIC's potential for criminality is general rather than precise. Due to the limits of the current risk prediction technology, it is impossible—even when using risk assessment instruments—to offer precise statements such as this: "Hank is at high risk to reoffend. His next criminal act will occur on Friday, May 26, at 9:00 P.M., in the parking lot of the Highlands shopping mall with his friends who sell drugs." Given that such precise estimates are unattainable, there is a need to merge clinical judgment with established science to assist in determining the likely outcomes for JICs.

Considering Outcome Imminence and Severity

The term *outcome imminence* refers to how soon a new criminal event might occur. Although this information may be of considerable importance to a variety of criminal justice stakeholders, determining the imminence of a criminal outcome with satisfactory accuracy can be difficult. This is due to the fluctuating nature of criminal risk domains (e.g., association or avoidance with certain peers, active or inactive substance use, variable employment status). One solution to determining outcome imminence is a synthesis of clinical information (any combination of test data, assessment information, behavioral observation, and a JIC's self-report). For example, a JIC with a history of substance abuse, anger regulation problems, and connection with criminal peers would be at *low* imminence if these factors were inactive or adequately managed. However, the imminence of a criminal event would rise dramatically if the JIC was acutely intoxicated, was in an angry state, and was socializing with antisocial friends.

Another consideration is the *outcome severity* (i.e., harmfulness) of a JIC's potential criminality. It can be phrased as a question: "What is the most serious act a JIC is likely to commit?" For example, two JICs may be at moderate risk to commit a new offense; however, their unique histories suggest that one is likely to commit shoplifting and the other assault. Both JICs are at the same risk level for a criminal outcome, but the second has greater outcome severity (assault is more serious than shoplifting). As with outcome imminence, there are no reliable assessment instruments that can effectively measure criminal severity, and thus using your clinical judgment to synthesize the available clinical information is the best solution.

Considering the Interrelationship of Criminal History, Dispositional Characteristics, and Opportunity

The types of actions exhibited by JICs in the past are indicators of their potential behavioral repertoires for the future. The presence or absence of specific environmental contingencies (i.e., opportunity) may facilitate or suppress a behavioral temptation to commit a similar crime in the future. For example, a man with a habit of retail theft may be walking down a street and see an item of interest in a store window. The store is locked, preventing him from entering and examining the item further; in addition, the store is in a popular tourist area, and there are several bystanders close at hand. In this situation, the opportunity for criminality is low. Alternatively, this man may be walking down the street and see an item of interest in an open window of a store in an area where virtually nobody else is around. In this situation, the opportunity for criminality is high. A key consideration in determining risk is to understand the situational circumstances connected to past criminal behavior.

There is often an interrelationship among a JIC's criminal history, dispositional characteristics (i.e., traits), and surroundings. As in the case described above, when certain dispositional characteristics (e.g., impulsivity, risk taking) and opportunity converge around a historical criminal pattern, the probability of criminal behavior is high. Conversely, consider a JIC with a history of driving infractions. In terms of traits and patterns, this person has reasonable self-control, a risk-adverse mindset, and no history of theft. The presence of an opportunity for a theft (e.g., a store display that is not well monitored) would have little influence, because there is a weak connection among this JIC's criminal history, dispositional characteristics, and opportunity. When you are formulating judgments about risk, it may be useful to consider the degree of opportunity to continue criminal patterns (e.g., a pedophile's exposure to children, a violent offender's continued involvement with a vicious street gang, a corporate criminal's ongoing access to sensitive financial information).

To summarize, JICs with severe problems across many of the criminal risk domains are considered at highest risk for future criminal behavior. The concepts of outcome imminence and severity are also elements to be considered in making judgments about risk, as is the complex interrelationship among established repertoires of behavior, traits, and opportunity. In practice, a thoughtful synthesis of assessment information can result in statements such as the following: "Jackie is considered to be at low risk for a criminal event, based on her score on an actuarial assessment instrument. It is likely, based on her history, that if Jackie commits another offense, she will engage in trespassing, joy riding, or disorderly conduct, which will be of low severity."

IDENTIFYING TREATMENT TARGETS

Your treatment efforts should directly target the relevant criminal risk domains for a particular JIC; this is the *need principle,* introduced along with the risk principle in Chapter 2. As noted earlier, judgments about risk level and treatment targets are linked: When a JIC's criminal risk domains change, his or her probability of engaging in further criminal behavior changes accordingly. We recommend a two-pronged approach to identifying treatment targets: (1) identifying the most salient criminal risk domains related to recent incidents of criminal behavior; and (2) identifying criminal risk domains that have an impact on general life functioning and serve as overall drivers of criminal behavior.

For some JICs, additional factors beyond primary criminal risk domains may need to be considered in case formulation. These factors may include acute symptoms related to mental health problems, transient life circumstances, or stable characteristics for a particular JIC (such as intellectual or physical disabilities). For example, it may become apparent that an insecure and dangerous housing situation that fosters criminal behavior will need to be addressed in treatment. Another possibility is the potential for active symptoms related to certain mental health conditions (e.g., paranoid ideation and manic episodes) to precipitate disorganized, violent, and criminal behavior. As discussed previously, such symptoms are not typically linked to criminal behavior; however, they sometimes can materialize as acute risk factors. In such cases, it is the active nature of symptoms that is of most concern, and the management of these symptoms may need to be given high priority in treatment, although the criminal risk domains will still need to be addressed at a later time. Table 6.1 presents a brief list of secondary domains that should also be considered in case formulation.

TABLE 6.1. Secondary Domains to Consider in Case Formulation

Secondary domains	Description
Intellectual disability	Deficits in general cognitive abilities, reasoning, and decision making
Presence of psychopathology[a]	Mental health problems (e.g., symptoms of psychosis; bipolar disorder; depressive, anxiety, and trauma-related disorders) and dysfunctional personality issues (e.g., prominent personality disorder features)
Physical health concerns	Chronic and acute medical conditions; overall physical health and stature (e.g., energy levels, ability to metabolize intoxicants, and/or ability to tolerate environmental insults)
Problematic housing	Unstable and/or dangerous housing situations; poor-quality living circumstances

[a]In the current context, *psychopathology* does not refer to substance use disorders or antisocial personality patterns, which are considered criminal risk domains.

Prong 1: Criminal Event Analysis

A good starting point for identifying treatment targets is to analyze past criminal events. This analysis can be done on the most recent offense(s), or any criminal incidents JICs have been involved with in the past. As a general rule, the more events analyzed, the greater the likelihood that patterns related to criminal behavior will become evident and as such, the stronger the conclusions. The purposes of our Criminal Event Analysis form (see Form 6.1 at the end of this chapter) are (1) to understand the relative influence of the criminal risk domains, as well as secondary domains, at the time of the offense(s); and (2) to determine whether these factors are still active, dormant, or extinguished. The Criminal Event Analysis will highlight critical areas to address in treatment. Examples of completed Criminal Event Analyses are shown in Figures 6.1 and 6.2 for the most recent offenses for Hank and Jackie, respectively.

When you are using this approach, it is important to stay focused on a single episode of criminal behavior, and also to be mindful of how it relates to the more general snapshot of risk domains and general functioning discussed below. It is also useful to determine whether a specific criminal event is a relatively isolated incident or represents a historical pattern of behavior. In many cases, the information gathered from your assessment (discussed in Chapter 5) will be adequate for completing this analysis. However, it is always important to seek as much information as reasonable to ensure that you have a good understanding of a criminal event, so follow-up questions may be necessary.

As can be seen in Form 6.1 and in Figures 6.1 and 6.2, the starting point in the Criminal Event Analysis is to record basic descriptive information about the JIC: name, age, gender, marital status, and criminal justice status (e.g., pretrial, probation, prison/length of sentence) in the box at the left. The box at the top, called Individual/Dispositional Domains, is used to identify all the individual/dispositional criminal risk domains relevant to the specific criminal offense. Whenever possible, you should include specific thinking patterns and substances that were involved at the time of the event, and identify secondary domains or other individual factors that may have also played a direct role. The box at the bottom, called Social/Contextual Domains, is used to identify all the social/contextual criminal risk domains relevant to this criminal event. These may include friends and family members that were part of the offense as well as additional factors that were directly related to the criminal behavior. The box at the right is used to document a brief description of the offense. Although the examples in Figures 6.1 and 6.2 reflect Hank and Jackie's most recent criminal incidents, it can be helpful to use this approach to sample a wider range of past criminal events, in order to understand potential recurring patterns of antisocial behavior (whether the JIC was arrested or not).

Prong 2: Criminal Risk Domains and General Life Functioning

The Criminal Risk Domains Worksheet (see Form 6.2 at the end of this chapter) is complementary to the Criminal Event Analysis and is used to identify treatment targets that are part of a JIC's current lifestyle (routines, relationships, and habits). The Criminal Risk Domains Worksheet is a simple overarching blueprint for developing a treatment plan that can be completed from the information obtained from the overall assessment and the Criminal Event Analysis. The worksheet consists of a circular schematic depicting two levels of interrelated components, with the concentric rings representing domains of functioning. The centerpiece consists of the criminal risk domains, and the outer circle represents the secondary domains listed in Table 6.1.

As mentioned throughout this treatment planner, the criminal risk domains constitute the core of the case plan, although the secondary domains may also be highly relevant for understanding the functioning of some JICs. Figures 6.3 and 6.4 provide completed examples of the Criminal Risk Domains Worksheet for Hank and Jackie, respectively. To use the worksheet, simply check the domains that are relevant for a particular JIC. From the completed worksheets for Hank and Jackie, a few observations can be quickly gleaned: Hank is a higher-risk case than Jackie, and each client has a unique constellation of factors that will become the focus of treatment.

FORMULATING A TREATMENT PLAN

The next step in case formulation is to assemble clinical information into a structured format for the purpose of developing a treatment plan. The Case Formulation Worksheet (see Form 6.3 at the end of this chapter) is intended to be used as an informal document to record and organize notes and assessment data across the domains assessed (including values and life priorities; see Chapter 4). Completed examples of the Case Formulation Worksheet for Hank and Jackie are presented in Figures 6.5 and 6.6, respectively.

As can be seen, the Case Formulation Worksheet has four sections. Sections I and II are titled Criminal Risk Domains and Secondary Domains, and each section includes three subcategories for each domain. The *Assessment Data* subcategory reflects the sources of information, such as test data, file retrieval, interview, and collateral sources. The *Relevance* and *Priority Level* subcategories reflect brief interpretations of the importance each domain plays in the JIC's overall criminal risk profile. Domains that have emerged in the Criminal Event Analysis should generally be viewed as

(text resumes on page 105)

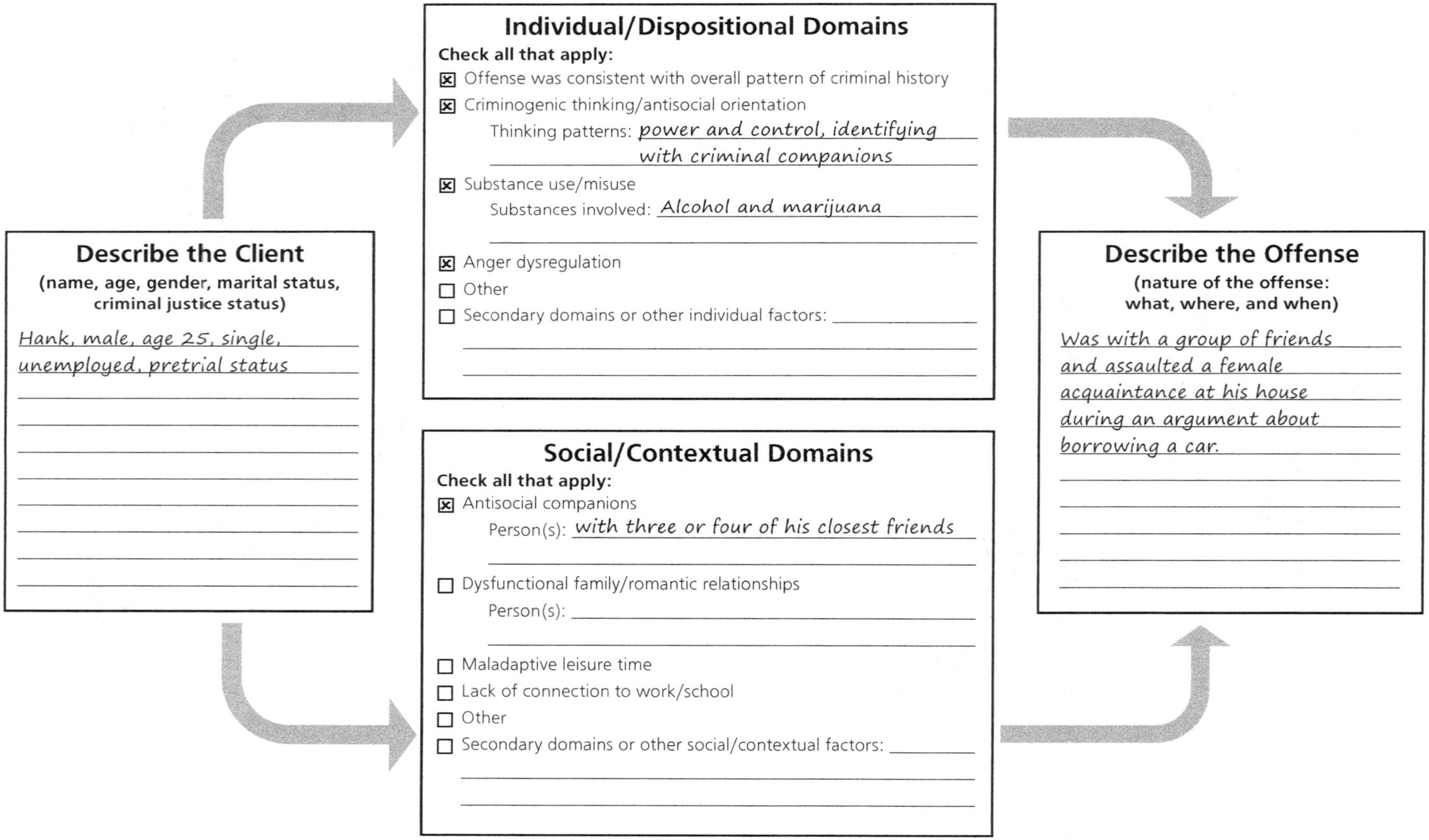

Individual/Dispositional Domains

Check all that apply:

☒ Offense was consistent with overall pattern of criminal history

☒ Criminogenic thinking/antisocial orientation

Thinking patterns: _power and control, identifying_ _with criminal companions_

☒ Substance use/misuse

Substances involved: _Alcohol and marijuana_

☒ Anger dysregulation

☐ Other

☐ Secondary domains or other individual factors: _____

Describe the Offense
(nature of the offense: what, where, and when)

Was with a group of friends
and assaulted a female
acquaintance at his house
during an argument about
borrowing a car.

Describe the Client
(name, age, gender, marital status, criminal justice status)

Hank, male, age 25, single,
unemployed, pretrial status

Social/Contextual Domains

Check all that apply:

☒ Antisocial companions

Person(s): _with three or four of his closest friends_

☐ Dysfunctional family/romantic relationships

Person(s): _____

☐ Maladaptive leisure time

☐ Lack of connection to work/school

☐ Other

☐ Secondary domains or other social/contextual factors: _____

FIGURE 6.1. Criminal Event Analysis: Hank's most recent offense.

94

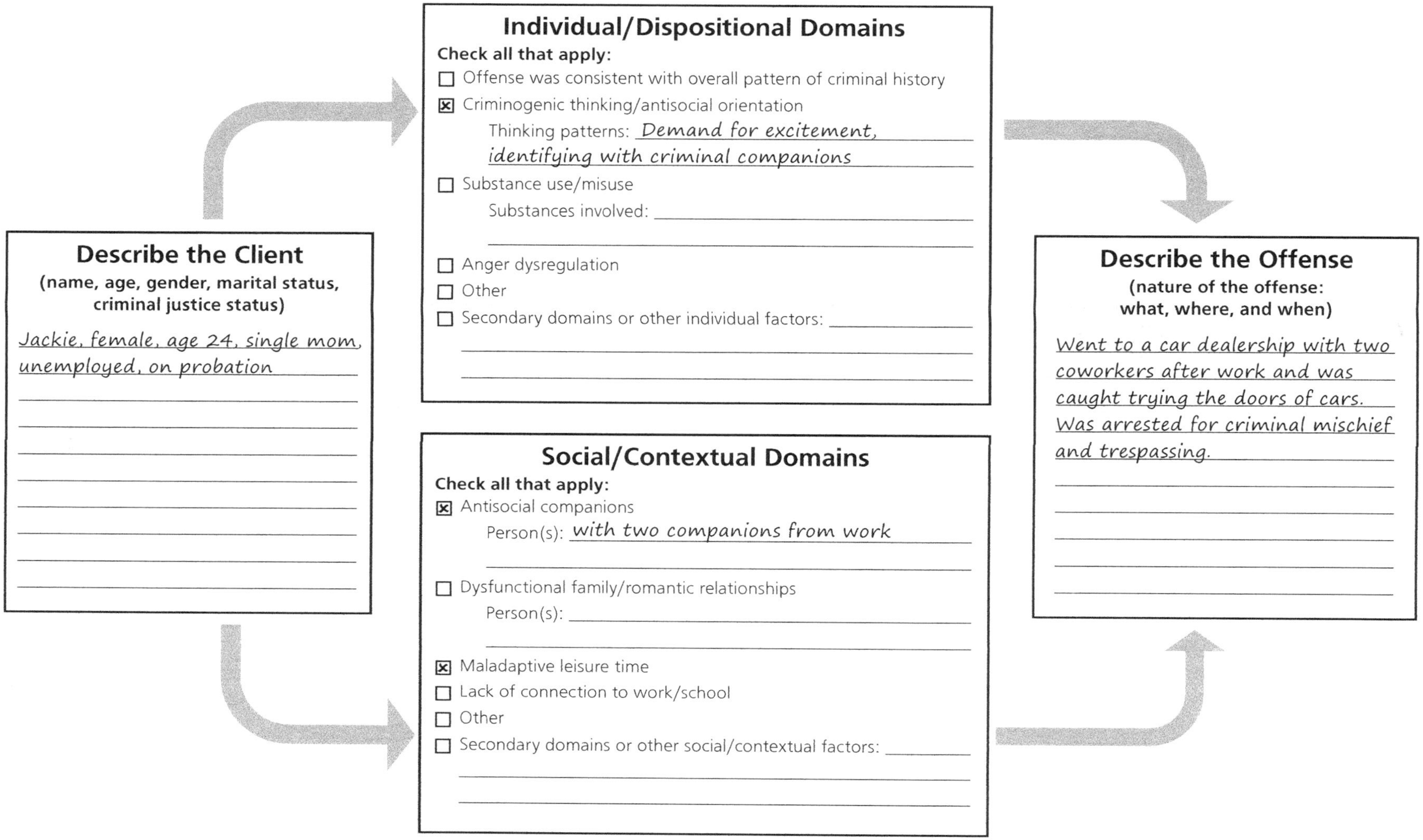

Describe the Offense
(nature of the offense: what, where, and when)

Went to a car dealership with two
coworkers after work and was
caught trying the doors of cars.
Was arrested for criminal mischief
and trespassing.

Individual/Dispositional Domains

Check all that apply:

☐ Offense was consistent with overall pattern of criminal history

☒ Criminogenic thinking/antisocial orientation

    Thinking patterns: _Demand for excitement,_
    identifying with criminal companions

☐ Substance use/misuse

    Substances involved: _____

☐ Anger dysregulation

☐ Other

☐ Secondary domains or other individual factors: _____

Social/Contextual Domains

Check all that apply:

☒ Antisocial companions

    Person(s): _with two companions from work_

☐ Dysfunctional family/romantic relationships

    Person(s): _____

☒ Maladaptive leisure time

☐ Lack of connection to work/school

☐ Other

☐ Secondary domains or other social/contextual factors: _____

Describe the Client
(name, age, gender, marital status, criminal justice status)

Jackie, female, age 24, single mom,
unemployed, on probation

FIGURE 6.2. Criminal Event Analysis: Jackie's most recent offense.

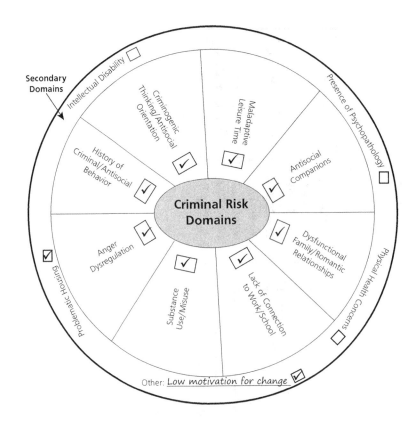

FIGURE 6.3. Hank's Criminal Risk Domains Worksheet.

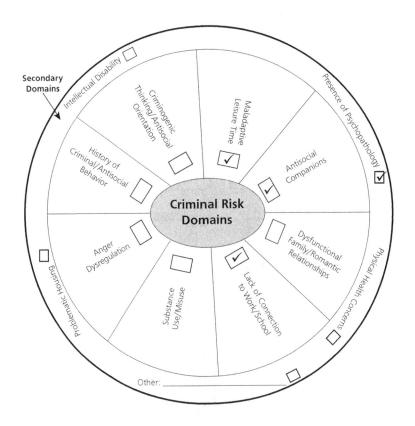

FIGURE 6.4. Jackie's Criminal Risk Domains Worksheet.

I. Criminal Risk Domains

History of Criminal/Antisocial Behavior	Criminogenic Thinking/Antisocial Orientation	Antisocial Companions	Dysfunctional Family/Romantic Relationships
Assessment Data: File and interview. • Referred for assault. • Hx. of drug selling (marijuana), DUI, and larceny. • Not involved with justice system for several years prior to recent arrest. • Unsuccessful on probation in the past, due to technical violations (failure to report; failure to complete mandated programming). • Served 1 year in prison; no disciplinary problems. • Has also been in fights for which he has not been arrested. **Relevance:** Based on overall lifestyle as assessed by structured interview, his current risk level seems high. His history of aggression and his current assault make his offense severity at least moderate. **Priority Level:** Static; history is not changeable.	**Assessment Data:** Interview suggests established criminal thinking patterns. His score on a specialized criminal thinking instrument indicates moderate level of criminal thinking (total score at the 79th percentile). **Relevance:** Prominent thinking patterns include: • Seeking dominance and control over others. • Identifying with, and seeking approval from, criminal associates. • Exploiting and manipulating situations/relationships for personal gain. **Priority Level:** Medium. Targeting criminogenic thinking can be incorporated in interventions addressing other risk domains, such as antisocial companions and employment.	**Assessment Data:** Interview confirms his alliance with antisocial peers and limited contact with prosocial companions. **Relevance:** Companions drink and smoke marijuana; also encourage fights and impulsiveness. **Priority Level:** High. Hank has a strong connection with antisocial companions. He is reinforced for his negative behaviors (such as aggression, drug use, and lack of employment). He has virtually no connection with positive peers who might offer alternative social reinforcement. Hank is unlikely to initiate or maintain changes unless he distances himself from antisocial companions. His most recent offense was committed with his friends present.	**Assessment Data:** Interview confirms that Hank's anger disrupts romantic relationships. Also, he has a negative attitude toward his family. **Relevance:** • Hank distances himself from his prosocial family (who could have a positive influence on him). • He gets involved in romantic relationships with women who use substances. • He has poor social skills, which means that his romantic relationships are volatile and risky. • Anger reactions damage healthy relationships. **Priority Level:** Medium. Over the longer term, Hank will need to repair relationships with prosocial family members, and he would benefit from skills for managing anger and improving his romantic relationships. There is less urgency about addressing this domain at the beginning of treatment.

FIGURE 6.5. Hank's Case Formulation Worksheet.

(continued)

Lack of Connection to Work/School	Maladaptive Leisure Time	Substance Abuse/Misuse	Anger Dysregulation
Assessment Data: File records and interview indicate weak interest in employment and limited job skills. **Relevance:** Hank lacks a pattern of stable employment. His poor involvement in work results in a shortage of money and provides him with excessive free time. **Priority Level:** High. Hank's lack of stable employment has a direct impact on other areas (such as excessive leisure time) and increases his exposure to criminal companions.	**Assessment Data:** Interview indicates that he lacks prosocial interests/hobbies. **Relevance:** Hank has excessive "free time" due to lack of stable employment. He has no structure and is aimless in his daily activities. **Priority Level:** Medium. Focus on employment first and address leisure time later.	**Assessment Data:** Interview confirms his positive view about substances and being intoxicated. Specialized testing indicates substance misuse (75th percentile). **Relevance:** • Hank uses marijuana and alcohol when available, and to excess when most times. • However, he is able to remain abstinent from marijuana when necessary (due to supervision), which is a positive sign. **Priority Level:** High. Hank's use of marijuana puts him in contact with criminal companions and makes him ineligible to pass preemployment drug screens. His use of alcohol fuels his anger reactions and increases aggressive behaviors. Hank was using substances during his most recent offense.	**Assessment Data:** Specialized testing indicates high levels of anger (95th percentile). Interview confirms that he is easily angered over minor perceived transgressions by others. **Relevance:** • Responds aggressively when provoked or when encouraged by friends. • Anger difficulties are likely to interfere with romantic and family relationships. **Priority Level:** High. His anger leads to aggressive and assaultive behaviors, which put him at risk for more justice involvement. His anger also interferes with his relationships. His excessive anger was a significant component of his most recent offense.

II. Secondary Domains

Intellectual Disability	Presence of Psychopathology	Physical Health Concerns	Problematic Housing	Other: Motivation
Assessment Data: Interview and review of records reveal no cognitive impairments. A general	**Assessment Data:** Specialized testing and interview indicate no symptoms of depression,	**Assessment Data:** No physical health problems or medical conditions were revealed.	**Assessment Data:** Interview indicates that he resides with a prosocial relative, but this is tentative	**Assessment Data:** • Specialized testing indicates low motivation for change.

screening measure of intellectual performance reveals average intellectual functioning.

Relevance: Hank has normal cognitive abilities and should have no difficulty responding to treatment and improving his lifestyle.

Priority Level: None.

anxiety, or more serious psychopathology.

Relevance: Mental health symptoms will not interfere with treatment of criminal risk domains.

Priority Level: None.

(he sleeps on couch).

Relevance: Hank's current living situation appears unstable; he is looking into living with a prosocial friend.

Priority Level: Medium. Currently staying with a relative. It is unclear how long the current housing arrangement will last.

Relevance: Physical health concerns will not interfere with treatment of criminal risk domains.

Priority Level: None.

• Interview reveals a limited awareness of the need for self-improvement.

Relevance:
• Hank is reasonably comfortable with his current lifestyle.
• He shows little motivation for change.

Priority Level: High. Lack of motivation has the potential to interfere with treatment. Motivational enhancement should be incorporated into all aspects of treatment.

III. Values and Life Priorities

Intimate and Family Relationships	Friends and Community	Career and Learning	Lifestyle
Hank values having a healthy dating relationship.		Hank values doing work that he finds rewarding and important, but he hasn't yet taken steps in the direction of developing a career path. He is interested in pursuing a career in commercial driving.	

FIGURE 6.5. (continued)

(continued)

IV. Treatment Targets, Interventions, and Change Indicators

Treatment Target 1:
- *Increase employment (which will reduce his free time and limit his exposure to criminal companions).*
- *Pursue commercial driving.*

Interventions:
- Enhance motivation to change by emphasizing his value of doing meaningful work.
- Restructure thinking about employment.
- Encourage pursuit of commercial driver's license.
- Encourage applications for obtainable jobs.

Change Indicators:
- More optimistic outlook regarding employment.
- Obtaining commercial driver's license.
- Eventual success in securing employment.

Treatment Target 2:
- *Reduce contact with antisocial peers.*
- *Address criminal thinking pattern of identifying with antisocial peers.*

Interventions:
- Engage in motivational conversations exploring the pros and cons of close friends and antisocial peers.
- Challenge thoughts about identification with criminal peers.
- Pursue behavioral steps for distancing from antisocial companions.
- Develop new connections with prosocial peers; enhance social skills.

Change Indicators:
- Monitor social contacts; improve balance between criminal and prosocial friends.
- Monitor thoughts related to friendships; increase positive thoughts related to prosocial companions.

Treatment Target 3:
- *Change patterns of substance use.*
- *Reduce frequency and volume of alcohol use.*
- *Eliminate marijuana use.*

Interventions:
- Engage in motivational and values conversations about substance use.
- Do cognitive restructuring of thoughts that facilitate substance use.
- Reduce time with substance-using companions, and develop relationships with companions less involved with substances.
- Engage in activities that do not involve substances.
- Let significant others know about change and solicit support.

Change Indicators:
- Monitor frequency, duration, and consequences of substance use.
- Monitor thoughts related to the use of substances.
- Achieve abstinence from marijuana, plus positive drug screens.
- Decrease use of alcohol; decrease episodes of intoxication.

Treatment Target 4:
- *Improve anger management (reduce both verbal and physical expressions of anger).*

Interventions:
- Engage in motivational conversations exploring the outcomes of anger episodes.
- Do cognitive restructuring focused on the theme of demandingness; develop a more flexible life philosophy.
- Build acceptance skills (the ability to have angry thoughts and feelings, but not give in to them).
- Improve problem-solving and assertiveness skills.

Change Indicators:
- Monitor frequency, intensity, and duration of anger episodes.
- Monitor consequences of anger episodes.
- Decrease conflicts and improve conflict resolution skills.

FIGURE 6.5. (continued)

I. Criminal Risk Domains

History of Criminal/Antisocial Behavior	Criminogenic Thinking/Antisocial Orientation	Antisocial Companions	Dysfunctional Family/Romantic Relationships
Assessment Data: File and interview. • Referred for arrest while intoxicated, trying to open doors at a car dealership. • Has one prior arrest for shoplifting a few years ago. • Currently on probation. **Relevance:** Jackie is a single mom who struggles financially to care for her 4-year-old son and her disabled mother. She does not have an extensive history of criminal justice involvements. Based on her overall lifestyle as assessed by structured interview, her current risk level seems low to moderate. **Priority Level:** Static; history is not changeable.	**Assessment Data:** Interview suggests the presence of several criminal thinking patterns associated with Jackie's most recent offense. Her score on a specialized criminal thinking instrument indicates a low level of criminal thinking overall (total score at the 25th percentile). **Relevance:** The thinking patterns she scored highest on were: • Demand for excitement. • Identifying with, and seeking approval from, criminal associates. • Justifying and minimizing. **Priority Level:** Low. Thinking can be restructured when other risk domains are addressed.	**Assessment Data:** Interview suggests that Jackie's recent friendships are problematic. Connections with prosocial friends have faded during the past year. **Relevance:** Jackie has been hanging out with her recent friends after work. Her work companions have a routine of drinking after a shift and selling marijuana. They have encouraged Jackie to join them. Jackie seems to have gravitated toward the men at work because of convenience: It's been easy to just stay for an extra hour or two after a shift, and it's helped offset the boredom of her job. **Priority Level:** High. Her recent offense was committed with this group of friends.	**Assessment Data:** • Interview confirms good relationships with her mother and siblings. • She had an abusive relationship with her father, with whom she no longer has contact. • She has a contentious relationship with her child's father. • She does not seem to have any romantic relationships. She describes this as due to a lack of time. **Relevance:** Lack of meaningful romantic relationships puts Jackie at high risk for "relationships of convenience." **Priority Level:** Medium. Over the longer term, Jackie would benefit from more meaningful romantic attachments.

FIGURE 6.6. Jackie's Case Formulation Worksheet.

(continued)

101

Lack of Connection to Work/School	Maladaptive Leisure Time	Substance Abuse/Misuse	Anger Dysregulation
Assessment Data: • File records and interview indicate limited job skills and transient work history. • Fired from current job due to recent arrest. • Earned high school diploma. **Relevance:** • Jackie lacks a career path. Her involvement in work that she finds unrewarding leaves her vulnerable to seeking excitement. • Her involvement in transient and unrewarding work potentially exposes her to criminally minded coworkers. **Priority Level:** High. Establishing a meaningful career path will eliminate most of the criminal influences from Jackie's life.	**Assessment Data:** Interview indicates that because she is a single parent and has a role in caring for her mom, there is little time for leisure activities. **Relevance:** Jackie seems to have a desire to seek out exciting activities when opportunities present themselves. **Priority Level:** Medium. Focus on employment first and address leisure time later.	**Assessment Data:** Interview suggests little interest in substance use. **Relevance:** Jackie will engage in occasional alcohol use in social situations. **Priority Level:** Low. Substance use is not a treatment target.	**Assessment Data:** Specialized testing indicates low levels of anger (27th percentile). Interview confirms that Jackie does not have difficulty controlling her temper, even in challenging situations. **Relevance:** Jackie shows good emotion regulation. **Priority Level:** Low. Anger management is not a treatment target.

II. Secondary Domains

Intellectual Disability	Presence of Psychopathology	Physical Health Concerns	Problematic Housing	Other: Motivation
Assessment Data: *Review of records and interview reveal no cognitive impairments.* **Relevance:** *Jackie has normal cognitive abilities and should have no difficulty responding to treatment.* **Priority Level:** *None.*	**Assessment Data:** *Specialized testing and interview indicate moderate depressive symptoms.* **Relevance:** *Her mood symptoms will likely diminish once she takes active steps to make improvements in her life. Mood symptoms are not severe enough to interfere with treatment.* **Priority Level:** *Low.*	**Assessment Data:** *No physical health problems or medical conditions were revealed.* **Relevance:** *Physical health concerns will not interfere with treatment of criminal risk domains.* **Priority Level:** *None.*	**Assessment Data:** *Interview indicates that housing is stable but finances are a struggle.* **Relevance:** *Housing seems stable.* **Priority Level:** *Low.*	**Assessment Data:** *Interview reveals motivation for change and a desire to put criminal justice problems behind her.* **Relevance:** *Jackie seems amenable to treatment.* **Priority Level:** *Low. Not much time will be required to address issues of motivation.*

III. Values and Life Priorities

Intimate and Family Relationships	Friends and Community	Career and Learning	Lifestyle
Jackie values staying involved with her family and wants to do a better job taking care of her mom.		*Jackie values engaging in work that is rewarding and challenging; she is frustrated by her own failure to pursue her education in recent years.*	

FIGURE 6.6. (*continued*)

(continued)

IV. Treatment Targets, Interventions, and Change Indicators

Treatment Target 1:
- Increase education and employment (which will provide meaning, reduce excitement seeking, and result in less exposure to criminally minded coworkers).
- Pursue community college.

Interventions:
- Explore her interests regarding a career path.
- Restructure thinking about employment.
- Improve time management.
- Encourage applications to community colleges.
- Encourage meaningful part-time employment.

Change Indicators:
- Develop more optimistic outlook regarding education.
- Begin taking college-level courses.
- Succeed in securing meaningful part-time employment.

Treatment Target 2:
- Reduce contact with antisocial companions from work.
- Address the criminal thinking pattern of identifying with antisocial peers.

Interventions:
- Challenge thoughts about identification with criminal peers.
- Pursue behavioral steps for distancing from antisocial companions.
- Re-establish old connections with prosocial peers.

Change Indicators:
- Monitor social contacts; eliminate contact with men from previous job; increase contacts with prosocial friends.
- Monitor thoughts related to friendships; increase positive thoughts related to prosocial companions.

Treatment Target 3:
- Restructure leisure time.

Interventions:
- Begin activity scheduling.
- Increase enjoyable activities.

Change Indicators:
- Increase presence of enjoyable activities in weekly routines.
- Decrease excitement seeking during leisure time.
- Begin to develop a dating life.

Treatment Target 4:

Interventions:

Change Indicators:

FIGURE 6.6. (continued)

having greater relevance and higher priority levels. Section III of the worksheet, Values and Life Priorities, incorporates information gathered in these areas.

Section IV of the worksheet is titled Treatment Targets, Interventions, and Change Indicators. *Treatment targets* are the specific domains on which clinical attention is focused. *Interventions* are the procedures used in addressing the treatment targets; these may include CBT change techniques, participation in structured community programs, individual or group counseling, and less formal activities. This section of the worksheet is designed so that specific (rather than vague) treatment targets and interventions are identified. It is best to prioritize targets according to their relevance to criminal conduct (the factors having the greatest influence on criminality should be addressed first, etc.), although this may not always be feasible for various reasons (e.g., some life areas may be more amenable to change than others). There are boxes for four treatment target areas, although it is conceivable that a JIC will have more than four treatment needs (which is especially likely with higher-risk clients such as Hank). Nonetheless, it is important to limit treatment targets to a manageable number. Keeping treatment as parsimonious as possible will allow you to pursue a focused approach, but it also prevents a JIC from becoming overwhelmed with excessive treatment requirements. Also, as noted in Chapter 2, criminal risk domains are synergistic, in that improvements in one domain will often have a positive ripple effect on others. Finally, Section IV also contains a subcategory for *change indicators,* which are markers reflecting treatment progress. These may include attendance at structured programs, pre–post change scores on tests, urine and drug screens, clinical comments by program delivery personnel, or the JIC's verbal self-reports of progress (e.g., reduced anger outbursts, job interviews obtained, time spent with certain friends).

AVOIDING BIAS IN CASE FORMULATION

Some of the opinions formed in forensic contexts will be accurate reflections of the functioning and status of JICs and will lead to good-quality decisions regarding treatment. Some opinions will be less accurate and produce less desirable outcomes. The accuracy of decision making is related in part to naturally occurring human judgment bias, as well as accuracy related to the technology of any assessment instruments that might be used (i.e., normal variance in assessment procedures and instruments). Given the potential consequences of inferior decision making (e.g., determination of supervision levels, suboptimal treatment, future criminality), it is important for you to be alert to the inherent biases that can make their way into clinical decision making, so that you will be better able to avoid potential pitfalls in JIC case formulation.

We now briefly discuss three main human judgment factors that are particularly relevant in the case formulation of JICs: *attribution bias, confirmatory bias,* and *base rate neglect.* For additional foundational source material related to forensic decision making, see Garb (1998) and Quinsey, Harris, Rice, and Cormier (1998).

Attribution Bias

It is rather natural for people to seek explanations for the causes of their own behaviors and that of others. Comments such as "The reason I did this or that was . . . ," or "Billy seems upset; I wonder if it is because . . . ," reflect the pursuit of explanation. Although this pursuit is natural and common, it seems that our explanation seeking is actually tainted. According to attribution theory, people have different casual explanations for their own behavior versus that of others. Specifically, people have a tendency to regard their own actions as based on contextual or situational influences, but to view the actions of others as based on personal traits or dispositions. In other words, explanations about ourselves are based on external causes, whereas as our explanations about others are based on internal causes. To use a sports example, a golfer who misses an easy shot is likely to blame his or her equipment or environment (e.g., "The ball had mud on it," "The sun was in my eyes"), while the playing partner may well attribute the missed shot to the person's skill level (e.g., "Tony is a poor golfer").

This issue has particular relevance for decision making in forensic contexts, as it relates to accurately assessing the personal characteristics or circumstances of JICs. Attribution bias can cause you to ascribe the reason for certain JICs' actions incorrectly (e.g., you may assume that a specific behavior is related to criminally relevant dispositional factors such as criminal attitudes, when in fact it may simply represent normal human functioning or be more influenced by situational factors). In the case of Hank, for example, Brenda may view his use of alcohol (which averages two drinks per day, although his use of illicit drugs is much greater) to be related to his "criminal nature," and may not even consider the fact that his consumption of alcohol may be within social norms and is relatively unrelated to his criminal patterns. Such attribution errors can have the unfortunate consequence of attracting clinical attention to issues unrelated to criminality.

Confirmatory Bias

People have considerable abilities to manage vast amounts of information related to a particular task by way of *cognitive schematic processing*—which is the unconscious organization of knowledge related to a specific topic. At the same time, however, people are amazingly susceptible at being selectively attentive to various pieces of information. *Confirmatory bias* is the human tendency to seek, retrieve, and analyze information that supports rather than challenges one's own opinion. The bias can become more pronounced in certain circumstances (particularly during periods of high emotion), to the point that false or illusory connections between information can be formed.

This bias, in either a *negative* or *positive* direction, can pose a threat to forensic decision making and contribute to faulty conclusions. For example, Brenda may view Hank's offense and lifestyle as particularly repugnant, and hence may fall prey to a bias toward seeking, interpreting, and analyzing information supporting her view that he is at high criminal risk (negative bias). On the other hand, if Hank is a young man with decent social skills, Brenda may be prone to downplay his role in negative events and to see him as at low risk for engaging in future criminal behavior (positive bias). If Brenda can establish a balance between confirming and disconfirming information, she will be more likely to develop an accurate case formulation.

Base Rate Neglect

Although it is unlikely that people working in professional decision-making capacities would regard themselves as soothsayers, they must devote a considerable amount of time and energy to predicting the clinical outcomes of clients across many care settings. In hospital settings, this may relate to predicting whether, and over what time span, a patient may recover from an illness. In forensic contexts, a primary focus of attention is determining whether a JIC will reoffend. Given the potential consequences of JICs' future behavior (criminality, harm to others, etc.), accurate prediction may be of particular importance. Human judgment research pertaining to prediction shows that people have a tendency to make consistent errors of prediction by, among other things, failing to integrate probability into their decision making.

Base rate neglect is the failure to consider the statistical probability of an event in making a prediction. In general, people form predictive opinions based on information that is readily available, and relatively proximal to an event, rather than considering the statistical likelihood. For example, most people estimating the chances of being struck by lightning will claim that these are very low, most of the time. Their estimate will change, however, if they become aware that someone they know has been struck by lightning.

In forensic contexts, base rate neglect occurs when practitioners disregard or misperceive (i.e., overestimate or underestimate) the statistical likelihood of a JIC's reoffending, which often results in an inaccurate case formulation and a suboptimal treatment plan. Perhaps the most obvious example in actual practice relates to the assessment and management of sexual offenders. The commonly referenced rate of sexual recidivism among sexual offenders is 13%, according to a comprehensive statistical review by Hanson and Bussiere (1998). To state this differently, 13 out of 100 sexual offenders would be expected to reoffend in a sexual manner, which may be regarded as low. It is common, however, for practitioners and correctional agencies to overestimate the statistical probability of any sexual offender's reoffending, and to mandate treatment or other rehabilitative activities that are incongruent with the risk level (i.e., to mismatch the risk with the treatment dosage).

Reviewing the information related to basic human judgment issues may give the impression that practitioners are weak at making clinical decisions. That is not the case, nor has it been our intention to suggest this in presenting this information. The point is that all humans are susceptible to errors of judgment. Being mindful of common errors that contribute to bias can greatly increase the accuracy of JICs' case formulations, treatment plans, and evaluations. As an aid to managing human bias in case formulation, it may be helpful to ask yourself the following questions:

1. *Which pieces of information are most important?* In many forensic contexts, there will be a variety of different streams of information available, some relevant and some not. A saying related to this notion is "Everything has purpose, but not everything has meaning." To use an example, a person may be walking on a sidewalk and then cross the street. There is certainly a purpose, or a reason, for this person to cross the street, but whether it is significant and therefore has meaning is unknown. If the person simply wants to cross the street for a change of scenery, then the behavior has no particular meaning. On the other hand, if the person crosses the street because he or she wants to examine a specific property to commit a burglary, or to follow a certain person for some nefarious reason, then the street-crossing behavior has meaning. You should determine what information has greater meaning for a particular JIC's case, and dedicate more time to those issues.

2. *What is the relative importance of each piece of the puzzle?* Each case will have different clinical facts from which to develop a case formulation. Sometimes there is voluminous information of a consistent nature, and sometimes there is sparse information of a divergent nature. Judgment is required as to what information has greater importance. In legal circles, discussions of the "weight of the evidence" are common and can be easily applied to forensic assessment. For example, the presence of problems within criminal risk domains should be of greater importance (and hence have greater "weight" in the decision-making process) than factors that are less risk-relevant (e.g., mental health symptoms).

3. *Is my clinical opinion biased in some way?* Although we may be mindful of the human judgment bias issues noted above, it can be easy to ignore these issues in the course of our clinical work. Constantly challenging your perspective regarding a particular case can be helpful. The self-talk phrase "Am I missing something?" can be a useful reminder. The process of case formulation is a blend of art and science and should be parsimonious.

KEY POINTS

- Practitioners must gather, interpret, and synthesize clinical information in order to form an opinion of the causes and maintenance of JICs' criminal behavior.

- Forensic case formulation consists of three components: (1) considering the likelihood of future criminal behavior; (2) pinpointing criminal risk domains to target in treatment; and (3) developing a treatment plan to reduce the risk of future criminality.

- Changes in functioning within criminal risk domains alter the probability of future criminal behavior.

- A first step in case formulation is completing a Criminal Event Analysis to identify the most salient criminal risk domains related to recent incidents of criminal behavior.

- A second step in case formulation is to understand how criminal risk domains affect general life functioning and serve as overall drivers of criminal behavior. The Criminal Risk Domains Worksheet can be used to develop this understanding.

- The Case Formulation Worksheet provides a structure for bringing together clinical information for the purpose of developing a treatment plan.

- Accuracy (and avoiding bias) in case formulation is important, so that treatment plans reflect the true needs of JICs.

FORM 6.1. Criminal Event Analysis

Describe the Offense
(nature of the offense: what, where, and when)

_____
_____
_____
_____
_____
_____
_____
_____
_____
_____

Individual/Dispositional Domains

Check all that apply:

☐ Offense was consistent with overall pattern of criminal history
☐ Criminogenic thinking/antisocial orientation
  Thinking patterns: _____
  _____
☐ Substance use/misuse
  Substances involved: _____
☐ Anger dysregulation
☐ Other
☐ Secondary domains or other individual factors: _____
  _____
  _____

Social/Contextual Domains

Check all that apply:

☐ Antisocial companions
  Person(s): _____
☐ Dysfunctional family/romantic relationships
  Person(s): _____
☐ Maladaptive leisure time
☐ Lack of connection to work/school
☐ Other
☐ Secondary domains or other social/contextual factors: _____
  _____

Describe the Client
(name, age, gender, marital status, criminal justice status)

_____
_____
_____
_____
_____
_____
_____
_____
_____
_____

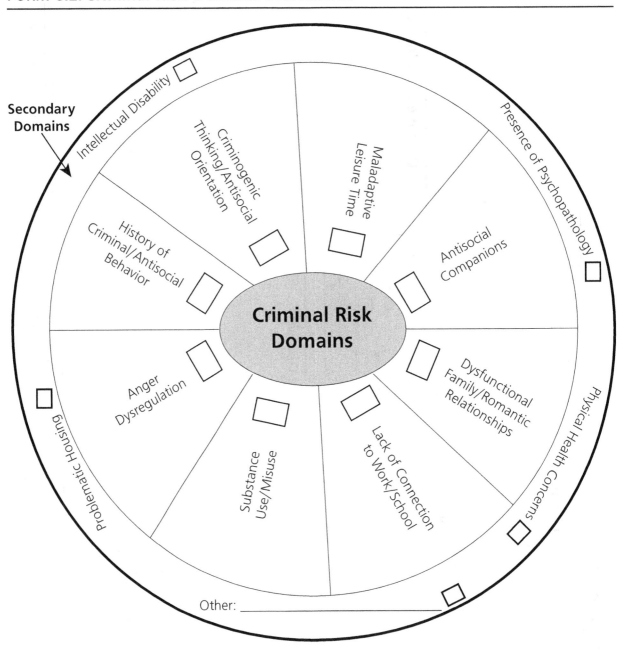

Secondary Domains

Intellectual Disability ☐

Presence of Psychopathology ☐

Criminogenic Thinking/Antisocial Orientation ☐

Maladaptive Leisure Time ☐

History of Criminal/Antisocial Behavior ☐

Antisocial Companions ☐

Criminal Risk Domains

Anger Dysregulation ☐

Dysfunctional Family/Romantic Relationships ☐

Substance Use/Misuse ☐

Lack of Connection to Work/School ☐

Problematic Housing ☐

Physical Health Concerns ☐

Other: _____ ☐

FORM 6.3. Case Formulation Worksheet

I. Criminal Risk Domains

History of Criminal/Antisocial Behavior	Criminogenic Thinking/Antisocial Orientation	Antisocial Companions	Dysfunctional Family/Romantic Relationships
Assessment Data:	Assessment Data:	Assessment Data:	Assessment Data:
Relevance:	Relevance:	Relevance:	Relevance:
Priority Level: *Static; history is not changeable.*	Priority Level:	Priority Level:	Priority Level:

(continued)

FORM 6.3. Case Formulation Worksheet (page 2 of 4)

Lack of Connection to Work/ School	Maladaptive Leisure Time	Substance Abuse/Misuse	Anger Dysregulation
Assessment Data:	Assessment Data:	Assessment Data:	Assessment Data:
Relevance:	Relevance:	Relevance:	Relevance:
Priority Level:	Priority Level:	Priority Level:	Priority Level:

(continued)

FORM 6.3. Case Formulation Worksheet (page 3 of 4)

II. Secondary Domains

Intellectual Disability	Presence of Psychopathology	Physical Health Concerns	Problematic Housing	Other
Assessment Data:	Assessment Data:	Assessment Data:	Assessment Data:	Assessment Data:
Relevance:	Relevance:	Relevance:	Relevance:	Relevance:
Priority Level:	Priority Level:	Priority Level:	Priority Level:	Priority Level:

III. Values and Life Priorities

Intimate and Family Relationships	Friends and Community	Career and Learning	Lifestyle

(continued)

FORM 6.3. Case Formulation Worksheet (page 4 of 4)

IV. Treatment Targets, Interventions, and Change Indicators

Treatment Target 1:	Treatment Target 2:	Treatment Target 3:	Treatment Target 4:
Interventions:	Interventions:	Interventions:	Interventions:
Change Indicators:	Change Indicators:	Change Indicators:	Change Indicators:

CHAPTER 7

Establishing Collaborative Goals and Focusing Conversations

As treatment progresses, Brenda and Hank develop a modicum of workable therapeutic rapport. Brenda soon decides it is time to negotiate with Hank about which areas of his life he may be interested in improving. From the assessment and her case formulation, she has come to realize that Hank's lack of meaningful employment, antisocial companions, use of substances, and excessive anger reactions make him vulnerable to experiencing future criminal justice problems. His demeanor certainly indicates that he is displeased with the consequences of his current actions—or at least with the results of "getting caught." However, Brenda is beginning to wonder if Hank's irritation stems not simply from dejection about dealing with the mandates imposed by the criminal justice system, but rather from a developing awareness of his deeper life problems. If this is true, then he may be experiencing the cognitive ambivalence typically accompanying the realization that change is needed. Whether Hank will channel his displeasure in a positive way and work to improve the risky domains of his life, or whether he will continue with his status quo lifestyle and end up in similar (or worse) circumstances in the future, is unknown. His trajectory is somewhat dependent on what insights into his lifestyle he gains from his interactions with Brenda, how he responds to those insights, and what steps he is willing to take to change the life areas that put him most at risk.

Focusing treatment on what matters most is not always straightforward. You will be required to bring up topics that can be embarrassing, can be difficult to discuss, and—if not handled skillfully—will engender defensiveness. Focusing becomes increasingly complicated when the clinical picture is chaotic and confused, and when JICs are uninterested in pursuing goals stipulated in court orders, mandated by community supervision conditions, or outlined by a program's mission. Therefore, two skills are essential for establishing collaborative goals in forensic treatment: (1) listening for JICs' own motivations for making changes, and (2) intentionally evoking and reinforcing those motivations. The two skills operate in tandem: Practitioners *listen for* statements by JICs that express (however ambivalently) some desire for change, and then *reinforce* those expressions and deliberately *elicit* from JICs additional reasons for change.

EVOKING MOTIVATION FOR CHANGE IN CRIMINAL RISK DOMAINS

Evoking is the process of supporting and encouraging JICs in voicing their own motivations for making changes in the criminal risk domains relevant to their lives. Despite the punitive contingencies that exist in most forensic environments, internal motivation for change is still necessary, and JICs who are successful in treatment go through a process of talking themselves into changing. Evoking rests on the premise that what JICs hear themselves say during interactions is more important than what practitioners say to them (Berg-Smith, 2010).

If you have received training in traditional CBT, you have been taught to pay attention to specific types of client verbalizations indicative of cognitive distortions, irrational beliefs, and dysfunctional schemas believed to be central to various forms of psychopathology. In MI (introduced in Chapters 2 and 3), a completely different constellation of language constructs is emphasized, related to motivation and subsequent change. It takes time to learn to identify, respond to, and elicit this specific form of client change language. It is like giving yourself a new antenna with which to listen to clients' verbalizations.

Two foundational terms are relevant for understanding evoking as a skill: *change talk* and *sustain talk*. Change talk is any client speech that favors movement toward and commitment to change, whereas sustain talk is client speech that favors maintaining the status quo or not changing (Miller & Rollnick, 2013). With JICs, sustain talk often takes the form of minimizations or justifications related to negative, risky, or criminal behaviors. In the case of a drug seller, an example of sustain talk would be "Selling drugs in my neighborhood isn't dangerous, because I know all my customers." This statement expresses a justification for continuing to sell drugs. Change talk from a drug seller, on the other hand, might sound something like "I'm getting a little tired of all the drug scene drama." Change talk may be quite subtle, expressing just a potential reason for change. It does not often involve a 100% commitment to suddenly stopping antisocial behavior and embracing a prosocial lifestyle. Also, both change talk and sustain talk will emerge in conversations, because it is quite normal for JICs (and people in general) to have two voices—one on each side of the equation (favoring change vs. maintaining the status quo)—bouncing around in their heads at the same time.

A key research finding in this area is that the ratio of change talk to sustain talk during practitioner–client interactions is an important marker for subsequent change and is associated with greater clinical improvement. A predominance of change talk predicts actual behavior change, whereas a higher proportion of sustain talk—or equal levels of sustain talk and change talk—are predictive of not changing (Moyers, Martin, Houck, Christopher, & Tonigan, 2009). Also, levels of client change talk and sustain talk can be influenced by a practitioner's response style (Glynn & Moyers, 2010). These findings indicate that a core skill in working with JICs is to facilitate and increase the expression of change talk.

Change Talk Subtypes

Change talk is organized across two levels and seven specific verbalization subtypes. The first level is known as *preparatory change talk* and consists of four change talk subtypes, which can be remembered by using the acronym DARN (*desire, ability, reasons,* and *need*). Preparatory change talk signals energy in favor of change. Here are some examples from Hank's case:

"I would really like to have a steady paycheck someday." [desire]

"I could probably look into schools for getting my CDL [commercial driver's license]." [ability]

"If I got a paycheck, I wouldn't have to keep hustling and looking over my shoulder all the time." [reasons]

"I can't do this forever. I've got to get some job skills and get my life on track." [need]

The second level, known as *mobilizing change talk*, consists of three change talk subtypes that can be remembered by using the acronym CAT (*commitment, activation,* and *taking steps*). CAT verbalizations by Hank would sound like this:

"Next week I will have information about three schools that offer the CDL." [commitment]

"I'm planning to buy the course materials so that I can get started." [activation]

"I looked on the internet and found the directions for getting to where the classes are held." [taking steps]

CAT verbalizations indicate a greater willingness or commitment to change.

Recognizing Change Talk

A first step in improving your evoking skills is "tuning your ear" to recognize change talk when it occurs. Read over the list of assorted JIC statements in Figure 7.1, and check the appropriate box to indicate whether each statement reflects change talk or sustain talk. Then go over the list a second time, and for those statements you have identified as change talk, try to identify the specific subtype and write it in the space provided. Answers are provided at the end of this chapter.

Responding to Naturally Occurring Change Talk

As you become more familiar with change talk, you will recognize much more motivation emerging in clients' conversations than you had previously noticed. Often change talk will bubble up naturally when JICs are ambivalent (at some level) about some of their current patterns. How you respond once change talk emerges will influence whether more change talk will occur.

For example, imagine that you hear statement 6 (from Figure 7.1). You could respond in the following ways:

"Sounds like being part of your son's life is a high priority for you." [reflection]

"Tell me, why it is so important for you to be a part of your son's life?" [open question]

"In spite of all the challenges you are facing, you really want to be a good father." [affirmation]

JIC statement	Change language		
	Change talk	Sustain talk	Change talk subtype
1. "I have my reasons for dropping out of school."	☐	☐	_____
2. "My family wants me to get a job and stop selling drugs."	☐	☐	_____
3. "I went to the employment group last week."	☐	☐	_____
4. "I might be able to cut down a bit."	☐	☐	_____
5. "There is no way to avoid gang activity in my neighborhood."	☐	☐	_____
6. "I want to be part of my son's life."	☐	☐	_____
7. "I plan to be more honest with my family."	☐	☐	_____
8. "I've got to stay out of prison."	☐	☐	_____
9. "I guarantee I'll make my court appointment."	☐	☐	_____
10. "I need to get high every day."	☐	☐	_____

FIGURE 7.1. Recognizing change talk exercise.

Any of these responses is likely to produce more change talk. As another example, you might respond to statement 8 (from Figure 7.1) by saying any of the following:

"You're willing to do whatever it takes not to end up back in prison." [reflection]
"If you do end up back in prison, what do you stand to lose?" [open question]
"How do you see your life unfolding if you are successful in staying out of prison?" [open question]

Of course, these responses utilize the OARS skills described in Chapter 3; however, they are now employed with a more strategic purpose—evoking more change talk. Also, when you are constructing end-of-session summaries, don't forget to include any change talk that has emerged during the session. Your goal is to consistently reinforce the most powerful arguments for change—those coming directly from JICs.

Actively Eliciting Change Talk

If change talk does not naturally emerge in a session, you can take steps to actively evoke it by asking strategic open questions. These are sometimes known as *change talk questions*, because the answers invite DARN CAT verbalizations (Berg-Smith, 2010). A list of generic questions that correspond to the change talk model is provided in Table 7.1. Feel free to create variations of these questions to fit a particular case.

TABLE 7.1. Questions Likely to Evoke Change Talk

Change talk subtype	Change talk questions
Desire	• "How would you like your life to be different?" • "Why would you want to _____ [insert a change related to a relevant criminal risk domain]?"
Ability	• "What gives you confidence that you could _____?" • "What strengths do you have that might help you in _____?"
Reasons	• "What might be the two most important reasons to _____?" • "What are the benefits of _____?"
Need	• "How important is it for you to _____?" • "What is at stake if you do not _____?"
Commitment	• "What do you see as the next step?" • "What is one specific thing you could do to _____?"
Activation	• "What are some things you might do to get ready to _____?" • "How could you start exploring how _____ would improve your life?"
Taking steps	• "What have you done so far in moving toward _____?" • "What are some things you have accomplished in prison [or on probation/parole] that can help you now?"

Responding to Sustain Talk

Sustain talk will also be naturally occurring during conversations. For those JICs who feel strongly that they have been coerced into treatment, levels of sustain talk may be particularly high. The good news is that sustain talk will often decrease over time with successful engagement. Keep in mind that it is important not to reprimand or punish JICs for verbalizing sustain talk, since it is a normal expression of ambivalence. Similarly, do not completely ignore sustain talk in hopes of extinguishing such statements. Because demonstrating that you grasp a JIC's perspective is critical, there will be times when you acknowledge the JIC's voices that are not in favor of change. In fact, failure to do so will damage your working relationship. However, as noted below, your goal is not to actively increase sustain talk, but rather to acknowledge it when it occurs.

Imagine that you hear statement 1 (from Figure 7.1). You might respond in the following manner:

> "Tell me about your reasons for dropping out." [open question]
> "Seems like you really gave it some thought before you dropped out." [reflection]

These responses demonstrate good listening about what is most important to the JIC. Although this may seem somewhat counterintuitive, if you avoid the impulse to offer advice or provide a lecture about the downsides of quitting school—and give the person space—change talk will often emerge naturally as the conversation unfolds. In the example above, confronting the JIC is likely to produce more sustain talk. Your task is to continue the conversation and listen carefully for DARN CAT verbalizations. If change talk does not bubble up naturally, you can make an active attempt to elicit it by using questions similar to the ones described above (e.g., "What concerns might you have about your decision to quit school?").

Additional Tips Regarding Change Talk

• *Change talk ebbs and flows.* The process of evoking change talk is not linear. Change talk will rise and fall naturally over the course of an interaction and across sessions. It is a mistake to believe that once change talk occurs, issues of ambivalence are in the past, and only DARN CAT verbalizations will exist moving forward. Even when JICs have voiced strong arguments in favor of change, sustain talk can sometimes follow. Expect this to happen, and continue to listen for and differentially reinforce change talk (over sustain talk) throughout the treatment process.

• *Change talk can be both positive and negative.* Attending to change talk will sometimes infuse conversations with an uplifting and optimistic quality, through revealing JICs' hopes and aspirations for a better life. This will be especially evident when you and a JIC are exploring the JIC's values and life priorities (Chapter 4). At other times, conversations will take on a negative and heavy tone, because the contents of discussions will be about regrets, losses, or outcomes JICs wish to avoid. Both tones are acceptable. For example, a common progression is for conversations to center first on the negative consequences of current life patterns, and then move to more positive anticipated outcomes that might result from making changes.

• *Avoid evoking sustain talk.* Because you are attempting to tilt the balance toward change talk and away from sustain talk, beware of asking questions likely to evoke sustain talk. Unfortunately, these types of questions are common among well-meaning forensic practitioners. Here are some examples of questions to generally avoid:

"Tell me why you can't just walk away from _____ [drugs, criminal friends, etc.]."
"Why are you not more motivated to change _____?"
"Why don't you stop _____?"
"Why won't you give up _____?"
"What are the pros and cons of changing _____?"

Such questions are ill advised because they will evoke sustain talk. The "pros and cons" type of question, also known as the *decisional balance technique,* will provide both types of talk but will not always guarantee a higher ratio of change to sustain talk. Although there may be times when such questions are useful in understanding a JIC's perspective and exploring potential roadblocks to change, overutilizing these types of questions will inadvertently increase levels of sustain talk during interactions. Think ahead in picking your questions. If the response to a specific question is likely to produce sustain talk, have a good rationale for asking it (Miller & Rollnick, 2013).

- *Give yourself a learning curve.* In conversations with JICs, there are often many statements that will attract your attention. It is important to be particularly attentive to change language. Tilting the balance in favor of change talk over sustain talk is a subtle art that you can excel at with effort and practice. If the concept of change language is new to you, then achieving higher levels of competency will require more support than this treatment planner can provide. MI training workshops, which are offered around the world, can provide a solid foundation of skills and opportunities to practice. (See Appendix B for a listing of practitioner resources.) Also, a series of self-guided exercises for recognizing, reinforcing, and eliciting change talk can be found in the excellent workbook by Rosengren (2018).

WHAT IS FOCUSING?

Following assessment and case formulation, you will have a good understanding of the most important targets to address in treatment. *Focusing* is the process of establishing agreement with JICs about treatment goals and clarifying a general strategic direction regarding the topics that will be discussed. Focusing helps set the stage for efficient sessions with JICs, while steering clear of nonstrategic interactions (e.g., "How's it going?") and chaos-driven sessions (i.e., sessions focusing on the "crisis of the week"). As a general guideline, focusing prematurely on a goal not currently shared by a client will most often result in disengagement, while goals identified collaboratively are more likely to hold intrinsic value to the JIC.

The focusing strategies we present are adapted from the MI model described by Miller and Rollnick (2013) and from agenda-setting strategies commonly used in CBT (Mitchell et al., 2015; Persons, 2008). As noted in previous chapters, clients suffering from traditional mental health problems ordinarily show up with some desire to reduce symptoms or solve the problems that brought them into treatment. When treatment starts off well, such clients will carry the greater part of the responsibility in identifying desired targets for change. In contrast, many JICs (like Hank and Jackie) lack awareness of how their functioning in certain life domains contributes to their ongoing difficulties and undermines their long-term well-being. Therefore, more active and skillful guiding in establishing a treatment direction may be required on your part. Collaboration in determining the focus of treatment with JICs will vary, and the proportion of your effort to a JIC's may be 60–40, 70–30, or 80–20, with you initially carrying the greater burden.

STRATEGIES FOR ESTABLISHING GOALS
AND FOCUSING CONVERSATIONS

We cover five strategies for establishing collaborative treatment goals and focusing conversations. Depending on the setting and the case, you may decide to identify several treatment goals at the outset, or to focus on one specific goal at a time and then engage in a new focusing discussion after progress has been made on the first goal. The skills of listening for, reinforcing, and eliciting change talk—discussed in the first part of this chapter—are integrated into all focusing discussions.

Focusing Questions

Perhaps the most straightforward strategy is simply to ask, in an open-ended manner, what the person considers the greatest concern or highest priority. Often, when asked directly, a JIC will identify a change that is consistent with a criminal risk domain. The benefit of focusing questions is that JICs themselves highlight the need for change, rather than being told by practitioners what is important. Of course, the disadvantage of this approach is that many JICs come to the table with entrenched thinking patterns that distort and interfere with their ability to accurately assess the long-term effects of their present lifestyles. Nonetheless, a direct approach is usually worth a try and at the very least will provide additional information about a JIC's level of awareness. Examples of focusing questions are provided in Table 7.2.

Be prepared for a wide range of answers to these types of questions. As you listen, your task is to reinforce any change talk that naturally emerges. Your overall strategy will involve matching the JIC's responses to any of the seven modifiable criminal risk domains (criminogenic thinking/antisocial orientation, antisocial companions, dysfunctional family/romantic relationships, lack of connection to work/school, maladaptive leisure time, substance abuse/misuse, and anger dysregulation) previously identified in your assessment and case formulation, and then guiding discussions toward those areas in subsequent meetings. If you try one or two of these questions and elicit change talk related to a criminal risk domain, congratulations! You are establishing a collaborative treatment goal. If not, then try one of the more directive strategies described below.

TABLE 7.2. Focusing Questions

- "What changes would you like to make?"
- "It looks like you are getting a lot of pressure from the court about the conditions of your probation. I would like to hear from you what you think is most important to work on."
- "If you were to make changes in your life once you get out of prison, what do you see as the first change you need to make?"
- "As you look at your life right now, what areas do you need to work on to make things better?"
- "In terms of changing something, what seems most urgent for you right now?"
- "If I were to run into you at the post office after your supervision period has ended, what would you want to tell me has changed in your life?"
- "When you think about your upcoming release date, what are you most worried about?"
- "Even though you feel like you are being forced to come here, what could we focus on that might be helpful for you?"
- "In order to avoid future legal problems, what do you need to do differently?"
- "What puts you most at risk for getting rearrested?"
- "What are the two most important things for you to work on so that you will not end up back in prison?"
- "Let's take a step back and consider together what is most important to focus on. What do you see as the highest priority?"
- "If I were to see you in the community a year after you are released, what kinds of things would you like to tell me are going well?"

Verbally Presenting a Menu of Options

Another strategy is for you to take the lead, describing several criminal risk domains that have emerged from the assessment and case formulation, and ask the JIC to pick what he or she views as most important. Several short focusing scripts are presented at the end of this chapter (Script 7.1). Feel free to use these scripts as a general guide, and to make adjustments or create variations that work best for your clients and setting.

Providing a Visual Stimulus of Criminal Risk Domains

A similar strategy is to provide a visual stimulus displaying a menu of options that can become the focus of treatment. Such stimuli can take the form of lists, charts, or figures that depict criminal risk domains, allowing JICs to choose from the options presented. For less verbal clients, simply identifying an area can be a starting point for more in-depth conversations. An example of a visual stimulus is provided in Form 7.1 at the end of this chapter. Script 7.2, also at the end of this chapter, can be used to introduce Form 7.1 and launch into the conversation.

Form 7.1 contains six of the eight criminal risk domains. Criminal history is not included because it is unchangeable (static). Also, because of its multifaceted nature, criminogenic thinking/antisocial orientation is not included in this form; it is difficult to capture the full range of thinking patterns with a brief label or description. A specific strategy for focusing conversations on criminogenic thinking patterns is presented next.

Asking Permission to Focus on a Relevant Criminogenic Thinking Pattern

Criminal thinking has been found to predict future criminality (Walters, 2012). As such, one of your primary goals in working with JICs is to alter thinking processes to improve decision making and reduce risky and self-defeating behaviors. It is important to discuss such patterns and make them focal points of treatment. In most cases, more than one criminal thinking pattern will exist; however, resist the temptation to address multiple patterns at once. Rather, put the focus on one pattern at a time. Once progress is made with one pattern, you can introduce the next at a later session.

There are two general steps in addressing thinking patterns with JICs. First, discuss the idea that for all human beings, thinking generally guides behavior. Also, with years of repetition, it is normal for thinking patterns to become automatic and for people to become less aware of how their thinking influences their actions. (See Script 7.3 at the end of this chapter for an example for how to frame meaningful conversations around thinking targets.) Second, present and describe to the JIC a specific thinking pattern that you have identified in your assessment. You will need to exercise a degree of finesse in using nonjudgmental language to describe relevant patterns. If you launch into the discussion with a pejorative tone (e.g., "You seem to have a tremendous disregard for others"), the conversation is unlikely to move forward productively. Consult Script 7.4 at the end of this chapter for ideas on how to introduce the full range of criminal thinking patterns; the patterns in this script correspond to the lists of criminogenic thinking patterns presented in Chapter 2 (Table 2.2) and Chapter 5 (Table 5.1).

Providing Feedback from Standardized Tests

Another way to focus treatment on relevant criminal risk domains is to provide feedback on standardized tests administered as part of the assessment (e.g., instruments assessing anger, criminal thinking, substance use; see Appendix A for recommendations). You can highlight areas of concern by sharing with JICs how their scores compare to those of others. Scores are usually presented in terms of percentiles, and the dimensions being measured are explained in easy-to-understand language. As a general guideline, limit your feedback to one or two scores representing the areas that are most critical, as opposed to providing too much feedback on all dimensions measured on an instrument. In addition, resist the temptation to convince a JIC to accept the feedback. Rather, provide this feedback as a platform to explore how relevant patterns might be negatively affecting the person's life. Feedback is presented as information for JICs to consider; they are free to reject it. However, most JICs are appreciative of the feedback if it is presented properly, even if it is uncomfortable to hear. Script 7.5 provides an example of presenting feedback on a standardized assessment (i.e., an instrument measuring anger); this can be used as a template for presenting information from assessments of other risk domain areas.

It is common for JICs to agree with high scores, since the tests accurately measure problem areas based on their own self-reports. Although there can be a variety of reactions to hearing how one's scores compare to those of a standardization group, these are almost always limited to a few themes. Table 7.3 provides typical reactions to feedback and corresponding sample practitioner responses. Even when a JIC does not agree with the feedback, open questions and reflections designed to explore the issue further and elicit change talk are usually effective. The one exception is when a JIC reacts with *confusion*. In this situation, your task is to explain the score again in another way that is likely to be understood. We recommend that when a client seems confused by percentiles, you simply use a descriptive label instead (e.g., "One area that you scored high in was . . .").

This style of presenting feedback works best for the kinds of human problems where people tend to minimize the consequences of their behaviors, or for which they have limited awareness regarding the longer-term consequences of such behaviors (e.g., anger, substance use, criminogenic thinking). It is not recommended for mental health problems that involve a tendency to obsess or ruminate about specific symptoms (e.g., anxiety and depression). For example, if significant anxiety is part of the clinical picture, saying to a JIC, "Your level of worry is greater than that of 95% of men your age," would probably be counterproductive and result in even more worry and rumination. However, if the JIC has little concern about using alcohol to manage his anxiety symptoms, we might present feedback on standardized testing results specific to alcohol use. Video examples of providing feedback in this style are available for substance use (Miller, Rollnick, & Moyers, 1998) and anger (Kassinove & Tafrate, 2014).

TABLE 7.3. JIC Reactions to Assessment Feedback and Practitioner Responses

JIC statements	Practitioner responses
"Yeah, my anger has always gotten me in trouble." [agreement]	• "Sounds like this is really on target for you." • "How have your anger reactions created problems in your life?"
"I didn't think my anger was that high. I thought I was like everybody else." [surprise]	• "This information is surprising. What do you think it means for you?" • "What have you noticed in everybody else?"
"I'm not sure it's a problem, because other people act the same way that I do." [minimizing]	• "It is hard to make sense of this information, because when you look around, it seems like your verbal reactions are just like other people you know." • "What have you noticed about how others handle their anger?"
"In my neighborhood you have to be tough. I have no choice; I have to say @#!$%& to people." [justifying]	• "So sometimes your anger reactions are strong, but you have your reasons." • "What usually happens when you angrily confront or yell at others in your neighborhood?"
"I don't have an anger problem. That score can't be right. Something is wrong with your test." [disagreement]	• "This score doesn't make sense for you." • "Let's put the test aside. How do you see your own anger in comparison to how others react?"
"Whatever . . . I don't believe in tests." [indifference]	• "You are not sure this information is relevant for you." • "Let's not go with what the test says. How do you see your anger reactions in comparison to others'?"
"Wow! Is 99% good?" [confusion]	• "Let's talk about what this score means." • "Let me draw a chart for you. When it comes to expressing your anger, here is where you stand compared to others. You are at the extreme high end, which puts you at risk."

WHAT IF I CAN'T GET AGREEMENT ON A FOCUS?

A collaborative agreement to work on one or more criminal risk domains can be established with the clear majority of JICs. Nonetheless, you will encounter occasional cases where a shared focus cannot be reached. Accept the fact that some JICs will not change their lifestyles and that their problems will sometimes worsen. Don't take such cases as evidence that you are failing in your work; you are likely to have a positive effect on many, but not all, JICs. In these cases, since it will be unproductive to move forward with the CBT strategies outlined in the next few chapters, we recommend that you take a step back and focus on engagement and discussions of values and life priorities (Chapters 3 and 4), leaving open the possibility that a collaborative focus will emerge with time.

KEY POINTS

- *Change talk* is any JIC language that favors change, as well as ideas for how change might happen. *Sustain talk* is expressed in JIC verbalizations that favor maintaining the status quo or not changing.

- Both change talk and sustain talk will naturally occur in conversations with JICs. The ratio between change talk and sustain talk is an important marker for subsequent change: A higher proportion of change talk predicts actual behavior change.

- Reinforcing naturally occurring change talk and actively evoking change talk, in the criminal risk domains most relevant to a JICs life, are core skills in forensic treatment. You want to be continually alert to tilting the balance in favor of change talk (over sustain talk) throughout the treatment process.

- *Focusing* is the process of establishing agreement with JICs about treatment goals and clarifying a general strategic direction regarding what topics will be discussed during sessions.

- The skills of recognizing, reinforcing, and eliciting change talk (with a general increase in change talk) are integrated into focusing discussions.

- Several strategies can be used to establish collaborative treatment goals: focusing questions, verbally presenting options, providing a visual stimulus of common criminal risk domains, asking permission to focus on a criminogenic thinking pattern, and providing feedback on standardized tests. It's OK to try several strategies to see which one works best with a specific case.

Answers to recognizing change talk exercise (Figure 7.1): 1, sustain talk; 2, change talk—reasons; 3, change talk—taking steps; 4, change talk—ability; 5, sustain talk; 6, change talk—desire; 7, change talk—activation; 8, change talk—need; 9, change talk—commitment; 10, sustain talk.

SCRIPT 7.1.   Examples of Focusing and Presenting Options

FOCUSING SCRIPT 1

"[JIC's name], I've really appreciated your honesty in the last few meetings about some of the problems you are facing. Let's take a step back for a moment and figure out together what is the most important issue to focus on first. Based on what you have said, I've created a list of areas we might talk about. Let's review the list, so you can tell me what jumps out as most important. Ready? Here they are: (1) finding work, (2) getting into a program to earn your GED, (3) staying away from your friends who drink, (4) stopping your marijuana use so you can pass your drug tests, and (5) getting your anger under better control. Which one seems to you like the top priority?"

FOCUSING SCRIPT 2

"Hi, [JIC's name], we have about 30 minutes for our meeting today. First, I would like to go over some of the areas of your life we might talk about, and then we can decide together where to go from there. We could talk about work—the kinds of jobs you are most interested in, what you see as options for employment, and resources that might be available to assist you. We could talk about your free time—what you see as the most productive ways to spend your time, and how to structure your daily routines so that you can accomplish your goals. Or we could talk about heroin use—the challenges you face in trying to stay clean, and some ways to make it easier. Which one of those things would you most like to talk about? What would you find helpful?"

FOCUSING SCRIPT 3

"[JIC's name], I have been thinking a lot about your case since we last spoke. I know you are feeling both excited and anxious as you get closer to your release date. Would it be OK if we focused our time today on some of the things that put you most at risk for ending up back in prison? [When they are asked for their permission in this manner, JICs usually say, "Yes."] OK, great. Here are some of the things you mentioned that could be a challenge: hanging out with your old friends; not having a paycheck and being tempted to sell drugs to get money; and living with your brother, who is still using. When you think about it, which one of these areas are you most concerned about?"

SCRIPT 7.2. Focusing on Criminal Risk Domains (to Be Used with Form 7.1)

"The bubbles on this chart contain different life areas that put people at risk for problems with the criminal justice system. If you take a look at the chart, you'll notice that the most common areas people struggle with are drugs and alcohol; having friends who are negative influences and who tend to get in trouble; having too much free time and a lack of structure; family problems; difficulties with work or school; and problems in managing anger. Based on our discussions, I have also written in _____ and _____ [these are any secondary domains you have identified from your case formulation, such as mental health symptoms, physical health conditions, and problematic housing]. Also, there are a few blank bubbles. In these, I would like you to write in some things related to your life that are not included, but that you think are important. [Allow the JIC some time to review the chart and write in additional factors.]. OK, great. When you look at the bubbles, which of these areas are most important for you to work on? [If the JIC chooses multiple areas, keep track of them, and then ask:] If you had to choose one, which one would you say is most important? OK, why did you pick _____?" [Reinforce change talk, and explore how making changes in the life area would be consistent with the JIC's values.]

SCRIPT 7.3. Focusing on Criminogenic Thinking Patterns (to Be Used with Script 7.4)

"[JIC's name], we are all guided by our thinking. As we go through life, we develop rules for how we interpret things, see ourselves, and react to others. With years of repetition, much of our thinking becomes automatic and inflexible, and we become much less aware of how some of our most important thinking patterns guide our everyday decisions. Of course, for all of us, our own thinking seems perfectly normal, because we have repeated many of the same thoughts in our heads for years.

"Unfortunately, some of the ways of thinking that people live by can cause problems for them. Part of our work together will involve creating an awareness of some of the thinking patterns that have developed for you. We will also explore the effect these patterns have had on your life. Only you can decide if a thinking pattern is working or not. Would it be OK if I shared with you one pattern I noticed? [When they are asked for permission in this way, JICs usually say "Yes."] One pattern that came up for you is a tendency to . . ." [Describe a specific thinking pattern, using the language provided from Script 7.4. Use some of the following questions to explore the pattern and elicit change talk.]

"Tell me more about this way of thinking and your tendency to _____."

"How has this way of thinking affected your life overall?"

"Looking back over your life, how has this thinking pattern sometimes worked against you?"

"What kinds of things have you lost in your life when you followed this way of thinking [Ask about areas such as relationships, jobs, money, health, freedom, respect, opportunities]?"

"What will keep happening if you continue to follow this way of thinking?"

"What is at stake if you don't change this way of thinking?"

"How does this way of thinking interfere with your value of _____ [mention a value the client has previously described as important]?"

"What is a new way of thinking that might work better for your life?"

SCRIPT 7.4. Describing Criminogenic Thinking Patterns to JICs (to Be Used with Script 7.3)

The following are suggestions for describing criminogenic thinking patterns to JICs. Try to avoid using the name of a thinking pattern (in bold); instead, highlight the description. The descriptions are meant to be honest, but nonjudgmental. Feel free to adapt these descriptions to emphasize the part of the thinking pattern that fits best for a particular JIC. Use Script 7.3 to introduce the conversation ("One pattern that came up for you is a tendency to . . .").

1. **Identifying with antisocial companions:** " . . . believe that you relate best to others who get into trouble or who have a lifestyle that puts them at risk for getting into trouble."

2. **Disregard for others:** " . . . look out for yourself and not think about how your actions affect others."

3. **Emotionally disengaged:** " . . . not show your emotions, because you think people will take advantage of you or it will make you look weak."

4. **Hostility for criminal justice personnel:** " . . . see all police officers, probation officers, judges, and so forth as enemies."

5. **Grandiosity and entitlement:** " . . . be overly confident; you expect things to go your way and you become angry when they don't."

6. **Power and control:** " . . . want to control other people and situations."

7. **Demand for excitement:** " . . . crave doing risky things just for the rush or the thrill, even though you know there are probably going to be bad consequences later."

8. **Exploit:** " . . . look for shortcuts, and have other people take care of things for you, or to use people for your own advantage."

9. **Hostility for law and order:** " . . . view rules as stupid and believe they don't apply to you."

10. **Justifying and minimizing:** " . . . think that even though something is illegal or harmful to others, you have reasons why it's sometimes OK to do it anyway."

11. **Path of least resistance:** " . . . believe that problems will take care of themselves."

12. **Inability to cope:** " . . . get overwhelmed and frustrated and give up when things get hard."

13. **Underestimating:** " . . . not think through the possible negatives that could result from your decisions, and then they take you by surprise later."

SCRIPT 7.5. Providing Feedback on Standardized Assessments

"[JIC's name], would it be OK if we spent a few minutes going over the scores on some of the paperwork that you completed in our last meeting? Great. This test measures different dimensions of anger. One of these dimensions is the level at which you verbally express your anger to others. The score on this dimension was high for you. You scored at the 96th percentile. This means that you express anger at a level greater than 95% of men your age. You are at the top 4% of scorers in terms of yelling, arguing, or having verbal conflicts with others when you are angry."

Use some of the following questions to explore the area and elicit change talk:

"What do you think?"

"How does this fit with how you see yourself handling your anger?"

"How has being so verbally expressive with your anger influenced your life?"

"Can you give me examples of some of the things you have lost because of your anger reactions [e.g., relationships, jobs, money, health, freedom, respect, opportunities]?"

"How have your anger reactions undermined your value of _____ [mention a value the client has previously described as important]?"

"Where do you see things headed if you do not get a handle on your anger?"

"How might your life be different if you made a change in how you dealt with your anger?"

"Thanks for your willingness to talk with me about this."

FORM 7.1 Life Areas That Put Me at Risk

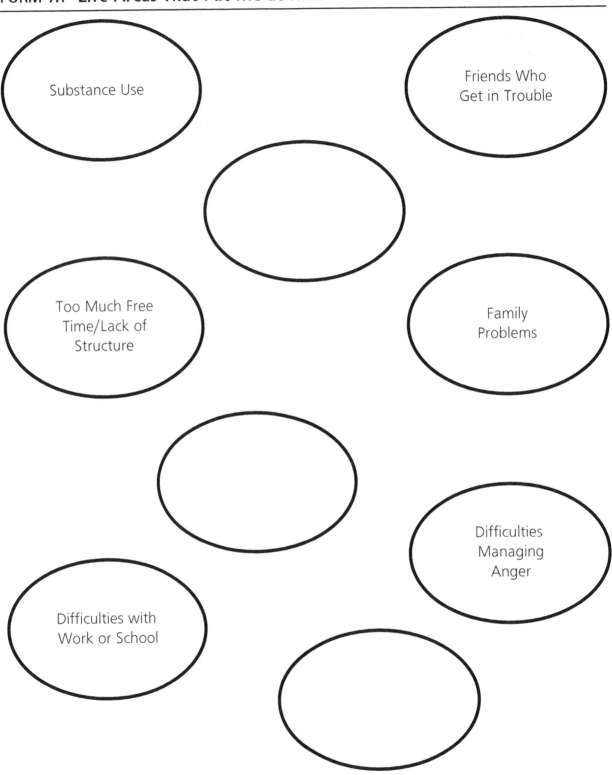

PART IV

DETAILED TREATMENT PLANS FOR CRIMINOGENIC THINKING AND ANTISOCIAL ORIENTATION

CHAPTER 8

Connecting Criminogenic Thinking to Decision Making in Criminal Risk Domains

From her assessment and from her conversations with Hank, it is clear to Brenda that Hank's current antisocial companions constitute a critical life area to target in treatment. She considers this criminal risk domain a treatment priority for multiple reasons: (1) Hank's primary companions engage in a great deal of partying associated with substance use and out-of-control behavior, both of which place him in risky situations; (2) his referring offense and several other incidents that did not result in arrest (but could have) were influenced by his companions; (3) his primary companions appear to possess an antisocial orientation and offer little in the way of prosocial modeling or stability; and (4) in fact, these companions encourage and reinforce some of his criminogenic thinking. Not surprisingly, Hank has a positive regard for his friends. To his credit, though, in an earlier focusing conversation, he has identified them as having a negative influence, in that they sometimes lead him into trouble. He also recognizes that spending time with his current network of friends is unlikely to help him establish a stable career and lifestyle.

Although Brenda and Hank have now reached some tentative agreement on what is relevant and important for improvement, the way forward is still unclear. It is unrealistic to assume that Hank can abruptly cut off all contact with his former friends; changing friends is not easy for anybody. Even if he were to do so, it is equally unrealistic to presume that the next friends he acquires will help him establish a more prosocial lifestyle. In fact, it is much more likely that the old patterns will simply resume with new acquaintances. So for Brenda, the question is, "Now that we've targeted a risk domain for change, how do I intervene?"

COGNITIVE VERSUS BEHAVIORAL COMPONENTS OF CRIMINAL RISK DOMAINS

A criminal risk domain that you and a JIC agree to target in treatment will probably have a cognitive component as well as behavioral components in need of change. The cognitive component encompasses the JIC's criminogenic thinking—most importantly, the client's thoughts related to decision making in the targeted risk domain. The behavioral components encompass behavior patterns, modeling, and/or situational reinforcement contingencies related to that risk domain.

The relative importance of the cognitive versus behavioral components will differ among JICs. For example, two probationers may both be assessed as "ranking high" or "in need of change" on substance abuse/misuse due to their occasional Ecstasy use, but *how* their use is related to their risk for a probation violation may be very different. For one JIC, the most important facet of the risk domain (substance abuse/misuse) may be primarily cognitive and connected with his incorrect belief that because he is not on probation for a drug charge, he could not possibly get a probation violation for positive drug tests. For another JIC, the cognitive component may be relatively unimportant; in fact, her thinking may be quite rational and free of distortion, and she may think of her Ecstasy use as self-destructive in her current situation. For her, the most salient aspect of the risk factor may be primarily contextual, in that she may live and work within a social network in which Ecstasy use is fairly normative, opportunities to obtain the drug are plentiful, and avoiding the club drug culture is difficult.

The chapters in Part IV of the book (this chapter and Chapter 9) are about the cognitive component; interventions that target behavioral components are discussed in Part V (Chapters 10, 11, and 12). Working with JICs on the cognitive component of the relevant risk domains of their lives involves changing the criminogenic thinking that underlies their decision making, and possibly a more general antisocial orientation. In this chapter and in Chapter 9, we review *connecting, monitoring,* and *restructuring* interventions to aid in that process. Connecting interventions help JICs make connections between their criminogenic thinking and their antisocial decision making. Monitoring interventions increase clients' awareness of their criminogenic thinking between sessions, and of the ways in which such thinking immediately influences their decisions. Restructuring interventions assist JICs in replacing their criminogenic thinking with thinking patterns and thoughts likely to lead to better outcomes.

LEVELS OF CRIMINOGENIC THINKING

As discussed in Chapter 2, criminogenic thinking is relevant at all three levels of cognition and belief (schemas, intermediate beliefs, and automatic thoughts). However, this treatment planner focuses on intermediate beliefs and automatic thoughts, due to their greater accessibility (as compared to schemas) and to the time-limited nature of court-mandated and correctional treatment. At the intermediate level of belief, what we refer to as *criminogenic thinking patterns* influence how JICs think, feel, and behave across different life areas, and produce the automatic *criminogenic thoughts* that arise in response to specific situations. For example, the criminogenic thinking pattern of exploit (the belief in manipulating situations/relationships for personal gain) may negatively affect multiple areas of JICs' lives by producing criminogenic thoughts that interfere with family and romantic relationships, frustrate the persons' probation officers, and derail the JICs from obtaining stable employment. The JICs may avoid making meaningful strides toward independence and instead exploit the generosity (e.g., sofa, finances) and patience of family members (e.g., "I don't need to look for my own place. My family should support me till I'm back on my feet"). The clients may view their probation officers as temp-agency employees who can be exchanged if unsatisfactory (e.g., "If my probation officer doesn't let me go out of state, I'll just ask to be transferred to another officer until I get one who will"). And they may think of employment as a backup plan rather than a necessity (e.g., "I'm going to see if I can hustle a disability claim like my friend did").

While treatment for traditional mental health problems often involves helping clients connect relevant intermediate beliefs and automatic thoughts with their emotional responses, our focus with JICs is on helping them connect their criminogenic thinking with their *decision making in relevant criminal risk domains*. This process involves (1) discussions connecting a specific criminogenic thought with a particular decision within a specific risk domain, and (2) tracing the impact of a more general criminogenic thinking pattern to decisions across multiple criminal risk domains (see Figure 8.1). We review strategies for both kinds of discussions in this chapter. As discussions about thinking unfold, you will notice that the OARS skills and evoking skills reviewed in previous chapters are used to elicit and reinforce healthier thoughts and thinking patterns.

In order to be successful in targeting criminogenic thinking, it is helpful to recognize how underlying thinking patterns are related to criminogenic thoughts. As noted in Chapter 2, the empirical literature that has developed on the assessment of criminal thinking provides a useful road map for some of the most common criminal thinking patterns (intermediate beliefs). Criminogenic thinking patterns can be identified through the use of criminal thinking instruments (see Appendix A for several examples) or through an assessment interview (Chapter 5), or they can be inferred through ongoing conversations with JICs. Table 8.1 expands upon the list of criminogenic thinking patterns presented in Chapters 2 and 5, and provides examples of criminogenic thoughts related to each thinking pattern.

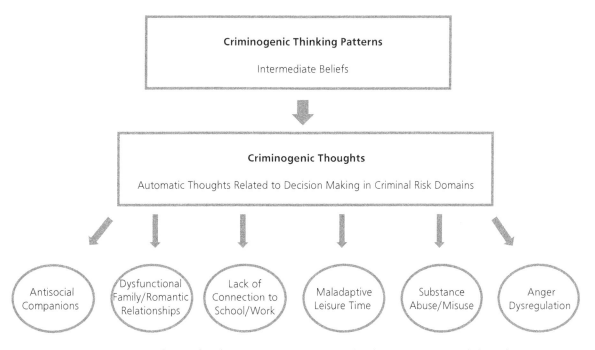

FIGURE 8.1. Relationship between criminogenic thinking patterns and thoughts.

TABLE 8.1. Criminogenic Thinking Patterns and Criminogenic Thoughts

Criminogenic thinking pattern	Description of pattern	Sample criminogenic thoughts
	Thinking patterns related to self and others	
Identifying with antisocial companions	Viewing self as being similar to, and relating best to, antisocial peers; seeing relationships with prosocial peers as unimportant	"I don't have anything in common with people who live a straight life." "I just can't say no when those guys come around to pick me up. We've been through so much together."
Disregard for others	Belief that the needs/rights of others are unimportant; antipathy/hostility to others; lack of empathy and remorse for hurting others	"There's no point worrying about people you hurt." "I don't give a shit about anyone else. Only the strong survive, so I have to look out for myself."
Emotionally disengaged	Belief that avoiding intimacy and vulnerability is good; lack of trust; fears about being taken advantage of	"I don't talk about personal issues. If I open up to someone, they will take advantage of me." "I don't let anyone know what's going on with me, unless I'm pissed."
Hostility for criminal justice personnel	Adversarial and suspicious attitude toward police, lawyers, judges, and so forth	"The cops are the real criminals." "Probation officers just want to violate you. That's why they always ask about your address—so they know where to find you when they want to arrest you."
Grandiosity and entitlement	Inflated beliefs about oneself; belief that one is deserving of special treatment	"I won't go to treatment unless you can find a facilitator smarter than me." "I'm not going to look for a job. Someone will see my talent and find me."
Power and control	Seeking dominance over others; seeking to control the behavior of others	"Nobody can tell me what to do. I tell other people what to do." "A family is not a democracy. I am the one who makes the decisions. That's how it is. As long as she cooks what I want, *lays* me when I want, and respects my authority, we won't have any problems."

Thinking patterns related to interacting with the environment

Demand for excitement	Belief that life should be focused on thrill seeking and risk taking; lack of tolerance for boredom	"There is no better feeling than the rush I get when stealing." "I felt happiest when I was on the run. It was a rush." "I enjoy taking risks. I've never backed down from one."
Exploit	General intent to manipulate situations or relationships for personal gain when given the opportunity	"Why should I pay child support? She has a rich boyfriend who can support my kid." "I don't have to come to your group program all the time. You said I can miss three sessions and still get the certificate."
Hostility for law and order	Animosity toward rules, regulations, and laws	"Laws are there to hurt you, not help you." "That's the way I am. I make my own rules."
Justifying and minimizing	Justification, rationalization, and minimization of harmful behaviors	"If I don't sell drugs in my neighborhood, somebody else will." "What I do isn't as bad as what the 'fat cats' on Wall Street get away with every day."
Path of least resistance	"Easiest way" approach to problem solving; a "no worries," "no plan needed," and "in the moment" style of life	"Everything will take care of itself." "I attended the first session and didn't see anything in the program that could possibly help me. I'll talk to the judge about getting the referral dropped."
Inability to cope	Giving up in the face of adversity; low frustration tolerance	"When I don't understand things, I give up." "All these programs and appointments you're making me do are stressing me out. I'd rather be back in jail."
Underestimating	Underrating the negative consequences of risky behaviors; overconfidence in decision-making skills	"What's the worst thing that could happen to me? Nothing!" "I won't go to jail for selling. I know all my clients."

CONNECTING CRIMINOGENIC *THOUGHTS* AND DECISIONS *WITHIN* CRIMINAL RISK DOMAINS

Connecting discussions generally explore two questions:

1. What is it about the JIC's thoughts in a particular criminal risk domain that lead to poor decisions?
2. How are the JIC's thoughts different when better decisions are made in this risk domain?

The answers to both questions are important, but for different reasons. The first question addresses the criminogenic thinking that we would like to see extinguished, while the second addresses the thinking we would like to see reliably installed in its place.

1. *What is it about the JIC's thoughts in this particular risk domain that lead to poor decisions?* As noted above, general functioning within criminal risk domains has a cognitive component as well as behavioral components, and these components will differ from JIC to JIC. Likewise, the criminogenic thoughts relevant to decision making in a given risk area will differ across JICs. For example, Hank and Jackie share a common risk area—antisocial companions. However, the way in which their criminogenic thoughts about their companions have influenced their poor decisions is strikingly different.

Hank, for example, got involved in a bar fight that could be more accurately classified as "companion-related" than "alcohol-related." He was not intoxicated and was just approaching the bar when another patron bumped into him and spilled portions of two drinks on Hank's pants. Hank was with two friends who, he knew, would "go nuts if I went off on the guy and made a scene . . . they would love it . . . high fives, free drinks." Anticipating their positive reaction to his "making a scene," and wondering about the snide comments he would get if he did nothing, Hank pushed and then punched the patron—who had, even in Hank's opinion, accidentally knocked into him. Yet Hank acknowledged that if he had not been with those friends, he would have acted differently: He would have interpreted the patron's drink spilling as an accident, accepted his apology, avoided aggressive action, and thought no more of it. Thus the trajectory of Hank's decision making was altered by the presence of his antisocial companions and his interpretation of *what his friends would think.* In sum, Hank's thoughts tipped his behavior in an aggressive direction.

In Jackie's case, she had been arrested with two older male friends from work when they were probing the doors of cars at an auto dealership late at night, hoping to find one that was unlocked. Unlike Hank, Jackie's behavior with these friends was not particularly influenced by a concern about what they would think if she did not acquiesce to their plans; nor was she especially concerned with pleasing them. When her friends suggested they go to the car dealership, Jackie thought that "it sounded like something kind of fun and exciting to do after a boring day at the car wash," and "it's not like we were looking to hurt anybody; it would just be fun to get into a car." Thus Jackie's friends suggested antisocial plans that were already appealing to her and that she was able to justify easily.

2. *How are the JIC's thoughts different when better decisions are made in this risk domain?* Although JICs may periodically make poor decisions, they do not *always* make poor decisions.

For instance, even a high-risk male JIC on probation who chronically spends time with criminal companions, violates his curfew, and smokes marijuana will sometimes make positive choices in these risk domains: He will sometimes avoid the negative influence of friends, understand the reasons and importance of abiding by his court-ordered curfew, and decline an offer to smoke pot. He thinks differently on some occasions, and we want to bring his attention to this different thought process.

For example, a few days after Jackie was arrested with her friends from the car wash, they called to see if she wanted to "drive around and have some beers." Although she was tempted at first, because "it was late and my son was in bed" and "the court would probably never know," she ended up declining the offer; her thoughts were that "nothing good can come of this" and "if the court does find out I left my son alone and I'm with them, that could lead to problems." We want JICs to make connections between their thoughts and productive and prosocial decision making, and to determine how these thoughts differ from their thoughts when they make destructive choices. These prosocial connections are then strengthened through the monitoring and restructuring activities described in Chapter 9.

Risks–Thoughts–Decisions Sequences

A structured connecting conversation about antisocial companions is provided below, and a sample script for this risk domain is provided at the end of this chapter (Script 8.1). We call this type of conversation a *risks–thoughts–decisions* (RTD) sequence. RTD sequences can be applied to the modifiable criminal risk domains. Additional scripts (Scripts 8.2–8.6) for sequences focused on the other remaining criminal risk domains can also be found at the end of this chapter.

Each RTD sequence should be applied uniquely to JICs that require attention in that criminal risk domain. For example, RTD–Leisure is best suited for JICs who struggle with constructive uses of free time. Alternatively, a JIC with vocational challenges should have his or her attention drawn to thoughts connected with prior job failures and successes (i.e., RTD–Work/School). The other scripts describe difficulties in family/romantic interactions (RTD–Family/Romantic), substance use (RTD–Substance Misuse), and dysregulated anger (RTD–Anger).

Although the focus of each RTD sequence is different, the underlying structure is similar. Each sequence is divided into two sections. The goal of the first section is to help JICs make connections between their thoughts and their antisocial decision making in a specific criminal risk domain. As noted earlier, the strength of these connections will vary from JIC to JIC; some may be quite automatic, long-standing, and ingrained, whereas others may be more malleable. The goal of the second section is to help JICs make connections between their thoughts and productive or prosocial decision making in the same risk domain. For some JICs, these connections may be less automatic, but are of significant importance in the change process. All of the sequences close with a summary highlighting differences in the thinking related to antisocial versus prosocial decision making, and a question for evoking change talk pertaining to better decisions in the future.

The recommendations that follow for conducting the RTD–Companions sequence are applicable to all RTD sequences. The beginning steps of each sequence are aimed at getting the JIC to talk about a specific criminal risk domain and a specific antisocial decision related to that area. If the JIC provides an example from the distant past, probe for something more current; in general, the more recent the example, the better. Script 8.1 provides a foundation for the conversation, but you may need to add follow-up questions, depending upon the degree of detail in the JIC's narration.

Once the JIC has presented a clear description of the circumstances surrounding the decision (e.g., what happened before, during, and after), attention shifts to the criminogenic thought that *preceded* the antisocial decision. Although questions that elicit thoughts can be very straightforward (e.g., "What were you telling yourself when . . . ?" or "What was going through your mind when . . . ?"), sometimes multiple attempts will be necessary to reveal key thoughts.

You may encounter several common obstacles when eliciting thoughts. The first is that JICs may state or describe what they *felt* (e.g., "I was really furious") rather than what they *thought* (e.g., "He shouldn't have talked about me behind my back"). In other words, they often confuse emotion with cognition. When this obstacle emerges, resist the temptation to move on to the next step. The JIC's emotional response to the situation can be acknowledged, but it is critical to be persistent in getting to the thoughts: For instance, "It sounds like you were feeling angry at the time. Feelings and thinking are two different things, though, so let's go back to your thoughts rather than your feelings. What was going through your mind before you acted?"

A second obstacle is that JICs may provide what they thought *after* their decision making rather than *before*. Thoughts that follow decisions usually take the form of regrets (e.g., "It was totally stupid what I did"), minimizations (e.g., "In looking back, it's not a big deal; nobody got seriously hurt"), and justifications (e.g., "I had no choice; I had to stick up for myself"). If you elicit thoughts that follow a decision, it is important to keep reframing questions until the JIC identifies his or her thoughts before the destructive decision was made. As noted in Chapter 2, the intent is to identify those "green light" moments when JICs give themselves permission to do something risky or self-defeating. For example, if the JIC expresses regret ("It was totally stupid what I did"), you might say, "So afterward, you thought you made the wrong decision, but what were you telling yourself beforehand?" A good way of making sure you have accurately captured the JIC's thoughts is to reflect them back (e.g., "It sounds like you were thinking you deserved a little fun and no one would know"). This also encourages the JIC to elaborate and provide more detail into his or her thought process at the time.

After a criminogenic thought is connected to a poor decision, each RTD sequence shifts to a search for a recent time when a prosocial (or at least not harmful) decision was made in relation to the same criminal risk domain, and to the identification of the thoughts that preceded the healthier decision. The same recommendations reviewed earlier apply to this stage of the sequence: Recent decisions are preferable to older ones; be persistent in capturing the JIC's thoughts rather than feelings; and help the JIC to identify thoughts prior to, rather than after, decisions have been made.

Each sequence is closed by summarizing for the JIC the key differences in the thoughts that were present prior to prosocial versus antisocial decisions and reinforcing better decisions in the future. This summary provides a natural transition to the monitoring and restructuring strategies discussed in Chapter 9. Brenda's RTD–Companions sequence with Hank provides an example of how these RTD sequences operate.

BRENDA: So it looks like we agree that it makes sense to spend some time focusing on the people you spend time with, because they may be having a negative influence on you by tempting you to do things that could get you into trouble with the criminal justice system. Tell me about a specific friend or acquaintance of yours who tends to get in trouble with the law, or who you think is probably a bad influence on you in some ways.

HANK: Just one? I can think of several.

BRENDA: Let's focus on just one or two. How about the one you have spent the most time with over the past couple of months?

HANK: OK. That would be Brendan and Jason. They're brothers. You can't be with one without the other.

BRENDA: What makes them a bad influence or seems to lead to trouble?

HANK: They're a little older than me. I've always kind of looked up to them and done things that I thought they would think were cool. They always seem to have something stupid going on, and I get caught up in that.

BRENDA: What's hard about avoiding their influence?

HANK: I've known them since middle school. We have a lot of history together.

BRENDA: And you want them to like you, even if it means . . .

HANK: I do things when I'm with them that when I look back, I know I shouldn't have done.

BRENDA: Give me an example of something you did with them recently that you think was probably a mistake.

HANK: I got into some trouble at this bar about a month ago. They were with me. We were walking up to the bar area and it was crowded, and this guy spilled his drinks and part of it got on me, and I ended up walloping him before the bouncers kicked us out.

BRENDA: What was the role of those brothers in this? How do they fit?

HANK: Right after the spill, they were, like, "Are you going to let him play you like that? What are you going to do about this? Show him what happens." Shouting stupid stuff like that from the sidelines, and I let it get to me, and took it to the next level.

BRENDA: What were you telling yourself before you got physical with the guy?

HANK: I was thinking, "These guys will go nuts if I go off on this guy and make a scene . . . they will love it . . . high fives, free drinks. They'll eat it up. They love this kind of stuff."

BRENDA: So, your actions were influenced by how you *thought* they would react?

HANK: Right. They weren't involved in the fight, but I did it because of them. If they hadn't been there, I would have accepted his apology, said, "No harm done," and gone about my business. But because they were there, saying those things, it went the other direction.

BRENDA: Give me an example of a recent time when you were able to avoid their influence and get out of a potentially bad situation with them.

HANK: A little while ago, they were telling me about this summer camp that was abandoned during the winter, and they wanted me to come with them to check it out and see what was there, if there was anything worth taking. I told them to go without me. There was no way I was getting involved in that.

BRENDA: What was going through your mind when you didn't go along with them?

HANK: I know where this leads, and I don't do jail any more, that's it. That's not my lifestyle.

BRENDA: So you can see yourself having a different lifestyle from them.

HANK: They are still doing things that are going to put them in jail, and I'm not about that any more.

BRENDA: So it sounds like when you're with Brendan and Jason, and you're thinking about making them happy or doing things you know they will like, it ends up in trouble, but when you are able to think about what's right for you, you end up making better choices. How can you continue to make better decisions when it comes to dealing with Brendan and Jason?

CONNECTING CRIMINOGENIC *THINKING PATTERNS* AND DECISIONS *ACROSS* CRIMINAL RISK DOMAINS

A connecting discussion that addresses a criminogenic thinking pattern (intermediate belief) is somewhat more complex than the sequences introduced above, because it involves analyzing the impact of a thinking pattern across two or more criminal risk domains. It also elicits the (automatic) criminogenic thoughts produced by that pattern. This type of discussion should help answer two important questions:

1. In what risk domains does this thinking pattern show up?
2. What criminogenic thoughts does it produce that precede antisocial decisions?

Script 8.7 at the end of this chapter provides guidelines for a connecting conversation known as the *thinking pattern impact* (TPI) analysis. The analysis begins with a guided discussion of the negative impact a thinking pattern has on decision making in two or more criminal risk domains. In the latter portion of the TPI, the discussion flows into an exploration of times when the JIC was able to "catch" him- or herself before acting on the pattern and made more constructive decisions, due to the ability to engage in healthier thinking.

We recommend that when you begin the TPI analysis, you choose just one criminogenic thinking pattern to discuss with the JIC. If there are multiple relevant patterns, address them in future sessions, rather than risk overwhelming the client with too much information. When you are describing the thinking pattern at the beginning of the analysis, remember to use the non-judgmental language described in Chapter 7 (see Script 7.4). For example, if you're targeting the criminogenic thinking pattern of justifying, describe it like this: "You have a tendency to think that even though something is illegal or harmful to others, you have reasons why it's sometimes OK to do it anyway," rather than "You have a tendency to make a lot of excuses for your criminal behavior."

As in the guidelines for RTD sequences, when you are eliciting an example of antisocial decision making, aim for a recent incident. A JIC who provides an example from the distant past should be encouraged to search for one that occurred more recently. Follow-up questions about the incident may be necessary, depending upon the degree of detail provided by the JIC.

Once the JIC has presented a clear narrative of the circumstances surrounding the decision (what happened before, during, and after), it's time to elicit the criminogenic *thoughts* that sprang from the criminogenic thinking pattern. As noted earlier, you will need to be persistent in the face of JICs who describe feelings rather than thoughts, or who describe their thinking *after* rather than *before* the antisocial decision. One way to help make sure that the relevant criminogenic thinking pattern has been captured is to reflect it back. This also heightens a JIC's awareness of the impact of the criminogenic thinking pattern on overall decision making (e.g., "Sounds like you didn't want to share your feelings with Simona, because it might have made you look weak"—emotionally disengaged).

After you have explored an example of the criminogenic thinking pattern's impact on one area of the JIC's life, search for *another* instance of the pattern in a *different* criminal risk domain. For example, if the JIC provided an example that did not relate to the criminal justice system, ask about the impact of the thinking pattern on the client's involvement with the law. If the JIC provided an example of the pattern's impact on substance use, ask about its impact on relationships with family or on the ability to find or maintain work. The goal is not to exhaustively explore every single instance of the thinking pattern's impact across the JIC's life; doing that could be demoralizing. Rather, try to identify two or three different risk domains in which the thinking pattern has emerged. The presence of the thinking pattern across a wider range of risk domains can always be revisited in a future session. Discussions about the impact of criminogenic thinking patterns on JICs' lives are ongoing in treatment and are not single-session endeavors.

The latter portion of the TPI analysis entails a search for a time (or times) when the JIC was able to avoid the influence of the thinking pattern. These are times when the client almost acted on it, but was able to exercise self-restraint and make a better decision. Although a criminogenic thinking pattern may often exert its influence, this is not always the case, and it is important to search for exceptions—those occasions when better decisions are made. There are times when the JIC "talks back" to the criminogenic voice, or sees things from a different perspective and consequently makes better choices. Repeat this process to probe for more than one example across risk domains when appropriate. Close the TPI analysis with a summary of the differences in how the JIC thinks and acts when the thinking pattern is allowed to predominate, versus when the client is able to avoid its influence. The summary should provide a natural transition to the monitoring and restructuring interventions discussed in the next chapter.

KEY POINTS

- *Criminogenic thinking patterns* are thoughts that influence how JICs think, feel, and behave across different life areas. *Criminogenic thoughts* are automatic-like thoughts that emerge during decisions in specific situations.

- Connecting discussions help JICs make connections between their criminogenic thinking and antisocial decision making. Such discussions are the first step in addressing the cognitive component operating within a criminal risk domain.

- *Risks–thoughts–decisions* (RTD) sequences are structured discussions that help connect criminogenic *thoughts* and decisions *within* a criminal risk domain. RTD sequences can be applied to the full range of criminal risk domains and identify thoughts that precede both poor and better decisions.

- The *thinking pattern impact* (TPI) analysis involves analyzing the impact of a criminogenic thinking pattern across two or more criminal risk domains.

- Conversations about criminogenic thinking are most effective when they are about recent incidents from the JIC's life, identify specific thoughts (rather than feelings), and elicit thoughts that precede (rather than follow) antisocial decisions.

SCRIPT 8.1. RTD–Companions Sequence

Step 1: Explore the high-risk FRIEND and the role the friend plays in high-risk behavior.

"Looking back over the past year, tell me about a friend or acquaintance of yours who tends to get in trouble with the law, or who you think is probably a bad influence on you in some ways."

"What is about this person that makes him [her] a bad influence or seems to lead to trouble?"

"What makes it hard to avoid spending time with him [her]?"

Step 2: Explore the risky DECISIONS connected with this person.

"Give me an example of some of the trouble you have gotten into with this person," or "Give me an example of something you did with this person that you think was probably bad for you, or self-defeating."

Step 3: Explore the THOUGHTS preceding the risky decisions related to this person.

"What were you thinking about or telling yourself when you agreed to [name of incident]?" or "What was going through your mind when you went along with [name of person]?"

Step 4: Explore a better DECISION related to avoiding this person's influence.

"Give me an example of a time when you were able to avoid this person's influence and get out of a potentially bad situation with him [her]."

Step 5: Explore the THOUGHTS preceding the better decision.

"What was going through your mind when you didn't go along with [name of person]?" or "How was your thinking different when you [name of positive incident]?"

Step 6: Summarize the contrast in THINKING that leads to the two types of decisions.

"So, to sum up the connection between [name of person] and bad outcomes, it sounds like you're thinking [reflection of JIC's negative thought], while the times you've made better decisions, your thinking was more like [reflection of JIC's positive thought]."

Step 7: Evoke change talk.

"How can you continue to make better decisions when it comes to _____ [name of person]?"

SCRIPT 8.2. RTD–Leisure Sequence

Step 1: Explore the connection between LEISURE and risk.

"When you have free time on your hands, how is that sometimes risky for you?"

Step 2: Explore the DECISION connected to a risky activity.

"Tell me a specific time when you were bored or had nothing to do and it led to a bad decision." [Make sure you are clear on the link between the JIC's leisure and how it increases risk before moving to Step 3.]

Step 3: Explore the THOUGHTS preceding the risky activity.

"At the time when you made the bad decision, what was going through your mind?"

Step 4: Explore the DECISION connected to a more productive activity.

"Now tell me about a time when you handled your boredom or downtime in a way that didn't turn out badly."

Step 5: Explore the THOUGHTS preceding the more productive activity.

"What was going through your mind when you [name of productive activity]?"

Step 6: Summarize the contrast in THINKING that leads to the two types of decisions.

"So, on the one hand, when you're bored or have nothing to do and think [reflection of JIC's negative thought], it leads to [name of risky activity]; on the other hand, when you're in that situation and think [reflection of JIC's positive thought], it leads to [name of productive activity]."

Step 7: Evoke change talk.

"How can you continue to make better decisions when it comes to your free time?"

SCRIPT 8.3. RTD–Family/Romantic Sequence

Step 1: Explore the high-risk RELATIONSHIP and the role it played in the JIC's recent offense(s).

"Tell me about a person in your family, or a person you are in a romantic relationship with, who has led you to get in trouble with the law."

"How has the relationship with this person caused problems for you?"

"What is about the relationship between the two of you that leads to problems with the court?"

Step 2: Explore a bad DECISION connected to this relationship.

"Give me an example of a time when something about this relationship resulted in your making a bad decision."

Step 3: Explore the THINKING connected to the bad DECISION.

"What was going through your mind right before you [describe the incident]?" [Make sure you capture the thinking that led to the specific behavior resulting in the incident.]

Step 4: Explore a better DECISION connected to this relationship.

"Now tell me about a time in this relationship when you almost made a bad decision, but ended up choosing something better."

Step 5: Explore the THINKING connected to the better DECISION.

"What were you telling yourself right before you decided to [describe the better behavior the JIC engaged in]?"

Step 6: Summarize the contrast in THINKING that leads to the two types of paths.

"So when you're thinking [reflection of JIC's negative thought], it leads to bad stuff like [describe the incident]; on the other hand, when you're able to think [reflection of JIC's positive thought], it leads to a better outcome like [describe the better behavior]."

Step 7: Evoke change talk.

"How can you continue to make better decisions when it comes this relationship?"

SCRIPT 8.4. RTD–Substance Misuse Sequence

Step 1: Set the agenda and explore the DECISION to engage in the substance use.

> "It has come to my attention that you have been using [insert alcohol or drugs, depending on the client's profile of use]. I would like to work on this with you."

> Or, "Can you tell me about a recent time you used [insert alcohol or drugs, depending on the client's profile of use]? Tell me about what happened. I'd like to hear what happened before, during, and after the use."

Step 2: Explore the THOUGHTS preceding the substance use.

> "What thoughts were going through your mind right before you used that time?"

Step 3: Explore a recent DECISION in which desire/opportunity for substance use was handled productively.

> "Now tell me about a time recently when you were in a very similar situation like we just discussed, but when you chose not to use."

Step 4: Explore the THOUGHTS preceding the productive decision.

> "So when you had this opportunity and didn't use, what was going through your mind? What were you thinking?"

Step 5: Summarize the contrast in THINKING that leads to the two types of decisions.

> "So, on the one hand, when you're in this mode of thinking [reflection of JIC's negative thought], it leads to use; on the other hand, when you're thinking [reflection of JIC's positive thought], it leads to not using."

Step 6: Evoke change talk.

> "How can you strengthen better decisions around this issue in the future?"

SCRIPT 8.5. RTD–Work/School Sequence

Step 1: Explore positive and negative WORK HISTORY. [Throughout this script, substitute school for work/job(s) if appropriate.]

"Tell me about a few examples where jobs went well. What were some of the best jobs you've had?"

"Tell me about a few work examples where things went badly."

"What are some of the problems you've had at work that led to you quit or get fired?" [Discuss until you've established any patterns connected to job or school failure.]

Step 2: Explore the THINKING connected with job success and failure.

[Success] "In the jobs that were going well, how were you thinking about the job on a day-to-day basis?"

[Failure] "When you worked at the [name of failed job] and it didn't go well, how were you thinking about the job on a day-to-day basis?" [Repeat for each failure discussed in Step 1.]

Step 3: Summarize the THINKING associated with job failure.

"So it looks like when things don't go well at work, you're thinking [reflection of JIC's negative thought]."

Step 4: Summarize the THINKING associated with job success (if it exists).

"So it looks like when things go well with work, you're thinking [reflection of JIC's positive thought]."

Step 5: Evoke change talk.

"In the future, how can you strengthen better thinking when it comes to work?"

SCRIPT 8.6. RTD–Anger Sequence

Step 1: Explore the connection between ANGER reactions and risk.

"Everyone gets angry from time to time. Tell me about when you get angry. How is that sometimes risky for you?"

[If necessary, follow up with:] "Tell me about one thing you've done recently when you became angry that could potentially lead to a problem with the criminal justice system." [Make sure you are clear on the link between the JIC's anger and how it increases risk before moving to Step 2.]

Step 2: Explore a recent bad DECISION connected with angry feelings.

"Tell me a specific time when you were angry and ended up doing something you later regretted." [Look for examples of aggressive behavior, negative verbalizations, substance use, police involvement, damaged relationships; get sufficient detail.]

Step 3: Explore the THOUGHTS preceding the anger-related behavior.

"At the time when you made the decision to [describe anger-related behavior], what was going through your mind? These thoughts might be very quick and automatic. Try and remember what you were telling yourself right before you [describe anger-related behavior]."

Step 4: Explore a recent better DECISION connected with angry feelings.

"Now tell me about a time recently when you handled your anger in a way that didn't turn out badly."

Step 5: Explore the THOUGHTS preceding the more positive or productive behavior.

"Even though you were angry, what was going through your mind when you [describe more positive or productive behavior]?"

Step 6: Summarize the contrast in THINKING that leads to the two types of decisions.

"So, on the one hand, when you're angry and think [reflection of JIC's negative thought], it leads to [name of regrettable behavior]; on the other hand, when you're angry and think [reflection of JIC's positive thought], it leads to [name of more positive or productive behavior]."

Step 7: Evoke change talk.

"In those moments when you become angry in the future, how can you strengthen the thinking that leads to better ways of reacting?"

SCRIPT 8.7. TPI Analysis

Step 1: Introduce a criminogenic thinking pattern, and probe for a specific instance of its impact on decision making.

> "Last time we met, one of the things we talked about was how you have a tendency to [insert description of criminogenic thinking pattern from Script 7.4]. I'd like to take that discussion a step further today and explore how this pattern has affected decisions across different areas of your life. Tell me about a recent time when you acted on this pattern, and it led to a poor decision or some trouble."

Step 2: Explore the specific thought connected with the incident.

> "What specifically were you thinking or telling yourself before you [describe the negative decision connected with the incident]?"

> "So it sounds like you were thinking [reflection of the JIC's thoughts at the time]."

Step 3: Explore the impact of the thinking in a different criminal risk domain.

> "Tell me about a recent time when you acted on this pattern and it led to a poor decision or some trouble with [name(s) of one or two other criminal risk domains that you think are relevant]."

Step 4: Explore the specific thought connected with the incident.

> "What specifically were you thinking or telling yourself before you [describe the negative decision connected with this incident]?"

> "So it sounds like you were thinking [reflection of the JIC's thoughts at the time]."

Step 5: Explore a time when the JIC was about to act on the pattern, but was able to "catch" him- or herself and make a better choice.

> "Now I'd like you to tell me about a recent time when you almost acted on this pattern, but were able to 'catch' yourself and make a better decision. That is, tell me about a time when this pattern almost influenced you, but you were able to think differently about a situation instead."

(continued)

Step 6: Explore the thoughts that emerged before the better decision.

> "What specifically were you thinking or telling yourself before you [describe the positive decision connected with the incident]?"

> "So it sounds like you were thinking [reflection of the JIC's thoughts at the time]."

Step 7: End the interaction with a summary that contrasts the decisions made when the JIC allowed the criminogenic thinking pattern to influence his or her behavior with the decisions made when he or she was able to think differently and not be influenced by this thinking pattern.

> "So, to sum up the connection between [name of criminogenic thinking pattern] and bad outcomes, it sounds like you're thinking [reflection of JIC's negative thoughts], while the times you've made better decisions, your thinking was more like [reflection of JIC's positive thoughts]. How can you strengthen the better thinking in the future?"

CHAPTER 9

Monitoring and Restructuring Criminogenic Thinking

We hope that the connecting sequences presented in Chapter 8 (the RTD sequences and the TPI analysis) have provided you with strategies to (1) heighten JICs' awareness of the link between criminogenic thoughts/thinking patterns and antisocial decisions; (2) help them recognize the thinking that produces more productive and prosocial decisions; and (3) enhance their motivation to challenge the influence of criminogenic thinking and embrace more prosocial thinking. The summaries that close the connecting sequences provide a natural transition to assigning JICs homework to monitor their criminogenic thoughts and thinking patterns.

MONITORING

Monitoring assignments serve the same purpose for JICs as for clients with mental health problems: They allow skill development to extend beyond treatment sessions into day-to-day life. In other words, such assignments provide in-the-moment opportunities for JICs to see how their thinking is linked to their behavior, as well as opportunities to practice alternative ways of thinking. The only significant difference between monitoring assignments for traditional mental health clients and those for JICs is the nature of the thinking that gets monitored. Whereas clients with depressive and anxiety disorders may be asked to monitor negative and anxious thoughts associated with changes in emotion, JICs are asked to monitor the criminogenic thoughts and thinking patterns associated with criminal conduct.

The Thinking Helpsheet, provided at the end of this chapter (Form 9.1), allows JICs to self-monitor their criminogenic thinking—both specific criminogenic thoughts and thinking patterns. This helpsheet has five sections (also referred to here as boxes). In the first section, Thought/Thinking Pattern, the practitioner writes down the specific thought or criminogenic thinking pattern being addressed. In the second box, Situation, the JIC relates details about the circumstances in which the thought or thinking pattern emerged. The third box, Immediate Thinking, is for the initial thoughts the JIC was aware of during the situation. In the Decision and Outcome section, the client records the actions and behavioral outcomes that occurred. Finally, the Better Thinking box is reserved for describing alternative thinking that could result in better decisions and outcomes.

It is best to use the Thinking Helpsheet after there is clarity regarding which thoughts or thinking patterns should be targeted. Conducting a thorough assessment and several connecting sequences will be particularly useful in this regard. The thoughts and thinking patterns discussed in the connecting sequences will most often become the targets for monitoring on the helpsheet.

Assigning the Thinking Helpsheet

To get started, in the top box of the Thinking Helpsheet, write an example of a criminogenic thought or criminogenic thinking pattern you want the JIC to monitor. For example, if you are having the JIC monitor a criminogenic thought, such as one that has come up in a connecting sequence, write in the thought (e.g., "I should act in ways that make my friends happy, even when I know it's destructive"). If you want the JIC to monitor a criminogenic thinking pattern, such as exploit, write down a description of the pattern in nonjudgmental language (see Chapter 7, Script 7.4): "A tendency to look for shortcuts, to have other people take care of things for you, or to use people for your own advantage."

The remainder of the Thinking Helpsheet is completed by the JIC, as thoughts or thinking patterns emerge during the days between sessions. It is important to instruct the JIC to use the helpsheet regularly, such as during a specific time each day, to reflect on any events that may be applicable to the thinking being monitored. In the Situation box, the incident in which the thought or thinking pattern emerged is briefly described; phrases capturing the basics of the situation (who, what, where, when) are fine. In the Immediate Thinking box, the JIC is asked to capture as accurately as possible his or her thinking during the situation. In the Decision and Outcome box, the JIC records what he or she did in response to the thought. Such actions might be self-defeating or destructive (the JIC acted on the thinking) or positive (the JIC did not act on the thinking). Finally, in the Better Thinking box, an alternative way of thinking is formulated that could have led to a positive outcome. Completing helpsheets provides a unique opportunity for JICs to examine the nature of their thinking and practice countering criminogenic thoughts with more prosocial thinking patterns.

Although the majority of the Thinking Helpsheet is completed by the JIC, we recommend that you work through an entire helpsheet together with a real-life example the first time it is assigned, so that there is minimal confusion regarding how to complete it. Script 9.1 (at the end of this chapter) provides instructions for describing and assigning the Thinking Helpsheet. Sometimes it is also useful to provide a refresher presentation about the helpsheet after the JIC has completed one or two, to serve as a reminder as to why the assignment is important and to ensure the task is being completed properly. Below, Brenda introduces the Thinking Helpsheet to Hank after they have gone through the RTD–Companions sequence.

"So we have talked about some of the thinking involved when you make poor decisions, and one example was a tendency to think that it's important to act in ways that make your friends happy, even when you know it's destructive or not good for you. Let's focus on that in more depth, and have you keep track of times when you have those kinds of thoughts. (*Brenda shows Hank the Helpsheet.*)

"This is called the Thinking Helpsheet. I'm going to give you enough copies to complete it on a regular basis, such as at the end of each day, or a time that works best for you. The more helpsheets you complete, the better it is for you in terms of learning about and improving your thinking.

"Let's go through it and complete one together this first time as an example. (*Brenda fills out the top box of the helpsheet.*) This is the thought I'd like you to focus on: 'I should act in ways that make my friends happy, even when I know it's destructive or might lead to a problem.'

"Over here, in the Situation box, you put down a real-life situation where this thought came up. For example, one event we talked about was the fight you got into at the bar, when you were with Brendan and Jason and the man spilled the drinks on you. Your friends began to say things encouraging you to get physical with him. (*Brenda fills in the Situation box.*)

"Then, in this Immediate Thinking box, you write down what went through your mind or what you said to yourself in that situation. For example, you mentioned that you thought those guys would really want you to get physical. You thought they would 'go nuts if I went off on the guy and made a scene . . . they would love it . . . high fives, free drinks.' So I'm going to write that down here. (*Brenda fills in the Immediate Thinking box.*)

"In the Decision and Outcome box, you write down what you did in response to the thoughts. In this case, you pushed and punched the man, so I'm going to write down 'Pushed and punched the person and got thrown out of the bar.' (*Brenda fills in the Decision and Outcome box.*)

"Finally, in this Better Thinking box, you write down a better way of thinking. In other words, you describe other thoughts that would lead to a better decision and outcome."

Brenda now encourages Hank to fill out this final box for himself:

BRENDA: So, in that situation, what would have been a better way of thinking in that moment?

HANK: Probably, it's not worth it to make them happy. They are just bored and trying to create drama. I shouldn't let them amp me up. I'm trying not to go to jail.

BRENDA: Exactly. (*Fills in the Better Thinking box.*) So, each night, I want you to reflect on what happened during the day and see if you can find examples where thoughts related to making your friends happy showed up. If they did, fill out a helpsheet, no matter what the outcome was. This may seem like a bit of work, but they are pretty easy to do. I'm hoping that the next time we meet, you will have a few examples from your life. That will be the starting point for our next session.

Homework Noncompliance

You might expect the likelihood of JICs' completing written homework like the Thinking Helpsheet to be low. Often JICs have not had successful experiences in school, and they may associate treatment homework with school homework. Yet we have been pleasantly surprised by the willingness of many JICs to complete the helpsheet. We suspect this is because, unlike traditional homework, the Thinking Helpsheet is about their real-world situations; in addition, it is relatively straightforward and nonjudgmental. Also, many JICs, at some level, want help and will seize the opportunity to do something to improve their own lives.

We are realists, however, inevitably there are times when JICs will fail to complete the homework. When this occurs, some practitioners choose simply to reassign it for the following appointment and move on to something else to cover in the session. We recommend that you avoid this option, as it can unintentionally reinforce a JIC for not following through with homework. Instead, it will be preferable to have the JIC complete the Thinking Helpsheet in the waiting room or in front of you during the session. Although this may seem rigid, it emphasizes the importance of completing homework, provides potentially useful material for the session, and (ideally) leads to greater diligence on the JICs part in future meetings.

RESTRUCTURING

One way of conceptualizing the cognitive restructuring process with JICs is that it gradually weakens the influence of their criminogenic thinking on decision making, while also strengthening the influence of their prosocial thinking on this process. Because both types of thinking are reflected in completed Thinking Helpsheets, we recommend using them as a protocol for restructuring strategies. In the restructuring strategies that follow, we assume you are reviewing Thinking Helpsheets completed by JICs. (These strategies can be adapted for use without the helpsheets, however.)

For a description and illustration of restructuring strategies, we return to the case of Jackie, who scored high on justifying on a criminal thinking instrument and who was assigned to monitor this pattern by using the Thinking Helpsheet. (She also scored high on identifying with antisocial companions and demand for excitement.) Jackie's completed helpsheet is presented in Figure 9.1. The situation Jackie has recorded concerns an argument with her sister that could have led to an arrest. The argument occurred when Jackie and her son were spending a few days visiting with her sister. Jackie's son had celebrated a birthday about a month prior to the visit, and Jackie's sister had apparently forgotten to get him a present. While Jackie's sister was at work, Jackie (without asking) took $100 in cash from her sister's dressing table and went shopping with her son to buy clothes, ice cream, and a video game. Her sister was furious when she discovered what had happened, which resulted in a shortened visit. Jackie's immediate thought before taking the money was this: "My sister didn't get my son anything for his birthday, so this will make up for that." Further discussion with Brenda indicates other justifications: a sense that her sister was easily able to afford the $100, and that taking the money was "not a big deal" because it was being spent on a member of the family. Despite Jackie's many justifications, she is eventually able to generate better thinking while completing the Thinking Helpsheet. Her better thought is this: "I should have asked her first. It's her money, and she can do with it what she wants."

Role-Playing Immediate and Better Thinking

Practitioners who are adventurous can strengthen prosocial thinking by engaging JICs in role-playing healthy thinking in response to criminogenic thinking. In Script 9.2, we present the steps for a restructuring role play we call Two Voices. Explaining the role play to JICs requires some time at first, but once they have done it, they will need only a brief reminder about how it works thereafter. It is ideally suited for use while reviewing a completed Thinking Helpsheet, but it can also be modified to follow a Connecting sequence. The role play uses personifications of Immediate Thinking and Better Thinking as two competing voices. During the role play, you play the role of the JIC's Immediate Thinking voice and feed criminogenic thoughts to the JIC. The JIC plays the role of the Better Thinking voice and must come up with prosocial thoughts that counter the criminogenic thinking.

The role play begins with a thorough review of a situation the JIC has captured on the Thinking Helpsheet. You then have the JIC describe their Immediate Thinking and Better Thinking in detail, going beyond whatever phrases or sentences have been written down on the helpsheet. Because you will be role-playing the Immediate Thinking voice (criminogenic thoughts), it will be particularly helpful if you have an in-depth understanding of how the JIC was thinking about the situation.

Thought/Thinking Pattern:

Coming up with reasons why it's OK for me to do something that could get me in trouble or be harmful to others.

Situation: Describe the situation where the thinking emerged (what happened, where, who was involved).

My sister's house, she was at work.

Took $100 from her dresser to buy my son something for his birthday—from her.

Immediate Thinking: Write a sentence or two that captures what was going through your mind during the situation.

"My sister didn't get my son anything for his birthday, so this will make up for that."

Decision and Outcome: Describe what you did as a result of the Immediate Thinking, and what happened then.

Bought clothes and video game for my son, went for ice cream.

Had a big blowout with my sister when she got home.

Had to leave her house.

Better Thinking: Write down another way of thinking that could lead to a better decision and outcome in this situation.

"I should have asked her first. It's her money, and she can do with it what she wants."

FIGURE 9.1. Jackie's completed Thinking Helpsheet.

Once you've discussed the situation and thinking to your satisfaction, explain the nature of the role play, using the Two Voices concept to refer to Immediate and Better Thinking. Explain that you would like to role-play those voices. You will be the Immediate Thinking voice and will verbalize some destructive thoughts consistent with that voice. The JIC will play the Better Thinking voice and try to counter those thoughts, just as the client did while completing the helpsheet.

Before starting the role play, give yourself a few seconds to think up several Immediate Thinking examples. Try to generate at least three examples that are at different levels of difficulty (easy, medium, hard) for the JIC to counter. Start with the easiest one. Provide your easiest Immediate Thinking example, and then ask the JIC to provide the Better Thinking to counter it. If the JIC can successfully counter your Immediate Thinking with Better Thinking, congratulate him or her (i.e., provide an affirmation), and determine whether you can move on to a more difficult example. If the JIC is successful in countering your next example, repeat the process, and go for a third or even a fourth round, at increasing levels of difficulty.

If the JIC cannot successfully counter your Immediate Thinking, try to avoid having the role play deteriorate or end abruptly. The goal is to have the JIC experience success and to strengthen his or her prosocial thinking. Give the JIC another opportunity to counter the Immediate Thinking example; if the client still struggles with a countering response, demonstrate how to counter the example, and then present a new Immediate Thinking example at a lower level of difficulty, so that the JIC can complete the role play with a successful experience.

Close the role-play session by (1) reinforcing the JIC's ability to generate Better Thinking and make better choices, (2) eliciting change talk about the importance of strengthening the Better Thinking voice, and (3) exploring ways of making the Better Thinking voice stronger. Let the JIC know that it's important to keep completing the Thinking Helpsheets, and that you will continue with the Two Voices role play in the future as the client brings in new helpsheets and real-life examples. Below is an example of Brenda's conducting this role play with Jackie.

BRENDA: (*After reviewing Jackie's Thinking Helpsheet*) So there are these two voices in your head for this situation. Let's be clear on what they sound like. You have this tendency to think of reasons why it would be OK for you to do things that could get you in trouble or be harmful to others, and in the situation you wrote about on the helpsheet, you told yourself: "My sister didn't get my son anything for his birthday, so this will make up for that." This led to an argument with your sister and could have led to your arrest. After the situation, when you completed the helpsheet, you were able to generate the Better Thinking voice, which is this: "I should have asked her first. It's her money, and she can do with it what she wants." Does that capture it pretty well? Or would you describe it differently?

JACKIE: No, that's good.

BRENDA: I'd like to try to something with you, then. I'm going to ask you to be a little bit of an actress for a few minutes. We're going to do a quick role play. I'm going to play the Immediate Thinking voice and present some ideas that come from that voice. I want you to be the Better Thinking voice and counter what I say. So we're going to role-play these two voices. I'm going to be the Immediate Thinking voice, and I want you to be the Better Thinking voice and see if you can counter my thoughts.

JACKIE: So you're the bad voice and I'm the good voice?

BRENDA: Right. Just give me a few seconds to think of what I'm going to say. . . . OK. Ready? "It's not that much money to her. She has a job and money coming in. It's not going to break her bank account." Now you counter that Immediate Thinking voice.

JACKIE: "But I can't just take it without asking. That's basically stealing. Ask first."

BRENDA: Good job. You countered that one nicely, so now I'm going to bump it up a notch. Ready? "Aunts should remember to get their nephews presents. She owes him this."

JACKIE: "She doesn't owe him. That's her money and her choice. She's allowed to do with it what she wants."

BRENDA: Very nice. How was that for you?

JACKIE: That was good. That was real.

BRENDA: I'm going to bump it up another notch. Ready? "My sister can be thoughtless and cheap. If she's too cheap to crack open her purse for her own nephew, I'll crack it open for her."

JACKIE: "It's not for you to decide. Ask her about getting him a present, and if she wants to do something for him, fine. If she doesn't, that's her right. But I have to ask."

BRENDA: You've done a really good job being the Better Thinking voice. What do you think would be different about your life if you paid more attention to that voice? How can you strengthen that better voice as you move forward?

Other Restructuring Strategies

The following four strategies are options that do not involve role play. They can be used in the same session or in isolation from each other. Like the Two Voices role play, they are ideally suited to follow a review of a completed Thinking Helpsheet, but can also be modified to fit nicely after a connecting sequence. Guidelines for each are provided at the end of the chapter in Script 9.3.

1. *Estimating the likelihood of problems.* One strategy for weakening criminogenic thinking while strengthening prosocial thinking is to use a completed Thinking Helpsheet as a stimulus for estimating the likelihood of the Immediate and Better Thinking to produce criminal justice involvement or other problems in the future. You can ask the JIC to estimate the likelihood, from 0 (unlikely) to 10 (very likely), that a future instance of the Immediate Thinking will lead to criminal justice involvement or other life problems. The JIC is then asked to estimate the likelihood that a future instance of the Better Thinking will lead to such problems. For example, in the case of Jackie, Brenda might say something like this:

"So if you have thoughts in the future like the one you wrote in the Immediate Thinking box, what do you think is the likelihood from 0 to 10, where 0 is unlikely and 10 is very likely, that such thoughts will lead you to have more problems with your family? What is the likelihood that these thoughts would lead to getting arrested?

"On the other hand, if you have thoughts in the future like the ones you wrote in the Better Thinking box, what do you think is the likelihood, from 0 to 10, that such thoughts will lead to more problems with your family? What is the likelihood that the Better Thinking thoughts would lead to getting arrested?"

Even if the JIC sees his or her Immediate Thinking as unlikely to result in a future negative outcome, the number the client estimates will most certainly be higher than that of the Better Thinking.

2. *Better thinking in similar situations.* Just as criminogenic thinking can generalize across situations, a more productive and prosocial way of thinking about one situation may be applicable to other risky situations. After discussing the Better Thinking box, you can ask the JIC to come up with several other real-life relationships or situations where the same type of Better Thinking may be helpful. In the case of Jackie, Brenda might say something like the following: "So, looking back, you think to yourself, 'I should have asked her first. It's her money, and she can do with it what she wants.' What is one other relationship you have where those kinds of thoughts may be helpful in the future?" Depending upon the JIC, the Better Thinking may be relevant to interactions with companions or family, use of substances, job searching, behavior at work, and so on. Encourage the JIC to articulate the applicability of the Better Thinking to the other situation(s) or relationship(s). Ask the client to walk you through how he or she might handle the other situations or relationship in the future.

3. *JIC-generated solutions.* Another way for JICs to strengthen the connection between prosocial thinking and decision making is for them to generate ideas about what would help them become more likely to act on the Better Thinking in the future. This may involve questions like "What's one thing you can do that will make you more likely to follow that Better Thinking in the future?" or "What would help you to make a decision based on the Better Thinking in the future?" Also, you can follow up and provide additional suggestions after JICs have had the opportunity to generate some of their own.

4. *Connecting better thinking to values and life priorities.* If you have already begun working on values and goals (see Chapter 4), you may find that the prosocial thinking JICs generate in their connecting sequences and Thinking Helpsheets is consistent with one or more of their underlying values. Thus you can strengthen productive and prosocial thinking by asking questions that highlight the importance of such thinking to living in accordance with values and goals. In the case of Jackie, Brenda might say something like this: "How might the Better Thinking relate to your value of staying involved with family members and taking care of your mother and helping her have a better life?" Brenda might also ask about ways in which the Immediate Thinking is not consistent with Jackie's stated values, or how underlying criminogenic thinking patterns interfere with important life goals (e.g., "How does coming up with reasons why it's OK to take something from a member of your family, without asking, interfere with your value of being involved with your family?").

As you try different restructuring strategies, do not be discouraged when JICs cling to a particular criminogenic thought or pattern. Restructuring a client's thinking is not a single-session undertaking. We can safely assume that entrenched criminogenic thoughts and thinking patterns are acquired over time, with repetition and practice. Extinguishing them and establishing more prosocial thinking will be gradual, and will require repetition and practice. Also, remember that it is not necessary to entirely eradicate or transform a JIC's thinking to achieve meaningful success. The aim is to reduce the impact of criminogenic thinking on the client's decision making. If you can reduce the strength or influence of criminogenic thinking sufficiently that its impact on decision making is negligible relative to that of prosocial thinking, this can be a significant change in the JIC's life. The bottom line is that JICs can—and we all can—have criminogenic thinking, but it does not have to guide our choices.

KEY POINTS

- The Thinking Helpsheet provides a structure for JICs to self-monitor specific criminogenic thoughts and thinking patterns between sessions.

- When assigning the Thinking Helpsheet, you help a JIC identify the criminogenic thought or thinking pattern to be monitored. The JIC then completes the remainder of the helpsheet (the Situation, Immediate Thinking, Decision and Outcome, and Better Thinking boxes) by using a recent real-life example.

- In the Two Voices role-play, the practitioner takes on the role of the JIC's Immediate Thinking voice, and the JIC practices countering criminogenic thinking by verbalizing the Better Thinking voice.

- Having JICs estimate the relative likelihood that Immediate Thinking and Better Thinking will lead to future problems is another way to reinforce more productive and prosocial thinking.

- Once more productive and prosocial thinking is identified, JICs can be asked to apply the Better Thinking to other risky situations or relationships.

- Another strategy to strengthen prosocial thinking and decision making is to elicit from JICs their ideas about what would help them act on the Better Thinking in the future.

- A final restructuring strategy is to highlight how criminogenic thinking undermines important values and life priorities, and how Better Thinking helps JICs live in accordance with important values and goals.

SCRIPT 9.1. Assigning the Thinking Helpsheet

Step 1: Introduce the criminogenic thought or thinking pattern that the JIC will be monitoring.

"So we have talked about some of the things that might get you into trouble. One of them is a tendency to . . . [for thinking patterns, see Chapter 7, Script 7.4]. And you have talked about how that has caused problems in the past. Let's focus on that."

Step 2: Introduce the Thinking Helpsheet.

"It is helpful for people to become aware of how their thinking influences decisions in their day-to-day lives. Here is a form I would like you to fill out at the end of each day, or whenever it is most convenient for you. It's called the Thinking Helpsheet. Let's go through it and fill one out together this first time as an example."

Step 3: Write down the description of the criminogenic thought or thinking pattern in the top box of the helpsheet.

"This is the thinking I'd like you to focus on. When this kind of thinking occurs in your life, fill in the rest of the Thinking Helpsheet."

Step 4: Explain the Situation box, and use an example from the JIC's life to illustrate.

"Over here in the Situation box, you describe the situation where the thinking influenced you." [Write down event.]

Step 5: Explain the Immediate Thinking box, using the same example.

"Over here in the Immediate Thinking box, you write down what went through your mind or what you said to yourself in that situation. For example, you mentioned that . . ." [Write down the JIC's words reflecting thinking that led to a poor outcome from the example discussed previously.]

Step 6: Explain the Decision and Outcome box, using the same example.

"Over here in the Decision and Outcome box, write down what you did and what the outcome was, whether it was positive or negative." [Write down the poor outcome the JIC has disclosed previously.]

(continued)

Step 7: Explain the Better Thinking box, using the same example.

"In the last box, you write down a better way of thinking that would lead to a better decision and outcome. For example, we discussed that a better way of thinking might be . . ." [Write down the JIC's own words for thinking that would lead to a better outcome. If the JIC has already made a good decision, ask:] "If you made a good decision, what can you do to strengthen that type of thinking in the future?"

Step 8: Ask whether the JIC has any questions.

"Do you understand what to do? Is there anything you are unsure about?"

Step 9: Give closing instructions.

"Each night, I want you to reflect on what happened during the day and see if you can find any examples where this type of thinking happened. If it did, fill out a Thinking Helpsheet, no matter what the outcome was. Please come in with a couple of these for next time, and we'll talk about them at our next meeting."

SCRIPT 9.2. The Two Voices Role Play

Step 1: Review the JIC's completed Thinking Helpsheet.

Positively reinforce the JIC for completing a Thinking Helpsheet. Have the JIC walk you through the helpsheet, providing specifics about the Situation, and elaboration on the Immediate Thinking and the Better Thinking.

"I'm glad you completed the Thinking Helpsheet. Now I want to you to walk me through the helpsheet. Tell me about the situation you wrote about. I want to hear about what happened before, during, and after the situation."

"OK, I've got a clear view of the situation. Now go over the Immediate Thinking with me. What was going through your mind at the time?"

"Now tell me about the Better Thinking. Try to describe it in detail for me."

Step 2: Summarize the JIC's Immediate Thinking and Better Thinking voices.

"It sounds like there are two voices in your head. Let's be clear on what they sound like. Sometimes you tell yourself [example of Immediate Thinking voice], and it leads to the difficulties we've talked about. At other times, you're able to tell yourself [example of Better Thinking voice]. Does that capture it pretty well? Or would you describe it differently?"

Step 3: Explain the role play.

Explain the nature of the role play, using the concept of the personified Two Voices.

"I'd like to try to something. I'm going to ask you to be a little bit of an actor for a few minutes. I'm going to play the Immediate Thinking voice and present some ideas that come from that voice. I want you to be the Better Thinking voice and counter what I say. In other words, I'm going to be the Immediate Thinking voice, and I want you to be the Better Thinking voice and see if you can counter my thoughts."

Step 4: Conduct the role play.

Now role-play the Immediate Thinking voice, and have the JIC role-play the Better Thinking voice. Give yourself a moment to think up several sample Immediate Thinking voice examples. Then say one of these to the JIC, and wait for the client to provide a counterargument in the form of the Better Thinking voice. Start at a low level of difficulty.

Positively reinforce the JIC's efforts and successes along the way. If the client does well, provide another example of the Immediate Thinking voice, at a slightly higher level of difficulty or complexity, and again have the JIC provide the counterargument in the form of the Better Thinking voice.

(continued)

"Good job. You countered that one nicely so now I'm going to bump it up a notch.

If the JIC does well with the second example, provide another example at an even slightly higher level of difficulty, and again have the JIC provide the counterargument in the form of the Better Thinking voice. Try to go through a total of three or four examples. If the JIC struggles, be supportive and try it again, or model an example of the Better Thinking voice.

Step 5: Debrief.

Reinforce the Better Thinking voice. Discuss ways to strengthen this voice. Finally, reinforce completing the helpsheets.

"Good job being the Better Thinking voice. What do you think would be different about your life if you paid more attention to that voice?"

"How can you make that voice stronger?" [It is OK to provide concrete and specific suggestions to the JIC if you have them.]

"What do you think are the chances that the next time you're in that situation, the Better Thinking voice will win out?"

"It seems like in situations such as [incident described on helpsheet], you can generate a Better Thinking voice that can lead to a better way of doing things. So I want you to keep doing these helpsheets for next time, so that we can keep strengthening healthier thinking and break some of the patterns that have led to problems for you."

SCRIPT 9.3. Guidelines for Other Restructuring Strategies

Step 1: Review the Thinking Helpsheet with the JIC.

Positively reinforce the JIC for completing the Thinking Helpsheet. Have the JIC walk you through the helpsheet, providing specifics about the Situation and elaboration on the Immediate Thinking and the Better Thinking.

"I'm glad you completed the Thinking Helpsheet. Now I want to you to walk me through the helpsheet. Tell me about the situation you wrote about. I want to hear about what happened before, during, and after the situation."

"OK, I've got a clear view of the situation. Now go over the Immediate Thinking with me. What was going through your mind at the time?"

"Now tell me about the Better Thinking. Try to describe it in detail for me."

Once you have gone through the Thinking Helpsheet, pick a strategy from Step 2a, 2b, 2c, or 2d below, and go through that strategy with the client.

Step 2a: Estimating the likelihood of problems.

"So if you continue in the future to act on thoughts like the ones you wrote in the Immediate Thinking box, what do you think is the likelihood from 0 to 10, where 0 is unlikely and 10 is very likely, that they will result in an arrest or other problems?"

"On the other hand, if you act in the future on thoughts like the ones you have in the Better Thinking box, what do you think is the likelihood, from 0 to 10, that they will result in an arrest or other problems?"

Step 2b: Better Thinking in similar situations.

"So, in this one situation, the Better Thinking you came up with is [reflection of JIC's Better Thinking]. Let's see if that type of thinking could also be helpful in other situations or relationships. What is one other possible situation or relationship where that thinking may be helpful in the future?"

"Tell me more about how it could be helpful in that situation [relationship]."

"So if this situation [relationship interaction] were to come up in the future, how do you think you would handle it, based on what we've discussed?"

(continued)

Step 2c: JIC-generated solutions.

> "What is one thing you can do that will make you more likely to follow that Better Thinking in the future?" or "What would help you to make a decision based on the Better Thinking in the future?"

> "How important is it for you to make decisions based on the Better Thinking?"

Step 2d: Connecting better thinking to values and life priorities.

> "How is the Better Thinking consistent with your value of [name of value]?" or "How can the Better Thinking make you more likely to succeed in your goal of [name of goal]?"

> "How is the Immediate Thinking really not consistent with your value of [name of value]?" or "How does this underlying thinking pattern of [reflection of criminogenic thinking pattern] really hurt you in your goal of [name of goal]?"

Step 3: Debrief.

Reinforce the Better Thinking. Discuss ways to strengthen the Better Thinking. Finally, reinforce completing the helpsheets.

> "What do you think would be different about your life if you paid more attention to the Better Thinking?"

> "How can you make the Better Thinking stronger?" [It is OK to provide additional concrete and specific suggestions to the JIC if you have them.]

> "What do you think are the chances that the next time you're in that situation, the Better Thinking will win out?"

> "It seems that in situations such as [incident described on helpsheet], you can generate Better Thinking that can lead to a different way of doing things. So I want you to keep doing these helpsheets for next time, so that we can keep strengthening healthier thinking and break some of the patterns that have led to problems for you."

FORM 9.1. Thinking Helpsheet

Thought/Thinking Pattern:

Situation: Describe the situation where the thinking emerged (what happened, where, who was involved).

Immediate Thinking: Write a sentence or two that captures what was going through your mind during the situation.

Decision and Outcome: Describe what you did as a result of the immediate thinking, and what happened then.

Better Thinking: Write down another way of thinking that could lead to a better decision and outcome in this situation.

PART V

DETAILED TREATMENT PLANS FOR HARMFUL LIFESTYLE PATTERNS

CHAPTER 10

Developing New Routines

Leisure Activities and Employment/Education

Brenda is sensitive to the fact that several factors contribute to both Hank's and Jackie's antisocial behavior, and that changes in aspects of their lifestyles are needed in order to reduce their risk for future criminality. Long-term treatment success relates to the integration of modified thinking and acting on a day-to-day basis—in other words, an improved lifestyle. We conceptualize a person's *lifestyle* as consisting of ongoing *routines* (discussed in this chapter), *relationships* (discussed in Chapter 11), and destructive *habits and patterns* (discussed in Chapter 12). As noted previously, the most important markers of success with JICs are a decline in criminal and self-destructive behaviors and an increase in positive behaviors. Therefore, assisting JICs in restructuring their lifestyles, in ways that introduce prosocial patterns and better decision making, is an important goal of treatment.

The interventions described in this chapter are designed to help JICs become less automatic in their day-to-day routines and take specific steps to activate prosocial lifestyle changes. To do this, JICs must replace risky activities with those that are more positive and productive. This is accomplished in three specific ways: reducing aimless use of leisure time, increasing education, and finding and sustaining meaningful employment. In this phase of treatment, emphasis is given to behavioral *movement* and deliberate *actions* JICs can take to improve their lives. Behavioral restructuring strategies are not single-session endeavors. A continued focus across sessions will be required for JICs to change entrenched lifestyle patterns.

We recommend that discussions about relevant criminal risk domains take place before the behavioral interventions described in this chapter (and Chapters 11 and 12) are implemented, so that JICs have some familiarity with the concept of criminal risk and its application to their lives. Since active participation is necessary, establishing some degree of engagement and having an agreed-upon focus are prerequisites for altering routines. A collaborative working relationship and shared goals will promote more investment from JICs in completing the homework and will result in more thoughtful discussions.

Regarding daily activities, JICs will be asked to reveal aspects of their lives that are possibly the riskiest. In regard to work and school, JICs will be asked to delve into past experiences that are often associated with disappointments and failures. Keep in mind that JICs may minimize the degree of risk associated with their existing lifestyles and may make external attributions regarding academic and vocational failures. These responses may be either intentional (i.e., they wish to present themselves in a positive light) or unintentional (i.e., they don't truly understand themselves). These are normal and common reactions among counseling clients in general (JICs and non-JICs alike), since people tend to minimize their self-defeating patterns, especially in interactions where others may judge them negatively or seek to change them. Therefore, lifestyle factors that are revealed as being associated with even a small degree of risk and failure will need to be thoughtfully explored. If you take a judgmental or punitive stance (e.g., "Haven't you learned that hanging out in your old neighborhood is a bad idea? The bottom line is if you keep making the wrong choices, you will be going back to prison"), the results will be less honesty and openness in the future. If you take an advice-giving stance (e.g., "You should spend more time developing your resume and adopt more realistic job expectations. That's what you need to do to find steady work"), the result may be a list of reasons from a JIC about why your advice can't be followed.

Several skills already presented in this treatment planner will be useful in discussing routines and potential lifestyle changes. Here are a few tips. First, look for opportunities to evoke change talk, as discussed in Chapter 7 (e.g., ask why certain activities or situations are risky, why some are more risky than others, and why change might be a good thing). Second, search for chances to reinforce the connections between potential lifestyle changes and JICs' personal values and life priorities that have previously been discussed (see Chapter 4). Third, it is important to affirm JICs' honesty when risky activities are revealed (e.g., "You seem to be serious about eliminating some of the risky behaviors that have caused problems for you in the past. That takes a lot of courage"). Fourth, keep it simple. It is a mistake to try to implement sweeping lifestyle changes in one meeting. It is best to end sessions with an agreed-upon, specific, and practical behavioral step that you are certain is achievable. Keep goals for each session modest, as you will be shaping lifestyle changes over the longer term. Finally, always look for opportunities during follow-up discussions to affirm JICs' efforts (e.g., "You really put a lot of time into looking for a job").

In a general sense, restructuring lifestyle factors will go hand in hand with the changes in thinking discussed in Chapters 8 and 9. People behave according to their thoughts—and they think according to their behaviors. For example, JICs who begin to change their criminogenic thoughts (e.g., from "My day doesn't really start until 11:00 P.M. That's when things get exciting" to "Hanging out all night isn't as fun as it used to be") will be more likely to alter their choices and activity patterns. Similarly, taking active steps to find meaningful work (e.g., developing new skills, trying a new job area) will challenge entrenched criminogenic thinking patterns and foster new thoughts (e.g., "I think I might be good at this. Maybe I don't have to hustle on the street any more"). A cognitive component can also be introduced by examining how JICs typically think when they are engaged in high-risk versus prosocial activities, or successful versus unsuccessful work or school experiences. To have the greatest impact over the longer term, your task is to focus treatment on changing both thinking and behavior.

LEISURE ACTIVITIES

Each week has a total of 168 hours, and knowing how JICs spend that time is essential to treatment success. If you work in an agency or program that has a public safety mandate, familiarizing yourself with the nature of JICs' daily routines becomes an even higher priority. Also, the vast majority of JICs will benefit from learning time management skills. We recommend *activity monitoring* as the first step for obtaining a snapshot of current routines. Depending on the typical time frame for your sessions, activity monitoring can usually be completed in one meeting. As always, if your sessions are brief, these steps can be covered across multiple meetings.

JICs may initially perceive the activity-monitoring process negatively and be hesitant or even reluctant to engage in it. That is, they may regard it as a method of supervision rather than self-improvement. It cannot be overstated that activity monitoring is not intended as a tool for detecting violations of probation, parole, or other community supervision! Using this tool to "catch" JICs in inconsistencies (e.g., "You said you were home with your daughter on Tuesday, so how come the cops were talking to you on the street corner?") will undermine its effectiveness and create an adversarial practitioner–client relationship. Similarly, activity monitoring will not be effective if it is presented as a tool for control (e.g., having JICs routinely complete and submit the activity-monitoring forms with no meaningful discussions; bureaucratically assigning forms every week for a 1-year period of probation just to have records in the file). Activity monitoring is designed to be implemented in a spirit of collaboration for reducing risk and shaping a better lifestyle.

Baseline Activity Monitoring

The first step in the activity-monitoring process is to determine the baseline routines of JICs—in other words, to find out what their lifestyles are like now. Form 10.1, provided at the end of this chapter, is an effective method of monitoring a JIC's routines during a typical weekday. The goal is to obtain a snapshot of what the client's life looks like during a normal 24-hour period. A parallel form (Form 10.2) is also provided at the end of the chapter, to monitor how time is spent on weekends. Have the JIC record employment, school, or other fixed obligations first, and then leisure activities. Use Script 10.1 at the end of the chapter to introduce these two activity-monitoring forms. Since this intervention is bound to be new for most JICs, inquire about any questions or concerns they might have. Reinforce the idea that understanding how one's time is spent is a first step in managing time more productively and making important life changes.

Rating Activities for Risk and Enjoyment

In the same or a subsequent session, ask the JIC to review the weekday and Saturday forms, and to rate each activity along two dimensions: (1) helpfulness in staying out of trouble (relative risk), and (2) level of enjoyment. Use Script 10.2 to introduce how to rate activities. Also, show the JIC Form 10.3, which provides written guidelines and examples for making ratings; again, both the script and the form are provided at the chapter's end. Ratings are placed in the boxes with the dotted lines on Forms 10.1 and 10.2.

For the first dimension (helpfulness in staying out of trouble; relative risk), activities can be rated either *positive, neutral,* or *risky.* Have the JIC place a P next to those activities that are viewed as generally helpful in avoiding possible criminal justice involvement, or that might otherwise be viewed as *positive* to self and others. For activities viewed as *neutral*—neither risky nor positive—ask the JIC to write in an N. These will usually be activities associated with obligations related to work and household chores, or things that the person does just to pass the time. Finally, have the

JIC place an R next to any activities that he or she believes might be *risky* in terms of increasing the likelihood of contact with the criminal justice system (e.g., hanging out with risky friends, being in an environment where people are using substances, being near triggers for anger outbursts, or pursuing dangerous activities). Have the JIC rate activities for potential risk, even if the activity does not always lead to a bad outcome.

For the second dimension (level of enjoyment), activities should be rated as *enjoyable, OK,* or *unpleasant.* Enjoyable activities are rated with an E, unpleasant activities with a U, and those in between are rated with an OK. Make sure the JIC understands that "helpfulness in staying out of trouble" and "level of enjoyment" are separate dimensions, and that each activity should be rated on both. It is likely that some activities will receive ratings of both P *and* E or R *and* E, as some positive activities will be perceived as enjoyable, and certain risky behaviors can also be associated with fun and excitement. It is likely as well that the JIC will rate some of his or her common risky activities as not particularly enjoyable (maybe an OK), and that some prosocial activities will be rated as ultimately enjoyable even though they are not particularly exciting.

Jackie's completed My Typical Weekday form (shown in Figure 10.1) reveals only one area of risk in her current routine: She reports that she gets bored around 9:00 P.M. and looks for something to do. If her son is spending the night at his father's apartment, she will go out with whoever is available, including her friends from the car wash. The remainder of her schedule is filled with activities that are relatively low-risk in terms of leading to problems. Jackie's enjoyment ratings indicate that she gets the most pleasure from exercising, spending time with her son, and talking on the phone with her mother or sister. Since she lost her job, however, her day lacks structure.

Review and Discussion of Overall Patterns

Once you have a snapshot of a JIC's routines and the nature of each activity, the next step is to use the activity-monitoring forms as springboards for a general discussion about lifestyle. Make sure to ask thoughtful questions about anything the JIC reveals as risky. Also, inquire about patterns that emerge in relation to enjoyable activities: the possible link between enjoyment and risk, a lack of fun in day-to-day life, and the connection between enjoyable activities and personal values. This conversation will reveal how JICs view the relative risk associated with various activities that are part of their lifestyles, and will highlight potential areas in need of change.

In some cases, no risky activities will be revealed. If this happens, ask JICs to speculate about the most risky activity on the forms or the activity that has led to the most problems in the past. Another option is to have JICs contrast their current routines with previous times when their lifestyles included more self-defeating and destructive activities. You might even ask JICs to complete activity forms depicting what their lives looked like when they were at their *worst* in terms of risk. In this way, you can highlight significant changes between their previous lifestyles and what is happening now.

Identifying Specific Behavioral Steps for Lifestyle Changes

Next, discuss a practical step for diminishing or replacing a high-risk activity with a new- less risky and prosocial alternative. Form 10.4 at the end of this chapter provides a structure for identifying a concrete and specific lifestyle change. After presenting Form 10.4, allow JICs time during

Time	Morning			Time	Afternoon		
6:00	Sleep	N	OK	12:00	Food shopping, make lunch	P	OK
7:00	Get out of bed; make breakfast for son	N	OK	1:00	Talk to Mom on phone	P	E
8:00	Get son to preschool	N	OK	2:00	Pick up son from preschool	P	E
9:00	Watch TV	N	OK	3:00	Hang out with son, talk	P	E
10:00	Watch TV	N	OK	4:00	Bring son to his father's	N	U
11:00	Go for a walk, exercise	P	E	5:00	Watch TV	N	OK

Time	Evening			Time	Night/Early Morning		
6:00	Make dinner	N	OK	12:00	Sleep	N	OK
7:00	Call Marissa (sister) on phone	P	E	1:00	Sleep	N	OK
8:00	Watch TV	N	OK	2:00	Sleep	N	OK
9:00	Bored, looking for something to do	R	U	3:00	Sleep	N	OK
10:00	Bored, watch TV	R	OK	4:00	Sleep	N	OK
11:00	Go to bed	N	OK	5:00	Sleep	N	OK

FIGURE 10.1. Jackie's completed My Typical Weekday form.

the session to consider each question and write their answers. In other words, this form serves to prompt an in-session conversation and is not meant to be completed by JICs in isolation. After the form is completed, discuss the responses and agree on a behavioral step to be taken before the next session.

Looking at Jackie's completed Questions to Ask Myself about How I Spend My Time form (Figure 10.2) suggests that she has a good understanding of at least one high-risk situation: She is aware that she will need to make plans for those evenings when her son is with his father. Jackie has come up with a short-term practical step and a longer-term goal she can work toward. In the short term, she can make plans to visit with her sister. For the longer term, she can look into

Questions to Ask Myself	Answers, Solutions, and Next Steps
What activities are most risky for me during weekdays? On weekends?	*Not having anything to do at night. If my son is staying at his father's apartment, I want to go out and do something fun, and I'll reach out to anyone I know is around. That sometimes leads to problems.*
What is at stake if I do not change these risky activities?	*I'll end up hanging out with Ted and Maurice, my car wash friends. They drink and other stuff. It ended badly at the car dealership.*
What new activities might replace these that would be more positive and healthy for me?	*I could try and make plans with my sister Marissa. Or maybe try and take a night class for college.*
What new activities would be more consistent with my values?	*The night class would help me get back to working on my college degree.*
What new activities might I enjoy?	*I would enjoy college classes.*
What is one practical step I could take to replace one high-risk activity?	*Make plans with my sister. Or look into the college course for next semester.*
I will know my plan is working if . . .	*I have less downtime at night. I have plans to get out of the house instead of acting out of boredom.*

FIGURE 10.2. Jackie's completed Questions to Ask Myself about How I Spend My Time form.

taking a college class in the evening. This will of course require more planning (e.g., enrolling in school, rearranging her son's visitation schedule with his father). The longer-term step is also consistent with Jackie's stated value of "doing work that is rewarding or important" and pursuing admission to a local community college.

Follow-Up and Review of Progress

In the subsequent session, you will review the JIC's progress on the step discussed in the previous meeting. If a new activity was successfully integrated into the daily routine that offset a risky one, it is important to affirm the JIC's efforts (e.g., "You did a good job in trying out something new this week. Let's talk about what you learned"). At this point, discuss ways to keep the change going—and, if appropriate, focus on another risky activity that could be altered for the next session.

In situations where JICs are unsuccessful in implementing the behavior change, focus the discussion on identifying obstacles such as low motivation, lack of opportunity to engage in the new activity, presence of criminogenic thinking patterns that interfere with the new behavior, or limited skills. These will be important areas to address as treatment moves forward.

Keep in mind that as routines begin to shift, new activities will need to be found that can fill the void left by activities previously associated with risk. New activities and routines that enhance happiness are preferred, as long as they do not increase risk potential. Remember, the long-term goal is to shape a more positive and prosocial use of time.

EMPLOYMENT AND EDUCATION

Education and job skills create a path to steady employment and a career; in turn, a good job provides the foundation for self-sufficiency and economic survival. Work also organizes daily routines and affords a social context that generally reinforces prosocial attitudes and behaviors. Not surprisingly, finding and keeping a job are predictors of reduced criminal involvement and subsequent JIC success (Cox, Bantley, & Roscoe, 2005; Rhodes, Dyouus, Kling, Hunt, & Luallen, 2013; Visher, Debus, & Yahner, 2008).

In most cases, addressing education and employment directly in treatment will be necessary, because this is a major problem area for this client group. For example, approximately 70% of high-risk probationers and those returning from prisons have not obtained a high school diploma (Cox et al., 2005). Unemployment rates vary across geographic regions and forensic settings, with estimates ranging from 30 to 35% for JICs on community supervision (Rhodes et al., 2013). For high-risk probationers, unemployment may be even higher, with estimates reaching up to 65% (Cox et al., 2005). For JICs reentering society after a period of incarceration, approximately 50–70% are unemployed a year later (Visher et al., 2008). Clearly, failure to meet basic educational benchmarks and job instability are common deficits among JICs.

To make matters worse, JICs who are unemployed (or underemployed) find themselves in one of the most competitive job markets in decades. Roadblocks to successful employment tend to cluster around a few common themes. First, having a criminal record adversely affects employment opportunities; those convicted of felonies are legally prohibited from entering certain professions (e.g., law enforcement, mortgage brokering) and may be disqualified from obtaining state licensure credentials for some occupations (e.g., as dentists, veterinarians, electricians, or plumbers). Perhaps more common are the stigma, prejudice, and general concern associated with hiring individuals with criminal backgrounds. Second, JICs' vocational histories make them less desirable in a competitive job market. Limited educational achievement, lack of marketable skills, and gaps in work history will often place JICs at the bottom of the applicant pool. Third, not having the required legal documents (e.g., copy of birth certificate, current driver's license, and proof of a stable address) can derail the hiring process. Fourth, a range of practical challenges often emerges, such as lack of appropriate interview and work clothing, a need for transportation, and unstable housing. Fifth, JICs may struggle with ongoing mental health, medical, and substance use problems that interfere with successfully maintaining employment. Sixth, internal obstacles such as pessimism about finding a job, lack of confidence, and negative beliefs about one's capabilities contribute to an ongoing cycle of academic and vocational failure. An excerpt from a recent interview with a JIC illustrates the many challenges faced in this area:

> "I realize that there isn't any help for ex-convicts returning into society, whether they are on probation or not. Because what I was faced with when I returned back into society after my incarceration period was homelessness, lack of work, and, you know, everything that falls under that—not having food, not having clothes, not having transportation, stuff like that. Because I was a grown man returning back into society after a period of incarceration, I have nothing but what I was released with. I feel like there should be more set up for people like that, especially when they are coming out being monitored by state probation. The actual issue here is the fact that I am human and I have nowhere to go."—Warren, JIC, age 26

Despite the many challenges, there is some good news. The vast majority of JICs, when asked, report a desire for stable and meaningful employment (Morani, Wikoff, Linhorst, & Bratton, 2011), which suggests that they are motivated for taking steps to improve the education and employment area of their lives. In addition, most U.S. states offer a variety of in-prison and community-based programs to support JICs in finding work. Although there is widespread recognition of the importance of such initiatives, the effectiveness of such programs has not been well documented (Visher, Winterfield, & Goggeshall, 2005). At the time of the writing of this book, another resource in the United States is the Work Opportunity Tax Credit (WOTC), which provides private for-profit employers with financial incentives for hiring individuals belonging to certain groups (e.g., a tax credit of $2,400 for each full-time employee hired; ex-felons, among others, qualify for the tax credit). The WOTC paperwork is minimal, and there is no limit to the number of JICs an employer can hire. This perk can sometimes get the attention of potential employers and tilt the balance in favor of JICs.

Depending on your role, you may take an active approach in assisting JICs in developing career and education plans, helping with job searches, and providing guidance for remaining employed. Or you may make referrals to designated outside agencies or programs that specialize in employment services and job support (e.g., job developers or employment specialists are on staff at some programs). Even when you are making referrals to outside services, however, it is still important to track and reinforce any positive steps JICs take in improving the academic and vocational areas of their lives. Equally important is to refrain from tactics that will unintentionally undermine JICs' efforts, such as scheduling probation or parole appointments at times likely to conflict with job interviews and work schedules.

A common error is to assume that a JIC has the skills to find, compete for, secure, and hold a job. Since JICs are a diverse group, you should tailor your approach to each case. As a starting point for individualizing your approach, have each JIC complete Form 10.5 at the end of this chapter and discuss the client's responses. Once you have a baseline understanding of the client's education and employment history and views, consider the list of more detailed treatment steps below.

In the case of Jackie, she seems to have developed an appreciation that a career path, rather than just another job, will be an important goal for reshaping her life (see Figure 10.3). Overall, she has realistic expectations about the amount of education required to become a nurse, and seems to be motivated to start taking courses. In terms of work, her ideal scenario would be to obtain a part-time job in the medical field. Since the beginnings of a career plan are starting to

Questions to Ask Myself	Answers, Solutions, and Next Steps
How satisfied am I with my current employment situation?	*Very unsatisfied. Don't like being unemployed.*
What would my ideal employment situation look like?	*I want to help people, maybe be a nurse.*
What type of education or training would help me get closer to my goal?	*College degree in nursing,*
What specific things can I do to get more education or job skills?	*Enroll in college classes.* *Get a part-time job at a medical office.*
What steps can I take to find a job, or a better job?	*My sisters might know someone who is hiring.* *Marissa has a good friend who is a doctor.* *Maybe even volunteer for a half-day to start.*
What can I do to improve my interview skills for new jobs?	*Practice interviewing.* *Get some experience so I have more confidence.*
Once I get a job I like, what are two things I can do to make sure I keep it?	*Show up on time.* *Ask questions.*
I will know my career plan is working if . . .	*I'm in school and working part-time in the medical field.*

FIGURE 10.3. Jackie's completed Questions to Ask Myself about Education and Employment form.

emerge for Jackie, useful steps in treatment would be to assist her in enrolling in college courses and finding part-time employment in the field where she seems most interested in working. Pursuing these goals will directly address two important criminal risk domains (lack of connection to work/school and maladaptive leisure time), and will set Jackie on a course more consistent with her overall values.

Understanding Education and Employment History

Understanding the details of a JIC's educational and employment history is a prerequisite to focusing on developing skills. For a JIC reentering the community after a period of incarceration, you will need to assess educational and employment history prior to incarceration, as well as any changes that have happened during time spent in prison (e.g., the JIC earned a GED or participated in a job skills program). Form 10.6 at the end of this chapter provides a simple checklist of basic questions related to education, employment, and marketable skills. Have the JIC complete this form independently, and follow up with a brief discussion to make sure you grasp the critical aspects of the person's educational and employment history. In addition, the questions in Script 10.3 will help identify important employment-related areas to work on, such as current attitude toward employment, recent job performance, conflicts with supervisors and coworkers, work attendance, terminations, and impulsive quitting. These questions are more in-depth than those presented in Chapter 5 for general assessment purposes. As always, these types of questions serve as a guide, so ask those that seem most relevant for a particular JIC.

Advancing Educational Achievement

Supporting JICs toward attaining further formal education has several practical benefits. First, it is likely to enhance their ability to compete with other job seekers in finding work. Second, attending classes provides an anchor point for structure and a meaningful use of leisure time. Third, education affords JICs opportunities to make new social connections and increases their circle of prosocial friends. Fourth, when successful, pursuing education challenges criminogenic thinking patterns and promotes prosocial thinking and a sense of self-efficacy.

For many JICs, obtaining further education will mean taking steps to earn a GED. For others, community college or technical programs are good starting points. There are certainly cases where higher levels of education make sense, such as completing a 4-year degree or even pursuing graduate-level work. Obviously, a thoughtful consideration of issues related to interest, motivation, and intellectual ability is required. Setting up JICs to fail is always counterproductive! Do not be surprised to see some JICs flourish when they pursue higher levels of education; deficits in educational achievement sometimes have much less to do with ability than they do with lack of past opportunities.

Enhancing Job Skills

Enhanced education, however, is not for everyone. For those who are unlikely to succeed in academic pursuits, it may be better to focus on enhancing job skills. Even though some JICs may possess strong intellectual abilities, it is possible that their interest and ambition is more related to vocational goals that do not require higher levels of education. The most common jobs for JICs are in construction, manual labor, maintenance, and factory work (Visher et al., 2008). Career paths can also be developed in other areas, such as automotive repair, cooking/other restaurant work, trucking/moving, carpentry, lawn care, and landscaping. Trades such as plumbing and electrical work may also be possibilities; however, certain types of convictions may limit JICs' ability to obtain full licensure in these trades in some states, as noted above. Job training programs, certificate courses, and apprenticeships should all be explored.

Finding Employment

Once consideration has been given to education and marketable job skills (work readiness), finding employment is the next step.

Practical Issues

As noted above, a range of practical issues will have to be addressed before JICs embark on job searches (see Figure 10.4 for a brief checklist). Your guidance and coaching may be necessary to resolve some of these common roadblocks to finding employment.

Positive Impressions and Interview Skills

Some thought should be given to how JICs are likely to present themselves to potential employers. Basic issues such as proper hygiene, grooming, and attire will sometimes need to be addressed (fingernails, facial hair, makeup, etc.). Having JICs pay attention to self-care will often go a long way toward improving first impressions. We have found that being direct is usually the best approach—provided that a positive and productive working relationship exists between you and the JIC. Below is an example of how to introduce the topic for discussion:

> "Mark, it's great that you are getting ready to go on job interviews. I wanted to focus today's session on how you might come across to potential employers. I'm sort of like a coach who is in your corner. So is it OK if we talk about things like hygiene and clothing? I want you to be successful."

☐ Proper identification documents
☐ Résumé
☐ Appropriate interview and work clothes
☐ Stable housing and legal address
☐ Contact information (phone number, professional voicemail, email)
☐ Transportation

FIGURE 10.4. Checklist of practical issues to address prior to job searching.

Although these types of conversations can seem awkward, JICs often appreciate the honest feedback. Very few people in their lives will be "up front" with them about such issues.

It will often take time for JICs to become competent in interviewing for jobs. Think of developing interviewing skills as more of a linear process than a series of disconnected one-time events. Failures are to be expected. Simulating job interviews during sessions, and providing coaching and feedback, can be helpful in building JICs' confidence and overall skills. Again, details such as eye contact, firm handshakes, appropriate speech volume and speed, and overall courteousness may need to be discussed and rehearsed during sessions. The aim is for JICs to convey a sense of competence, dependability, and reliability to potential employers. Also, after an interview takes place, taking time to review things that went well (and things that did not) will allow JICs to learn from experience.

Another skill that requires practice is providing accurate answers to difficult questions. Inquiries about criminal history are generally the most challenging (e.g., "Do you have a felony conviction?"). Some JICs will feel the need to share intimate details regarding their criminal histories with potential employers they are meeting for the first time. This is usually a mistake. Encourage JICs not to lie or embellish, but to handle the question in a matter-of-fact manner by adhering to the following guidelines:

- Disclose the nature of the offense and when it occurred.
- Convey responsibility for mistakes.
- Describe the sentence and current criminal justice status.
- Mention any programs that have been attended or completed (even if these are mandated by probation or parole), or any positive steps taken.
- Say when the probation or parole period ends.
- Reiterate that it was a mistake that is now being used as a learning experience.

An example might sound like this:

"When I was younger, I got involved in selling drugs. In 2015, I was convicted of a felony for the sale of narcotics. It was foolish, and I should have known that the fast money was not the way to go. I also regret that I may have hurt a lot of people with the drugs I sold. I was sentenced to 3 years in prison and served 2½ years. I am on probation for the next 2 years and taking advantage of several rehabilitation programs. Looking back, I realize I made a huge mistake. I lost almost 3 years of my life because of it. I am a different person today. I'm using it as a learning experience as I try to move forward and do positive things in my life."

Responses should be tailored to a JICs unique history and circumstances. Once a response is developed, it should be rehearsed until it becomes effortless. JICs often feel a sense of relief once they have a genuine and coherent response that reflects their own personal story.

Time Management and Job Search Strategy

JICs who are actively searching for employment are likely to be more successful if they structure their activities toward the goal of getting a job. The activity-monitoring procedures described in the first part of this chapter can provide a snapshot of how much time is being devoted to finding employment. Discussions can focus on ways JICs can alter their routines to increase job-searching activities.

A good starting point is to connect JICs to programs that specialize in job placements for ex-offenders. Practitioners who work in such programs are often familiar with local employers who hire JICs; they usually have lists of specific contacts at local businesses and know which organizations are currently hiring. Other strategies for finding work include asking friends, family members, and relatives about potential job leads. Examining "help wanted" advertisements online, on social media, and in print can also be useful. For some businesses, JICs can apply in person to get their applications on file, so that they can be called at a later time if a job opening should materialize. Finally, offering to be a volunteer will help build relevant work experience, cultivate potential references, expand a JIC's professional circle, and provide more connections to job leads.

Keeping a Job

Even when employed, many JICs can benefit from some degree of job monitoring, support, and ongoing skills building. Here are a few areas that commonly need attention.

Time Management Skills

JICs are not always good time managers. This will be especially true for individuals newly released from prison, who may have significant deficits when it comes to directing their own lives. At the most basic level, check to make sure that some type of accurate alarm clock is in place, to prompt getting up at a consistent time in the morning. Most mobile phones have alarms that can be used for this purpose. Developing a structure for weekly schedules, reminders, and "to do" lists will also be important for job success. Lastly, encourage JICs to be on time for work obligations by being 10 minutes early for everything!

Communication Skills

Depending on the job, specific types of communication patterns may be the focus of ongoing skills building. These will usually involve face-to-face interactions and telephone conversations. As always, details such as tone of voice, body language, facial expressions, and gestures are important. Coaching can also be directed toward improving skills related to professional electronic communications, such as emails and text messages.

For many JICs, asking for clarification or help in performing work tasks can be something that does not come easily or naturally. Encourage JICs to recognize when help is needed, rather than waiting too long to ask. Reinforce the idea that asking for help and guidance demonstrates responsibility and not failure. Have JICs practice making such requests.

Maintaining a Focus on Honesty and Integrity

Because of their histories, JICs are not usually given the benefit of the doubt when things go wrong. Slight missteps that may be overlooked for other employees may be met with greater suspicion for

JICs. Therefore, it is important for JICs to pay particular attention to honesty and integrity across all interactions with supervisors, coworkers, and customers. Here are a few behaviors to reinforce:

- Give accurate information when communicating.
- Take the time to get the right answers; if necessary, promise to get back to people.
- Do not take any supplies, materials, or equipment for personal use.
- Use work time for work and not personal business.
- Take leave for appropriate reasons only.
- Document work time accurately.

Accepting Feedback

Feedback and criticism from supervisors or colleagues can sometimes be received poorly (e.g., interpreted as disrespect) and trigger negative reactions from JICs. With repeated practice, such situations can be handled skillfully. It is important to discuss with JICs that feedback is essential for growth in any job.

In-session role plays are helpful for developing new skills, especially in situations where a JIC has experienced recent difficulties when receiving feedback. Start by having the JIC take on the role of the supervisor; you play the JIC. Once the JIC (as the supervisor) delivers the feedback, model actively listening to what the supervisor is saying. Then respond in a way that is constructive and not defensive. Next, switch roles, and observe how well the JIC does in duplicating your response with his or her own style. Provide feedback, and repeat with several rounds of practice. You can also escalate the level of difficulty by taking on a harsher tone and being more demanding. Make sure to let the JIC know that you are increasing the difficulty level (e.g., "John, let's try it again. This time, I'm going to raise my voice and shout at you. Try to respond the way we practiced"). A sense of humor while practicing new skills is often helpful. The quality of the interaction should be playful and positive, not punishing. Finally, discussions can focus on modifying how the JIC interprets employer feedback, with the goals of not taking such communications so personally, letting things go, and not holding grudges.

Handling Disagreements and Conflicts

Working as part of a team will inevitably lead to disagreements, and JICs may have poor skills at handling such situations. If conflicts and anger outbursts are ongoing problems, see the section on anger management in Chapter 12 for additional ideas. Below is a short list of behaviors to reinforce in treatment:

- Never use physical means, threats, or intimidation to resolve conflicts.
- Think before speaking.
- Actively listen to the other person's perspective.
- Apologize when wrong.

The in-session role-play strategy described above is also useful in practicing skills for responding to challenging coworkers.

Moving Up the Ladder or Making a Transition

In situations where a JIC seems like a good fit in a current job, the client may wish to explore opportunities for advancement. One way to do this is for the JIC to consider learning more than the current work role and to ask his or her employer for cross-training in other areas of the business. This will broaden skills, make the JIC more valuable to the current employer, and set the stage for advancement.

A JIC who is not content with the current employment situation runs the risk of impulsively quitting out of frustration. In such a case, it is important to be supportive and to validate the JIC's perspective, explore what is not going well in the current job, and help the JIC develop a plan for finding a new job. Planned exits are always better than quitting in a fit of anger.

KEY POINTS

- Understanding how JICs spend their time is an essential component for successful treatment. *Activity monitoring* is the first step in obtaining a snapshot of current routines.

- Once a list of current routines is established, activities are rated by JICs along two dimensions: (1) relative risk, and (2) level of enjoyment.

- After discussing routines, the next step is to begin to replace high-risk activities with new, less risky alternatives. The long-term goal is to shape a more positive and prosocial use of time.

- Education and job skills are important for establishing a career. In turn, a good job organizes daily routines, provides a social context that generally reinforces noncriminal attitudes and behaviors, and is necessary for economic survival.

- Limited educational achievement, lack of marketable job skills, and employment instability are major deficits for this client group.

- In most cases, advancing educational achievement and enhancing marketable job skills will have to be addressed directly in treatment.

- Assisting JICs in finding employment often involves attending to a range of practical issues (e.g., résumé, work clothes, transportation), improving positive impression and interview skills (e.g., hygiene, eye contact, rate of speech, answering questions about criminal history), and developing time management and job search strategies.

- Ongoing coaching may also be required to support JICs in keeping a job. Common treatment activities include improving skills in the areas of time management, responding to negative feedback, handling disagreements, and maintaining a high degree of integrity and honesty.

SCRIPT 10.1. Introducing Activity–Monitoring Forms (My Typical Weekday/My Typical Saturday)

"[JIC's name], we all have activities in our lives that involve different situations, people, and places. As we go through life, many of our activities become automatic, and we no longer think much about them. Some of our activities help us achieve important goals and move forward with our lives. Other activities create risk for problems and interfere with what we value most. Also, some activities are enjoyable, while others feel more like obligations. Our routines, and how we spend our time, shape how our lives turn out.

"Part of our work together will involve looking at how you spend your time, to see if your daily activities are leading you to the kind of life you want. Of course, you are the one who gets to decide how you want to spend your time—because it's your life.

"This form is designed to take a snapshot of a typical weekday. [Show Form 10.1.] It's an important step in understanding and learning how to manage your time. Here is how it works. Pick a typical weekday, from the past few days, and list the things you did during a 24-hour period. We will go through it together, and it will only take a few minutes. [Have the client fill in work, school, and other obligations first, and then add other activities around those.] For example, in the morning section, list all the things you did between 6 A.M. and 11 A.M. So if you got up at 8:30 A.M., write that here. If you went for a walk to the store at 1 P.M., write that in the afternoon section. Complete it the same way for the night and early morning sections of the form. For example, if you went out with a friend at night, indicate the amount of time you spent with your friend. Also, list the time you went to bed.

"Do you have any questions?"

[After this form is completed, introduce Form 10.2.] "I would also like you to complete this form for a recent Saturday. It's the same idea, and we will do it together. Try to remember your activities. [Have the client fill in work, school, and other obligations first.]

"Thanks for sharing a bit about what your life looks like with me."

SCRIPT 10.2. Script for Rating Activities

"[JIC's name], let's go over the activities on both of these forms [Forms 10.1 and 10.2] to get a deeper understanding of your life and how you spend your time. Here are some instructions for rating each activity. [Show Form 10.3.] First, we are going to look at which activities help you stay out of trouble and which ones create risk for problems. Look over all the activities, and pick out the ones that you view as positive and healthy. Then place a P next to each of these activities in the upper box with the dotted lines. P stands for *positive*. You know, things that keep you physically healthy, activities that keep you centered, activities that help you achieve your goals, things that are consistent with your values, and activities that keep you out of trouble.

"OK, next go over the list and put an N next to each of those activities that are essentially *neutral*. These would be the kinds of activities that are not positive or risky; they are just things that are part of your life. They may be obligations or parenting responsibilities. They may be things you do just to pass the time. Again, put your ratings in the box with the dotted lines.

"The next step is to identify those activities that might put you at risk for having more problems with the criminal justice system. Even if these activities did not cause a problem for you during the typical day you wrote about, think about whether they have risk potential. These activities would involve people, places, events, or situations that have led to poor decisions or problems in your past. These might be the kinds of activities that, if you continue doing them, are likely to create problems in the future. Put an R next to each of these activities. R stands for *risky*.

"Now we are going to look at your life from a different perspective and have you consider the level of enjoyment you get out of each activity. Put an E next to anything that brings you joy or pleasure. The E stands for *enjoyment*. Put this rating in the second box with the dotted lines. You may find that some activities you enjoy overlap with activities that you view as healthy; other activities that are fun may overlap with ones that are risky. This is normal for most people, since some positive activities can be enjoyable, and some risky activities can also be exciting.

"OK, next go over the list and put a U next to those activities that are *unpleasant*. These are things that you dislike doing. You know, things that are boring or just negative. Again, put your ratings in the second box with the dotted lines. Lastly, put an OK next to those activities that are medium in terms of enjoyment. These would be the kinds of activities that are not really fun, but are not unpleasant; they are just part of your normal life. These activities may be obligations or things you do just to pass the time.

"Let me know if you get stuck on an activity and are not sure how to rate it."

SCRIPT 10.3. Questions to Ask JICs about Work

PERCEIVED INTEREST AND VALUE IN EMPLOYMENT

"How do you feel about working?"

"How important is it to get a job?"

[If JIC is working:] "How important is your job to you?"

"How important is it for you to maintain employment?"

"Tell me about your career goals."

[If JIC is working:] "Do you see yourself going further with this job?" [If so:] "How far?"

[If JIC does not seem that interested in work:] "Tell me why work is not important to you."

EMPLOYMENT ACHIEVEMENT

"What was the best thing about your last job?"

[If JIC is working:] "What is your favorite part of your current job?"

"What positive recognition have you received in this job or other jobs you have had in the past?"

"Have you been promoted or earned awards through your current job? How about other jobs you have had in the past?"

"What has been your biggest struggle with work?"

"What feedback have your bosses given you about your performance?"

CONFLICTS WITH SUPERVISORS

"How well do you generally get along with people in authority at work?"

"How well do you get along with your boss(es) or supervisor(s)?"

"In the past, who has been your favorite boss? Why?"

"How often do you have disagreements with your bosses or supervisors?"

"Tell me about the biggest disagreement you have had with a boss or supervisor."

[If JIC is working:] "Have you had any conflicts with your current boss?" [If yes:] "Tell me what caused it, and how you resolved it."

(continued)

CONFLICTS WITH COWORKERS

"How well do you get along with the other people at work?"

"Do you consider any of your coworkers friends?"

"What coworkers have you had issues with?"

"Tell me about any significant arguments that you have had at work with coworkers—you know, like yelling, screaming, or threatening."

[If yes to arguments:] "What happened? What did these arguments look like?"

"Have you ever had a physical fight or altercation with a coworker at work?"

WORK ATTENDANCE AND UNEXCUSED ABSENCES

"In general, do you miss work days and sometimes not show up?"

[If JIC is working:] "How many times in the past year have you missed work?"

"What are the reasons you miss work?"

"Where do you go when you miss work?"

"How do your supervisors react when you miss work?"

"Have you gotten into trouble because of absences?"

TERMINATIONS AND IMPULSIVE QUITTING

"Have you been fired or let go from a job in the past?"

[If yes:] "How many times?"

"What was the reason given for you being fired or let go?" [Explore each incident.]

"Have you ever quit a job out of frustration or anger?"

[If yes:] "How many times?"

"Did you give notice?"

"Why did you quit the job?"

FORM 10.1. My Typical Weekday

Pick a recent weekday, and briefly list how your time was spent for each period of the day: morning, afternoon, evening, and night. Be specific and honest in describing your life, and list the people and places that were part of each activity. This is an important first step in organizing your time more productively and taking control of your life.

Morning	6:00							
	7:00							
	8:00							
	9:00							
	10:00							
	11:00							
Afternoon	12:00							
	1:00							
	2:00							
	3:00							
	4:00							
	5:00							
Evening								
Night/Early Morning								

FORM 10.2. My Typical Saturday

Pick a recent Saturday, and briefly list how your time was spent for each period of the day: morning, afternoon, evening, and night. Be specific and honest in describing your life, and list the people and places that were part of each activity. This is an important first step in organizing your time more productively and taking control of your life.

Morning	6:00						
	7:00						
	8:00						
	9:00						
	10:00						
	11:00						
Afternoon	12:00						
	1:00						
	2:00						
	3:00						
	4:00						
	5:00						

Evening							
Night/Early Morning							

FORM 10.3. Looking at My Life and Rating My Activities

Look over the forms you have completed for your activities during a typical weekday and Saturday. Consider each activity you listed, and rate it on two dimensions: (1) the degree to which the activity is helpful in staying out of trouble, and (2) the degree to which the activity is enjoyable. Use the guidelines below to make your ratings. When you're done, each activity should have two ratings next to it.

1. Helpfulness in staying out of trouble: Classify each activity as P, N, or R, based on the descriptions below.

Positive and healthy. Place a P next to activities that you believe are *positive and healthy* for you. These would be the kinds of things that are good for you physically, bring you inner peace, enhance your future, are consistent with your personal values, and/or keep you out of trouble. Examples: "Took a walk to clear my head," "Looked for a new job," "Read my daughter a story," "Exercised," "Meditated," "Volunteered at church," "Read a self-help book," or "Was at work" (if you see your job as a positive thing in your life).

Neutral. Place an N next to activities that you believe are *neutral.* These would be the kinds of things that are part of your life, but are not necessarily either healthy or problematic. These types of activities are often obligations or things that you do just to pass the time. Examples: "Drove an hour to work," "Watched TV," "Played video games," or "Attended a class."

Risky. Place an R next to any activities that you believe are *risky* and might lead to more problems with the criminal justice system. Be honest about your life. Even if the activity did not lead to a bad outcome on the day for which you are rating it, put an R next to any activity that has led to problems in the past, or that you think has the potential to create problems in the future. Examples: "Went to a party where people were using," "Got in an argument with my baby's mother," "Missed my court appointment," "Hung out with John and his friends," or "Got drunk with Jennifer."

2. Degree of enjoyment: Classify each activity as E, OK, or U, based on the descriptions below.

Enjoyable. Place an E next to activities that you find *enjoyable.* These would be the things in your life that are fun and bring you pleasure. Some of these activities may be things you have already rated as *positive.* This is OK, since many positive activities can be enjoyable. Some activities might also be things you have already rated as *risky.* This is also normal, because some risky activities can also be exciting.

OK. Place an OK next to the activities that are in between *enjoyable* and *unpleasant:* They aren't enjoyable, but they aren't unpleasant either. These are activities that you don't mind doing, but that you probably rarely look forward to. These activities could have been rated as *healthy, risky,* or *neutral* when you've considered how helpful they are in staying out of trouble.

Unpleasant. Place a U next to the activities that you find *unpleasant* or do not enjoy. These are activities that you would be willing to go out of your way to avoid doing. These activities could have been rated as *healthy, risky,* or *neutral* when you've considered how helpful they are in staying out of trouble.

FORM 10.4. Questions to Ask Myself about How I Spend My Time

Write your answer to each question below with a short sentence or two. Be prepared to discuss potential solutions or next steps that you might come up with.

Questions to Ask Myself	Answers, Solutions, and Next Steps
What activities are most risky for me during weekdays? On weekends?	
What is at stake if I do not change these risky activities?	
What new activities might replace these that would be more positive and healthy for me?	
What new activities would be more consistent with my values?	
What new activities might I enjoy?	
What is one practical step I could take to replace one high-risk activity?	
I will know my plan is working if . . .	

FORM 10.5. Questions to Ask Myself about Education and Employment

Write your answer to each question below with a short sentence or two. Be prepared to discuss potential solutions or next steps that you might come up with.

Questions to Ask Myself	Answers, Solutions, and Next Steps
How satisfied am I with my current employment situation?	
What would my ideal employment situation look like?	
What type of education or training would help me get closer to my goal?	
What specific things can I do to get more education or job skills?	
What steps can I take to find a job, or a better job?	
What can I do to improve my interview skills for new jobs?	
Once I get a job I like, what are two things I can do to make sure I keep it?	
I will know my career plan is working if . . .	

FORM 10.6. Education and Employment History Checklist

What is your highest level of education?

_____ Some high school

_____ Completed high school or equivalent

_____ Some college, but did not complete degree

_____ Completed undergraduate or college degree

If yes, what degree? _____

_____ Some graduate school

_____ Completed graduate degree

If yes, what degree? _____

_____ Some trade or technical school

If yes, what area? _____

_____ Completed a certificate in a trade or skill

If yes, what skill? _____

_____ Other formal education (please specify) _____

What is (or was) your current legal occupation? _____

_____

What is (or was) your approximate yearly income? _____

_____

On what basis are you currently employed?

_____ Full-time (35 hours or more per week)

If yes, what type of job? _____

_____ Part-time (less than 35 hours per week)

If yes, what type of job? _____

_____ Stay-at-home parent

_____ Student

_____ Unemployed, looking for work

If yes, for how long have you been unemployed? _____

_____ Unemployed, not looking for work

If yes, why are you not looking for work? _____

What skills, training, or talents do you have?

_____

CHAPTER 11

Restructuring Relationships

Friends and Family

Both Jackie and Hank are social individuals; they have regular contact and ongoing relationships with other people. Unfortunately, some of their respective relationships influence them in negative ways (e.g., encourage antisocial actions and discourage prosocial behaviors) and may undermine efforts to change their lifestyles. In this chapter, we present strategies for exploring and restructuring close friendships and family relationships.

Restructuring social networks will often vary from one JIC to another, because of the unique characteristics and the contextual issues related to each person's life. Although the specific social target (i.e., close friendships, family relationships, romantic partners, or a combination of these) may differ across JICs, the approach to modifying maladaptive social connections is similar and generally follows six steps:

1. Identifying high-risk relationships
2. Distancing from high-risk individuals
3. Strengthening existing positive relationships
4. Reestablishing positive relationships that have been dormant
5. Developing new social connections
6. Improving social skills (when necessary)

In Chapter 10, we have described some general principles for modifying JICs' routines related to leisure and employment, and many of these same principles are relevant for restructuring relationships. The strategies described in this chapter should be implemented in a collaborative spirit and should honor JICs' freedom of choice in their relationship decisions. Like the forms and strategies/techniques presented in Chapter 10, the ones presented in this chapter are not intended as tools for detecting violations of probation, parole, or community supervision, but rather for lifestyle improvement. Effectiveness can be undermined if conversations become judgmental in tone (e.g., "You should know by now that nothing good comes from spending time with Tony"). Changes in thinking (from "My boys have my back" to "My current friends are dragging me down") can drive important changes in behavior such as relationship choices. Conversely, taking behavioral steps to change relationships (e.g., approaching new people) will often combat criminogenic thoughts and foster a healthier perspective on social connections (e.g., "I have more in common with Jen's family than I thought"). A sustained focus across sessions will be necessary to have enough of an impact on both thinking and behavior to result in less risky relationship patterns.

ALTERING CLOSE FRIENDSHIPS

Associations with like-minded criminally oriented peers is one of the major criminal risk domains to be targeted in treatment (Cottle, Lee, & Heilbrun, 2001). For JICs in community settings, existing social connections can undermine efforts in treatment to change problematic routines (e.g., aimless use of leisure time) and destructive habits (e.g., substance use), if the existing peer group reinforces criminal thinking patterns and behaviors. For JICs reentering the community from prison, friends can set the stage for a return to substance use, drug selling, gang activities, and other illegal acts (Martinez & Abrams, 2013).

A good first question to consider is "To what extent is the overall pattern of antisocial behavior occurring in the presence of friends (10%, 50%, 80%)?" Once it has been determined how involved friends are in a JIC's pattern of criminal behavior, a good follow-up question to ponder is "How are friends influencing antisocial behaviors?" For example, some JICs admire and respect criminal friends, and will take the lead in engaging in criminal behaviors simply to obtain approval from such individuals. Some JICs will follow others and go along with criminal activities just to fit in and be accepted. A relative isolation from prosocial influences (even in the absence of criminal peers) can also increase risk, because there is no one in an isolated JIC's life to actively express concern about criminal and self-defeating behaviors, and no one to model healthier patterns. As noted in Chapter 8, Hank's antisocial decision making has been strongly influenced by his thoughts about what his friends will think, and this has resulted in a pattern of destructive actions. Jackie, on the other hand, has spent time with friends who suggest antisocial plans that seem exciting to her and that she can easily justify.

A range of other factors affect JICs' choices of persons to spend their time with, and these concerns will also need to be considered. For example, JICs who live in high-crime areas, gang-infested neighborhoods, or isolated rural communities may have limited opportunities to improve their social connections. Similarly, JICs who are incarcerated will certainly have a narrow range of people available for new prosocial friendships; however, decisions about reestablishing friendships with people in the community will become critical when these JICs are making the transition from a prison setting. Some JICs enter treatment with significant impairments (e.g., mental health problems, intellectual disabilities) and limited skills (e.g., lack of concern for others, poor listening), any of which can make forming new friendships challenging or unlikely. You will need to be realistic about the extent to which JICs' relationship patterns can be altered.

Adding another layer of complexity is the fact that different social patterns often emerge among JICs with similar offense histories. For example, some adult sex offenders may have intimacy deficits and may seek out relationships with teenagers; others will find like-minded adult peers who are accepting of deviant sexual practices that society considers criminal (e.g., sex with children). Some drug-involved JICs may spend time with those whose lives center around obtaining or using illicit substances; others may surround themselves with individuals in recovery. Ideologically motivated violent JICs (e.g., terrorists of various political persuasions) may actively seek out and spend time with those who share similar beliefs.

Baseline Monitoring and Rating of Close Friendships

As noted above, a first step is to understand the nature of JICs' close friendships. Script 11.1 and Form 11.1, both provided at the end of this chapter, are useful templates for introducing the topic and providing instructions for describing friendships and making ratings. Here are a few guidelines:

1. Keep the focus current, and ask about close friendships that have been most important and influential during the past year.
2. Emphasize "face-to-face" friends, and not friends with whom JICs mainly interact via social media (Facebook, Instagram, etc.).
3. It is acceptable to include people JICs live with, such as roommates, but do not include close relatives.
4. There may be situations where some family members (such as cousins) may also be considered as close friends, but only if they do not live in the house. Any relative living in the house should be considered someone with whom a JIC has a family relationship; these relationships are discussed in the next section.
5. In those cases where JICs report having numerous close friends (e.g., 30 or 40), ask them to discuss their closest friends (10 at most).
6. Have JICs who are incarcerated fill out Form 11.1 based on (a) people they had relationships with before they were incarcerated, and with whom they have maintained some contact with during their period of custody; and (b) the friends in prison that they expect to maintain after their release.

In the case of Jackie, examining her completed Looking at My Close Friends form (Figure 11.1) reveals a mix of positive and negative influences. On the negative side are the car wash coworkers she was arrested with, as well as a neighbor who, as it turns out, tends to be impulsive and engages in shoplifting and binge drinking. Jackie spends time with this neighbor only when she is bored. On the positive side are a married couple who have a child approximately the same age as Jackie's son, and who have reached out to her for help with child care, play dates, and dinners. Jackie also has a few longer-term prosocial friendships with people who maintain steady work or go to school, who are not involved in high-risk activities, and who have been supportive and helpful to Jackie in the past. Unfortunately, Jackie has let these friendships lapse over time, and particularly during the past year; she has failed to reciprocate offers to get together, and at times has even avoided them. She recognizes that changes in this area could be helpful.

Discussing Behavioral Steps for Restructuring Close Friendships

Once you have a snapshot of a JIC's inner circle of close friends, it is time to discuss potential steps the JIC can take to weaken (distance) or strengthen specific relationships, as well as the possibility of making new friendships. It must be emphasized to the JIC that altering existing relationships

Friend	Description	Rating (+/−)
Ted	At work—got arrested with him. Was in contact almost every day because of work.	−
Maurice	At work—got arrested with him. Same as above: Was in contact almost every day because of work.	−
Gail	Neighbor. Shopping/dancing/movies. Hanging out and drinking. One or two times a week.	−
Timothy & Sara (married)	Neighbors. Child care/movies/dinner One or two times a month.	+
Maya	Friend since high school. Used to go dancing/movies/dinner/shopping/vacations.	+
Sonya	Friend since high school. Same as above: Used to go dancing/movies/dinner/shopping/vacations.	+
Paulina	Friend since middle school. Used to do lots of things together: church/dinners/shopping/etc.	+

FIGURE 11.1. Jackie's completed Looking at My Close Friends form.

is not an easy task, but it is a necessary step to a more positive lifestyle. Eliminating or reducing contact with familiar people (even though they may have a negative influence) and developing new social connections take time and energy.

Present Form 11.2 (provided at the end of the chapter) during a session, allowing the JIC time to consider each question and write each answer. After the form is completed, discuss the responses. For situations where distancing from close friendships is identified as the best course of action, reinforce the JIC's reasons for doing so by eliciting change talk. Discuss specific behavioral steps the JIC can take to gain some distance from high-risk individuals, and troubleshoot potential challenges. Coaching may also be necessary regarding what the JIC can say when such individuals are encountered. There is also the possibility that pulling back from some relationships (e.g., gangs, paranoid individuals) will pose special challenges; JICs may believe that they will be stalked or threatened if they try to remove themselves from these relationships. Such challenges may warrant attention, discussion, and thoughtful planning.

In cases where JICs have a history of prosocial friendships but no current contacts, the focus may involve identifying and then reestablishing prosocial friendships that have been dormant for several years. It is not uncommon for JICs to have had prosocial friends with whom they have gradually lost contact as they've gravitated toward an antisocial lifestyle. Reaching out to a friend with whom there has been no dramatic falling out, but just a natural "drifting away," can be a daunting—but energizing—step for a JIC who is dissatisfied with his or her current lifestyle.

In cases where JICs have no close friendships at all, the first step will be to determine why the person is a "loner." If the person has weak social skills in relating to others, then the task is to make improvements in such skills. These may include maintaining appropriate (or at least not overtly odd) personal hygiene/appearance, posture, eye contact, personal space, verbal tone/inflection, and gestures; decreasing complaining; becoming more reliable; positively reinforcing others; and learning skills for opening conversations, perspective taking, and active listening. If JICs have sufficient social skills but have no close friendships, the task shifts to methods of exposing them to relationship opportunities. You might encourage JICs to attend various prosocial activities, such as a fitness club or hobby-oriented events/meetings (e.g., cards, pottery, cooking, book clubs), with the aim of exposing them to potential new friendships.

Jackie's completed Questions to Ask Myself About My Close Friends form (Figure 11.2) reveals that she is aware of the individuals she needs to distance herself from and those with whom she can more easily reconnect. The most problematic relationships are with the car wash friends she has been spending the most time with over the past year, but they are also relatively recent. Her prosocial friendships are of longer duration but largely dormant. Her challenge in these latter cases is reestablishing contact. She is aware that the lapse in these friendships is largely her own doing, and she desires to change this pattern. The longer she has been out of contact, however, the more difficult she finds it to reach out to her old connections. As a concrete next step, calling Paulina, her oldest friend, is agreed upon as a homework assignment. During the session, addressing Jackie's concerns about how she will be received, rehearsing what she will say, and setting up an approximate day and time to make the call can help make it more likely that Jackie will follow through and successfully complete the assignment.

Questions to Ask Myself	Answers, Solutions, and Next Steps
What friendship puts me at most risk for future problems?	*Ted and Maurice from work.*
What are the most important reasons to distance myself from T & M ____ ?	*Don't want to get arrested again.* *Don't want to waste any more time doing the kind of stuff they do.*
How important is this friendship to me? What will tempt me to spend time with T & M ____ ?	*Not that important right now.* *They were fun and didn't judge me.* *They were nice.*
What specific things can I do, or say, to distance myself from T & M ____ ?	*Don't call or return texts.* *Stay away from the places I know they hang out.*
If I decide to not spend time with T & M ____ , what will I do instead?	*Spend more time with my son.* *Get back in touch with my real friends.* *Move forward with my life.*
What is one specific step I can take to improve my relationships with my positive friends?	*I have to reach out and get in touch. That's on me.* *I could call Paulina and invite Tim and Sara over.*
If I wanted to have more positive friends in my life, where would I find them? What steps would I take?	*I know where they are. I just have to get in touch.*

FIGURE 11.2. Jackie's completed Questions to Ask Myself About My Close Friends form.

Follow-Up and Review of Progress

In subsequent sessions, you will review how well JICs did in taking the steps discussed in the previous meetings (e.g., distancing, strengthening, reestablishing, making new friendships, or practicing basic skills). In cases where JICs are unsuccessful in implementing changes related to their close friendships, identify obstacles such as poor social skills and lack of opportunities for developing new social connections. Remember that relationship change is a process requiring continued focus, so be realistic regarding the time required for successfully altering social networks. For many JICs, restructuring close friendships will be a worthwhile endeavor that will ripple out and significantly reduce a large element of risk inherent in their current lifestyles.

CHANGING FAMILY DYNAMICS

Although family relationships serve important functions in all of our lives, there is no "perfect" family. For most people, a certain degree of family dysfunction is the norm. However, the family lives of JICs tend to be particularly messy and fraught with criminality, mental health problems, substance abuse, and significant intrafamily conflict. Family factors consistently emerge as predictors of recidivism for both men and women (Barrick, Lattimore, & Visher, 2014; Visher, 2013), and therefore offer a promising target for treatment. In terms of risk for future justice involvement, a primary concern is family and romantic relationships that ignore, reinforce, or model criminal behavior. In cases where JICs are enmeshed with family members involved in criminal and other antisocial activities, separation/distancing from or avoidance of specific family members may become a reasonable treatment goal.

Family and marital/romantic relationships may also lack nurturance, or even worse, become sources of ongoing conflict, which can lead to police involvement. Even when the family circle contains "healthy" individuals, JICs themselves often cause significant damage to these relationships. Therefore, repairing key "healthy" family relationships may also be a worthwhile treatment objective (strengthening and reestablishing). In some cases, looking beyond the immediate family, at extended family members, will be necessary for finding more positive relationships (developing new connections).

Baseline Monitoring and Rating of Family/Romantic Relationships

The first step in the intervention process is to get an overview and understanding of current family and romantic relationships. Use Script 11.2 to launch into the discussion and to introduce Form 11.3 (both of these are provided at the end of this chapter). JICs are asked to list their closest family members and current romantic partners (up to 10) and to indicate, for each person, the presence of problems (criminal justice, drugs/alcohol, mental health, and conflict). Each family member and romantic partner is then rated in terms of being generally positive or risky.

In the case of Jackie, her completed Looking at My Family and Romantic Relationships form (Figure 11.3) reveals a small network of family members, but a family with many strengths. She has identified two aunts, one uncle, her mother, her son, and her sisters as her current family relationships. She has also identified her son's father as a previous romantic partner who is still involved in her life. Apart from an aunt with alcohol and behavioral control problems, Jackie describes her family network as generally hard-working, nurturing, and supportive. Jackie's lack of educational and occupational achievement relative to her sisters is a source of friction, however, and her mother's health problems have been an area of concern for all. Jackie's arrest and behavior over the past year have alarmed the family and have led to a few arguments with one of her sisters. The most potentially antisocial and destructive member of the family—her biological father, who had drug and criminal justice issues—abandoned the family when Jackie was very young and has been out of touch for many years. She has cousins who have been involved in the criminal justice system for drug selling, but she has not had contact with that side of the family since she was younger. Her son's father, who has problems with alcohol, remains an ongoing source of conflict. Jackie has not had any other romantic partners in the past year.

Family Member/Romantic Partner	Problem Areas				Rating (+/−)
	Criminal Justice	Drugs and Alcohol	Mental Health	Family Conflict	
1. Mom					+
2. Marissa—sister					+
3. Karla—sister				✓	+
4. Ben—uncle		✓ (years ago)			+
5. Naomi—aunt					+
6. Riley—aunt		✓	✓	✓	−
7. Elliot—son (age 4)					+
8. James—ex, son's father		✓		✓	−
9.					
10.					

FIGURE 11.3. Jackie's completed Looking at My Family and Romantic Relationships form.

Restructuring Family Relationships

Once you have a detailed understanding of the family dynamics, it is time to discuss potential steps JICs can take to alter specific family and romantic relationship patterns: distancing, strengthening, and/or reaching out to family members who are more positive. Use Form 11.4 (provided at the end of the chapter) to structure the conversation.

Distancing involves reducing the amount of time spent, or eliminating contact altogether, with the family members or romantic partners most associated with risk. The steps JICs might take to distance themselves from certain family relationships will be straightforward in some circumstances, but can pose serious challenges in others. Depending on the nature of the relationships and the living situation, some relationships are just easier to distance oneself from than others. For example, an adolescent JIC living with a parent who has criminal justice, substance abuse, and conflict problems may want to distance him- or herself, but will have limited opportunities for doing so. In cases where certain family relationships cannot be altered in the present or near future, the discussion should focus on limiting exposure to that family member and their influence. Reinforcing JICs' autonomy and decision making will be helpful over the longer term. Even though JICs may be forced to live with disturbed or criminally oriented family members, they can still decide their own paths in terms of what they want their lives to be about. They may also be able to choose how much of their leisure time they will spend at home.

Strengthening includes plans to increase contact and spend more time with positive family members and romantic partners. Again, it is not uncommon for JICs to have damaged their connections with healthy family members as they have drifted into criminally oriented lifestyles. Reestablishing such family connections may require effort. In more complicated scenarios, a longer-term plan to repair the damage JICs have caused to healthy family relationships will need to be developed. As a rule, it takes a significant amount of time to rebuild trust in family relationships—and only an impulsive or unfortunate moment to tear it down.

In cases where no or only a few positive family relationships are available, widening the search to include extended family members may provide avenues for positive relationships. Improving social skills (see the discussion of these in the previous section) may apply equally to JICs who are seeking to rebuild family relationships or who want to find more positive romantic partners.

For Jackie, improving family relationships is less about avoiding relationships and more about repairing positive relationships (see Figure 11.4). The most antisocial influence in her family network (an aunt) is one she already avoids as much as possible. Even though Jackie shares parenting responsibilities with her former romantic partner (her son's father), Jackie has also taken steps to distance herself from him as much as possible. Although she has not often demonstrated it recently, Jackie wants to help her mother and spend more time with her, and opportunities to do so are ever present. A useful next step, therefore, is for Jackie to take a greater role in her mother's life by spending one night per week doing an activity with her. Jackie's behavior toward her sisters, which is sometimes resentful, irritable, and impulsive, can be improved by examining the thinking patterns associated with those relationships (see Chapters 8 and 9), as well as rehearsing in session more constructive ways of engaging and responding to her sisters. Despite the friction in these relationships, Jackie values and looks up to her sisters, and they are potentially powerful resources for her in developing a more prosocial lifestyle.

Questions to Ask Myself	Answers, Solutions, and Next Steps
Which people seem to have the most problems? Which have the fewest?	*Aunt Riley has the most: She drinks a lot, she has an anger problem, and she loses control.* *James also drinks and is difficult to deal with.* *Marissa has the fewest: She has a good job, her own place, she makes good decisions.*
Which relationships put me at most risk for future problems?	*James: We argue a lot.* *Karla: We fight and get on each other's nerves, even though we love each other.* *Aunt Riley: She gets into trouble with everyone.*
What are the most important reasons to distance myself from risky family members and romantic partners?	*Aunt Riley can be trouble. She is loud and attracts attention, especially when she is drinking. She gets into real fights.* *James is someone I do not want to spend time with, because we do not get along.*
What specific things can I do or say to distance myself from risky family members and romantic partners?	*I don't have to go out with Aunt Riley to any bar or restaurant. I just keep my time with her to family get-togethers.* *Talk to James less. Only communicate with him when things come up about my son.*
In what ways can I help my family members who have problems?	*My mom needs help with daily stuff—I can help her. I want to do more for her.*
What family and romantic relationships are most healthy for me?	*My mom, my sisters, my Uncle Ben and Aunt Naomi—they are good people.*
What is one specific step I can take to improve my relationships with positive family members and romantic partners?	*I can do more to help my mother—I have to talk to my sisters about that.* *I have to stop arguing with my sisters, especially Karla.*

FIGURE 11.4. Jackie's completed Questions to Ask Myself about My Family and Romantic Relationships form.

Follow-Up and Review of Progress

In moving forward, you will continually review the steps JICs take in altering family and romantic relationships, and troubleshoot difficulties that arise. Since few people get to pick their families, this can be a challenging area to change. Nonetheless, even a small shift in how a JIC relates to one or two specific family members, or a change in a romantic relationship, can alter the JIC's risk profile for the better.

KEY POINTS

- Strategic relationship changes can significantly diminish an influential element of risk inherent in the lifestyles of JICs. Such changes will typically involve relationships with close friends, family members, and romantic partners.

- Understanding the social context of JICs' lives begins with baseline monitoring and risk ratings of existing relationships.

- A critical step in restructuring relationships is to develop awareness about the negative impact of high-risk relationships on JICs' lives and to foster motivation for change.

- Practical steps JICs can take to distance themselves from high-risk individuals are then developed collaboratively.

- Equally important is to develop awareness, motivation, and practical steps for strengthening existing positive relationships, or healthy relationships that have been dormant.

- Ongoing coaching aimed at improving social skills may be necessary for assisting JICs in creating new friendships and romantic relationships.

SCRIPT 11.1. Discussing Close Friendships

"[JIC's name], today I want to talk about the people you hang out with. Most of us have a few people we consider to be close friends. Close friends are people you can reach out to, share your problems with, and put your trust in. The people we spend time with often influence our lives in significant ways.

"You do not have to tell me their full names; you can use nicknames, initials, or first names. Think about your closest friends—people you hang out with the most. List first names or initials in this first column here. [Show Form 11.1.] You do not have to fill in all the spaces; if you just have a few, that's OK. Just a reminder: This is about your friends and not your family.

"In the second column, for each person you listed, briefly describe how you met this friend and the kinds of things you do together. [Get information for each friend listed.]

"In the last column, put a plus sign [+] next to a friend's name if you think that this friend helps keep you out of trouble and generally helps you to make good decisions. If you think that spending time with this friend puts you at risk for future criminal justice problems, place a minus sign [–] next to the friend's name. For example, these would be people you have gotten in trouble with in the past, friends who try to get you to do risky things, people who use drugs and drink heavily, or friends you know who make really poor decisions."

[Ask about each friend listed.]

"Tell me a little about _____, and why he [she] gets a minus. Tell me a little bit about _____, and why he [she] gets a plus.

"Thanks for sharing with me what your inner circle of friendships look like."

SCRIPT 11.2. Discussing Family Relationships

"[JIC's name], every family has problems and struggles. Today let's talk about the types of problems your family has experienced. Think about the family members who are part of your life right now. List them on this form. [Show Form 11.3.] You can list parents, your own children, brothers or sisters, uncles and aunts, nieces and nephews, and cousins. Also, list any romantic partners who are currently a significant part of your life. If you have a big family, you can list up to 10 members. If you have only a few family members, list as many as you can think of.

"Think about the family members and current romantic partners you've listed. As far as you know, which ones have had criminal justice involvement? You know, like being convicted of a crime, being on probation or parole, spending time in prison, or having ongoing problems with the police. Put a checkmark next to each family member or current romantic partner who has experienced these kinds of difficulties. [For each family member or romantic partner where justice involvement has been identified as a problem, explore the details related to the person's criminal history—e.g., "What exactly occurred? When did this happen? How has their behavior influenced you?"]

"Which of your family members and current romantic partners have experienced problems with addiction to alcohol or other drugs? Again, put a checkmark next to each. [Ask for more detail regarding drug and alcohol problems—e.g., "What is your understanding of his or her problem? What are the drugs? How has substance use affected this person's life? What effects has it had on you?"].

"Which of your family members and current romantic partners suffers with a serious mental health issue that you might be aware of? Again, place a checkmark next to each. [Explore the nature of the mental health problems for each person identified—e.g., "What is your understanding of his or her problem? What effects has this problem had on your family? How have you dealt with this?"]

"How do the members of your family generally get along? [If applicable:] How do you get along with your current romantic partner? Who argues or fights the most among your family members? Place a checkmark next to the name of each person who seems to have ongoing conflict with other family members or with you. You know, like major arguments, fights, or long-term grudges. [Explore the nature of family or interpersonal conflict for each person listed—e.g., "What are the arguments or fights with this person like?" Search for aggressive verbal behaviors, such as noisy arguing, yelling, screaming, and insulting; destruction of property, such as throwing objects and breaking doors or walls; and physically assaultive behaviors, such as pushing, shoving, and hitting. Ask: "How bad do arguments get? How much are you usually involved in these arguments or fights? Have family or romantic partner conflicts led to criminal justice problems? Which persons in your family, or in your current romantic relationships, have you had the most trouble getting along with in the past year?"].

"Now look at the chart and consider the overall influence that each family member or current romantic partner has on your life right now. In the last column, put a plus sign [+] for each family member or current romantic partner who has a positive influence on you. You know, people who are there for you when you need them, help you in positive ways, help keep you out of trouble, and generally help you make good decisions. If you think that the person's influence is negative, and spending time with this family member or romantic partner puts you at risk for future criminal justice problems, place a minus sign [−] next to that person's name.

"Thanks for sharing with me what your family and romantic relationships look like."

FORM 11.1. Looking at My Close Friends

Close friends are people you can reach out to, share your problems with, and trust. To get a deeper understanding of how your close friends are influencing your life, fill in the information below for each close friend. In the column labeled Friend, list the first name or initials of each close friend. In the column labeled Description, provide a couple of phrases about each person and your relationship with this person (e.g., how did you meet the person, what types of things do you do together, and how often are you in contact with the person?). In the column labeled Rating, put a plus sign (+) next to each friend who is positive (e.g., keeps you out of trouble, makes good decisions). Put a minus sign (−) next to each friend who is negative (e.g., puts you at risk for trouble, makes poor decisions).

Friend	Description	Rating (+/−)

FORM 11.2. Questions to Ask Myself about My Close Friends

Write your answer to each question below with a short sentence or two. Be prepared to discuss potential solutions or next steps that you might come up with.

Questions to Ask Myself	Answers, Solutions, and Next Steps
What friendship puts me at most risk for future problems?	
What are the most important reasons to distance myself from _____?	
How important is this friendship to me? What will tempt me to spend time with _____?	
What specific things can I do, or say, to distance myself from _____?	
If I decide to not spend time with _____, what will I do instead?	
What is one specific step I can take to improve my relationships with my positive friends?	
If I wanted to have more positive friends in my life, where would I find them? What steps would I take?	

FORM 11.3. Looking at My Family and Romantic Relationships

To get a deeper understanding of how your family is influencing your life, fill in the information below about the family members and romantic partners who are part of your life right now. In the column labeled Family Member/Romantic Partner, list the first name of each family member and describe how this person is related to you. Also, list any current romantic partners who are a significant part of your life. In the column labeled Criminal Justice, check the box if this person has ever been convicted of a crime, on probation or parole, incarcerated, or had ongoing problems with the police. In the column labeled Drugs and Alcohol, check the box if this person has ever experienced significant problems with drugs or alcohol. In the column labeled Mental Health, check the box if this person has ever experienced serious mental health problems. In the column labeled Family Conflict, check the box if this person engages in serious and ongoing conflict (e.g., disagreements, fights) with you or other family members. In the column labeled Rating, put a plus sign (+) next to the name of each person who is positive (e.g., is there if you need help, keeps you out of trouble, helps you make good decisions). Put a minus sign (–) next to the name of each person who is negative (e.g., puts you at risk for more problems).

Family Member/Romantic Partner	Problem Areas				Rating (+/–)
	Criminal Justice	Drugs and Alcohol	Mental Health	Family Conflict	
1.					
2.					
3.					
4.					
5.					
6.					
7.					
8.					
9.					
10.					

FORM 11.4. Questions to Ask Myself about My Family and Romantic Relationships

Write your answer to each question below with a short sentence or two. Be prepared to discuss potential solutions or next steps that you might come up with.

Questions to Ask Myself	Answers, Solutions, and Next Steps
Which people seem to have the most problems? Which have the fewest?	
Which relationships put me at most risk for future problems?	
What are the most important reasons to distance myself from risky family members and romantic partners?	
What specific things can I do or say to distance myself from risky family members and romantic partners?	
In what ways can I help my family members who have problems?	
What family and romantic relationships are most healthy for me?	
What is one specific step I can take to improve my relationships with positive family members and romantic partners?	

CHAPTER 12

Managing Destructive Habits

Substance Use and Anger Reactions

In this chapter, we discuss behavioral steps for changing problems related to substance use and anger reactions. Although these topics may seem at first like strange bedfellows for a chapter, there is frequent comorbidity between anger and substance use problems. Moreover, JICs' verbal and physical anger reactions can develop into habitual and destructive patterns, in a manner much like the misuse of substances. In addition, JICs are often initially resistant to suggestions to change their anger and substance use patterns. Therefore, building awareness and motivation are critical in addressing these criminal risk domains.

CHANGING SUBSTANCE USE PATTERNS

As noted in Chapter 6, Brenda has identified substance use as a treatment target for Hank (but not Jackie). Although Hank's substance use does not rise to the severity of physiological dependence, his use of substances is certainly linked to his legal problems (e.g., he has used substances abusively, has been involved in alcohol-related arrests, and is subject to routine drug testing while he is under criminal justice supervision). Brenda has also identified dysregulated anger as a treatment target for Hank (but, again, not for Jackie). In fact, Hank's most recent offense and several of his previous problems with the law have been the result of anger-related aggressive responses.

Substance Use in the Justice–Involved Population

The focus of this treatment planner as it relates to substances is on the relationship between JICs' substance use on the one hand, and their offending potential and involvement in the criminal justice system on the other. To that end, several facets of the empirical literature on substance use in justice-involved populations are highlighted. First, although estimates of the rates of substance abuse and dependence (as defined in editions of DSM prior to DSM-5; DSM-5 now refers to these diagnoses as mild and moderate/severe substance use disorder, respectively) among justice-involved populations vary significantly from study to study, they are consistently higher than those found in the general population (Staton-Tindall, Havens, Oser, & Burnett, 2011). For example, rates of alcohol abuse or dependence among male inmates have ranged from 18 to 30% (depending upon the study), while rates of other drug abuse or dependence have ranged from 10 to 48% (Fazel, Bains, & Doll, 2006). Among female inmates, rates of alcohol abuse or dependence have ranged from 10 to 24%, while rates of other drug abuse or dependence have ranged from 30 to 60% (Fazel et al., 2006). In community settings, the majority of probationers and parolees have been in substance abuse treatment at least once, and almost 20% report three or more treatment experiences (Substance Abuse and Mental Health Services Administration, 2011). The overall implication is that if you work with JICs in prisons or the community, you can expect that substance use problems will be common among a relatively large percentage of your cases.

A second area of relevant research concerns the causal connections between substance use and criminal/other antisocial behaviors. In a survey of federal and state inmates, almost 20% reported that they committed the offense for which they were incarcerated in order to obtain money to purchase drugs (Karberg & Mumola, 2006). A survey of probationers found that 14% reported being on drugs when they committed their offenses (Bonczar & Mumola, 1998), while a survey of federal and state inmates found that over 25% reported being under the influence at the time they committed the offenses for which they were incarcerated (Karberg & Mumola, 2006). The treatment implications from this literature are that substances (1) can serve as a driver for criminal behavior (linking substance *dependence directly* to criminality), and (2) can operate as a mechanism by which judgment becomes impaired and offending results (linking substance *abuse indirectly* to criminal and antisocial behavior).

A final area of relevant research concerns the frequency with which JICs use substances while they are under criminal justice custody or supervision. Although drugs can be difficult to obtain in prisons, recent studies have found rates of use during incarceration in the double digits and as high as 40% (Andia et al., 2005; Rowell, Wu, Hart, Haile, & El-Bassel, 2012). Similarly, about 30% of probationers reported using drugs within the past month (U.S. Department of Health and Human Services, 2012). Thus many JICs may be actively using substances (abusively or recreationally) at the time they come to treatment, in spite of their criminal justice supervision.

Although treatment of substance dependence (or moderate/severe substance use disorder, as now defined by DSM-5) is beyond the scope and aim of this treatment planner, CBT resources for such treatment are available (see Bishop, 2001, 2014; Marlatt & Donovan, 2005; Wanberg & Milkman, 2008, 2014), as are CBT-oriented self-help programs (see *www.smartrecovery.org*). Also, having your own referral list of professionals in your institution or community who provide intensive services for substance dependence will be invaluable. Our focus in this treatment planner is on substance abuse and misuse, by which we mean substance use placing JICs at risk of further involvement in the criminal justice system.

Is All Substance Use among JICs a Problem?

Although prevalence rates of alcohol and other drug abuse/dependence are reasonably high among those who are justice-involved, obviously not all JICs have a pattern of drug or alcohol misuse. Does this mean that a JIC's regular drinking, occasional marijuana use, or infrequent use of hard drugs is OK? Probably not. Traditional mental health clients who report drinking a few beers a week, who smoke marijuana a few times a month, or who uncommonly use harder drugs may never have their substance use become a part of their treatment plan. However, alcohol and especially drug use that might be regarded as somewhat normative or nonharmful for a traditional mental health client must be understood in a different context during work with JICs, because of the restrictive conditions often imposed by the criminal justice system in correctional and community settings.

Any alcohol use by those who are incarcerated is illegal. A JIC who brews *pruno* (prison hooch) in a cell, or who obtains alcohol from the outside, is risking disciplinary action and new criminal charges. The fact that the amount consumed might be within the World Health Organization's (Babor & Higgins-Biddle, 2001) guidelines for nonharmful drinking is irrelevant. Similarly, any drug use in prison is illegal. Even in states where marijuana use has been decriminalized or legalized, inmates engaging in marijuana use are risking acquiring new criminal charges.

Substance use among community-based JICs (on probation or parole) must also be placed within the context of the restrictions imposed by the criminal justice system. Probationers and parolees typically have prohibition clauses as part of their conditional release and are subjected to regular testing to ensure compliance. Failure to remain abstinent from drugs or alcohol can result in a technical violation and a subsequent return to custody. Thus even low levels of use of any illicit substance can put these JICs at risk for a criminal justice sanction. Alcohol use, even for those over 21 years old, can be restricted by parole and probation officers and is routinely forbidden at halfway houses and other transitional housing programs. For JICs who are living in their own residences, a home visit by a probation or parole officer that reveals the presence of alcohol (e.g., beers in the refrigerator), while not resulting in a violation, is not going to be viewed positively and is going to be a source of concern for the officer.

Finally, even what seem like nonharmful levels of illicit substance use can increase a JIC's risk for further justice involvement through subtle social mechanisms that can be easily overlooked by practitioners. For example, JICs who use marijuana must purchase it, which puts them in contact with drug sellers and a network of antisocially oriented individuals. Cannabis use is also very likely to occur in a social environment, increasing contact with companions likely to have some degree of criminal risk potential. The more frequent the use, the less time spent on more productive activities with prosocial influences. Lastly, the physical presence of marijuana, detected by way of urinalysis testing, may prevent JICs from passing preemployment drug testing.

Overall, a conservative approach to substance use is the best course of action for JICs in terms of reducing their risk for reoffending and further justice involvement. In this regard, the less they use the better, and abstinence may be best of all. For JICs who are unwilling to consider abstinence, successfully completing their period of criminal justice supervision will probably require a significant reduction in the frequency or quantity of substance use and changes to the situations in which they use. It is important to point out, however, that most JICs will eventually be discharged from their correctional supervision requirements (i.e., released from custody, terminated from probation or parole), at which time they are free to do as they please. Overall, the plan should be to educate and support JICs toward a degree of substance use that does not create problems in life functioning, whether this is abstinence or controlled use.

In developing alcohol treatment goals with a JIC, you may want to consider the guidelines for nonharmful alcohol use released by the World Health Organization (Babor & Higgins-Biddle, 2001): (1) no more than three drinks per day on average for men, and no more than two drinks a day on average for women; (2) no more than four drinks on any one occasion; (3) no drinking in situations that could lead to social harm (e.g., problems at work or with finances) or damage to physical health (e.g., fetal effects in pregnant women, liver problems); and (4) abstaining at least 1 day per week. Establishing similar goals with respect to drug use is more difficult, especially for JICs who are being drug-tested. For JICs who are reluctant to pursue abstinence from drugs even while being drug-tested, conversations about the impact of a given substance on their decision making and criminal justice involvement can be helpful.

Regardless of the particular goal, we offer several overarching recommendations for implementing behavioral interventions focused on substance use:

1. *Do your homework first.* Behavioral interventions are implemented after an assessment and case formulation have been conducted (see Chapters 5 and 6), and after a focusing session (see Chapter 7). When sufficient time is devoted to the assessment and focusing process, a collaborative relationship and shared goals in this area are much more likely to emerge, resulting in less defensiveness and greater engagement and motivation for change.

2. *Don't neglect relevant criminogenic thoughts and thinking patterns.* Behavioral interventions are intended to supplement, not replace, work on criminogenic thinking patterns (see Chapters 8 and 9). Addressing the thought processes that precede substance use are crucial, especially when that use occurs during treatment and under circumstances in which JICs are being tested for alcohol or drugs, or in which the use could have led to further antisocial and criminal activity. Behavioral interventions provide a natural next step after cognitive restructuring. For example, a productive discussion that addresses a JIC's tendency to underestimate the likelihood of violating his or her probation with a positive drug test for marijuana can be followed up with practical behavioral steps that can be taken to replace the marijuana use with an enjoyable prosocial activity.

3. *Integrate values into the discussion.* Substance use that is destructive or that can lead to criminal justice involvement is probably inconsistent with whatever values JICs have verbalized (see Chapter 4). Incorporating the identified values from previous conversations into substance use discussions will help JICs set behavioral steps for change, face setbacks productively, and stay motivated to persist in making changes in this criminal risk domain.

Working with Clients Who Are Reluctant to Address Substance Use

As we have mentioned in prior chapters, it is common for JICs to minimize past and potential future harm associated with their substance use. For example, an alcohol-related fight is described as having been started by "the other guy"; an arrest for DUI is attributed to "cops having to write tickets"; and marijuana use is "something that's legal in Washington State, so I shouldn't be arrested for it here." JICs whose referring offenses were not explicitly alcohol- or drug-related may be particularly resistant to addressing their substance use; they are likely to see any conditions imposed by the criminal justice system as blatantly unfair and disconnected from their legal problems.

Taking a judgmental stance or tone, or one that is intended to "cut through the bullshit," is likely to result in further resistance and defensiveness. Similarly, offering advice is likely to result in rationalizations that support maintaining current use patterns. In addition, in a court-mandated or correctional context, a JIC who believes that his or her disclosure about substance use will lead to further sanctions is unlikely to discuss the subject honestly.

Our recommendation for avoiding these pitfalls is to remember that your role is not to convince JICs that change needs to happen. Rather, your role is to guide JICs into exploring the impact of their substance use on their decision making, and the possible consequences of continuing this pattern while being involved with the criminal justice system. The hope is that such an exploration will allow JICs to convince themselves of a need for change. Many of the skills discussed in Chapters 3 and 7 provide the foundation for doing this. Eliciting and reinforcing change talk, and affirming positive changes as they occur, will be more effective than threats and advice giving. Make an effort to elicit change talk (e.g., "How could changing your marijuana use make a difference while you're on probation?" or "How might your relationship with your son look if you changed your drinking?"). Also, take advantage of opportunities to reinforce naturally occurring change talk ("So what you're telling me is that smoking pot right now is pretty self-destructive," "It seems like you're coming to the conclusion that there would be far less conflict in your relationship if you weren't drinking"). When JICs move in a positive direction, affirm those steps ("You've come a long way on this goal in the past few weeks," "Changing was harder than you expected, but you've persevered").

Form 12.1 (presented at the end of this chapter) is intended to provide a structure for enhancing awareness and motivation. A completed example of this form for Hank is provided in Figure 12.1. In the column on the left in Form 12.1, JICs record the types of substances they have used in the past year. For each one, they check the box indicating whether the use could lead to more criminal justice involvement or a potential problem in other life areas. After the form is completed, use open-ended questions to explore the reasons behind the boxes that have been checked. As always, take advantage of emerging opportunities to evoke and reflect change talk. Follow up with questions like the ones below in order to work on establishing a goal:

"Given your current situation, what's the best goal for you in regard to substance use?"
"What would that goal look like?"
"What might be challenging about achieving that goal?"
"At times in your life when you have had a less risky pattern of use, what were you doing differently than you are doing now?"
"What do you stand to lose if you do not get a handle on your use?"

As suggested above, JICs may be hesitant to complete paperwork related to substance use for fear of negative consequences by criminal justice personnel. It is crucial to emphasize that monitoring substance use patterns (see below) is an important step toward a more positive lifestyle.

Monitoring Substance Use

A practical step in making changes to a JIC's use of substances is to have the JIC keep a log to record this use. Initially, the log will help you get a snapshot of the frequency and context of use.

Substance	Problem Areas				
	Criminal Justice	Interpersonal Conflict	Work/School	Emotional	Behavioral
1. Alcohol	✓	✓		✓	✓
2. Marijuana	✓	✓	✓		✓
3.					
4.					
5.					
6.					
7.					

FIGURE 12.1. Hank's completed Looking at My Substance Use form.

It also provides an opportunity to increase awareness of a habit that may have become automatic, and to be mindful of its impact. Over time, the log also provides a gauge of progress in this criminal risk domain. Like activity monitoring (see Chapter 10), substance use monitoring is not intended to be a tool for detecting violations of probation, parole, or other community supervision. It must be presented in a spirit of collaboration, with the intention of helping the JIC make changes that can keep him or her out of the criminal justice system.

To start, ask the JIC to record each use of alcohol and drugs between the current and next appointment (see Form 12.2, provided at the end of this chapter). In the Description column, the JIC provides a snapshot (by jotting down phrases) of each episode of use for that day: the type of substance used, the amount, and the situation in which it occurred. In the Rating of Enjoyment column, the JIC writes an E if the substance use was experienced as *enjoyable,* a U if the use was *unpleasant,* and an OK if it was somewhere in between. The purpose of rating enjoyment is to provide you with a marker of how important and reinforcing the substance use is to the JIC. Substance use that is routinely rated as enjoyable will require a much more challenging search for alternative activities that are equally or more enjoyable. Conversely, if a JIC sees that the ratings of use are primarily OK or even unpleasant, it can enhance motivation to make changes, and reduce the sense of such substances' importance in the client's life.

In the Rating of Risk column, the JIC writes an R next to each episode of use that could have resulted in criminal justice problems. This may include use during a period of drug testing, or drinking to the point where there was a loss of control over behavior. The JIC writes an N next to episodes of use perceived as safe or neutral in terms of likely legal problems. The purpose of the risk rating is to enhance awareness about the connection between use and further criminal justice or life problems. A script for introducing Form 12.2 is provided in Script 12.1 (also provided at the end of the chapter).

When a JIC brings a completed log to treatment, reinforce the client for completing the homework assignment, and then review the material on the log. Start by discussing each episode of substance use in the Description column, exploring the details about the context in which the use occurred. This should be helpful in identifying the problematic companions, family members, leisure activities, or emotional states that facilitate use. This process can also be helpful in identifying any criminogenic thoughts associated with use (which can be addressed through the cognitive restructuring activities discussed in Chapters 8 and 9). After reviewing the material in the Description column, discuss the ratings. If substance use has been rated as enjoyable, brainstorm other activities the JIC might possibly engage in that are equally enjoyable, but do not involve substances. If substance use has been rated as risky, inquire about what made the use risky, and reinforce any change talk that emerges. If an episode of use that strikes you as risky has been rated neutral, try to capture the thought process that made the substance use seem neutral to the JIC. This may reveal a relevant criminogenic thought that you can address in a cognitive restructuring discussion. For substance use that is rated as OK or unpleasant, and also risky, highlight the JIC's perception of costs relative to the lack of benefits, and identify alternative behaviors the person can engage in during similar situations. If the log reveals that progress has been made in changing substance use patterns from the prior session, close the discussion with a new goal for next session (or a commitment to continue working toward the current goal). Continue to use the completed logs to provide a gauge of progress.

Identifying Specific Behavioral Steps for Changing Substance Use

A review of Form 12.2 can set the stage for a discussion of practical steps to reduce and/or replace substance use. Form 12.3 provides a structure for JICs to articulate the specific activities and people that facilitate their substance use, and to consider approach and avoidance goals to change existing patterns. Like the Questions, Answers, and Next Steps . . . forms in previous chapters, this form is not intended to be completed as a homework assignment. It should be completed and reviewed in session. The conversation it generates is intended to lead to one or more behavioral steps to be taken before the next session. This process starts with a JIC generating possible alternative activities, as well as different individuals with whom the JIC can spend time that will facilitate the changes the client is working toward. In discussing these activities and individuals, you can focus on those changes the JIC seems most interested in pursuing and those the JIC perceives as the most rewarding; ideally, you are looking for activities that are more rewarding than the JIC's current pattern of use. In discussing next steps, you should feel free to provide suggestions if the JIC seems stuck, and scale back next steps that seem unrealistic. As with other behavioral homework assignments, next steps should be those you are confident the JIC can achieve.

Hank's completed Questions, Answers, and Next Steps for My Substance Use form is presented in Figure 12.2. The answers to his first three questions reveal some challenges in making changes in this area. First, Hank identifies a number of people who would probably interfere with his plan to reduce his alcohol use and stop smoking marijuana (at least while he is under supervision). Second, the number of people who would support the change in his use is significantly smaller, and he's been disconnected with them for a long time. Third, his initial ideas about next steps are vague (e.g., "get another Friday night activity") and unrealistic (e.g., "move, get a new phone"). Clearly, Hank and Brenda will need to give further attention to his network of friends (see Chapter 11 for behavioral steps focused on altering companions) before meaningful steps can be taken in this area.

However, Hank's responses to the last two questions provide an opportunity for immediately implementing some small next steps that have a high likelihood of success. In reply to the question about possible new activities, Hank has listed three that he may be interested in trying out—weightlifting, reading, and detailing cars. Further discussion reveals that reading is of relatively low interest to Hank, while detailing requires technical training and coursework. Weightlifting, on the other hand, is of high interest, due to a neighbor who has invited Hank to lift "any time." A next step of getting in touch with the neighbor to lift weights is established for the next session. For the question about old activities, Hank lists running and small engine repair. He was on the track team in high school and genuinely enjoyed running, but let it go as he got older. He has an interest in getting back in shape. A next step of calling Tony (a former friend and track teammate, who is also listed as one of the people who may encourage his change in substance use) to go for a run is also established for the next session. Hank has previously demonstrated some skill in repairing small motors for neighbors and friends for small amounts of money; how he might reestablish this former activity is a topic for a later session.

In subsequent sessions, you will review the JIC's progress on the step discussed in the previous meeting, along with the newly completed Log of Weekly Substance Use. If a next step has been successfully completed and has led to the expected change in substance use, remember to affirm the JIC's behavioral change, and discuss ways to keep the change going. If appropriate, set a new goal in the same area for the next session.

Question: In what situations is my use most likely to lead to trouble?

Answer: *Spending time with Brendan and Jason after they get off work on Friday—always drinking, smoking, looking for trouble.*

Next Step: One step I can take right away to avoid those situations is *get another Friday night activity or stay home.*

Question: Who are some people I know who might hold me back in changing my pattern of use?

Answer: *Brendan, Jason, Andre, Kelly, Ashley, Tina.*

Next Step: One step I can take right away to avoid those people is *move, get a new phone, tell them I need to change some things about how I live so I can stay out of trouble and get back on track.*

Question: Who are some people I know who will probably encourage me in changing my pattern of use?

Answer: *Tony, Amy.*

Next Step: One step I can take right away to spend more time with them is *to reach out to them— we haven't talked in a long time.*

Question: What are some *new* activities that I could try out when I would otherwise be using?

Answer: *Weightlifting, reading, auto detailing.*

Next Step: One step I can take right away to try these new activities is *get together with a friend who does weightlifting in his garage.*

Question: What are some *old* activities that I used to enjoy (but haven't been doing lately) that I can try again?

Answer: *Running, small engine repair.*

Next Step: One step I can take right away to do these activities is *stretch and run tomorrow.*

FIGURE 12.2. Hank's completed Questions, Answers, and Next Steps for My Substance Use form.

If the JIC has been unsuccessful in implementing the next step, review what went wrong. Look for low motivation, lack of opportunity, a criminogenic thinking pattern, and/or lack of skills. Do not reassign the next step until you think you have successfully addressed the problem and are reasonably certain the client will be capable of carrying it out. Scale back the next step if necessary; you are looking to establish a pattern of success and sense of accomplishment when it comes to homework assignments. This often means starting small.

Announcing Change and Soliciting Support

Imagine that you frequently indulge in pastries—the fatty, creamy, highly unhealthy, but thoroughly enjoyable type. In order to stem your rising cholesterol levels, you decide to cut back on your intake of these delicacies, and you tell your closest friends about this new change in your diet. The simple act of telling your friends about this planned change may set off a series of changes in their behavior toward you—changes that are seemingly innocuous, but not inconsequential. First, they may express support for your intentions and praise you for taking a healthy step forward. Over the days and weeks ahead, they may refrain from casually offering you a rich pastry when you meet them for coffee, and if they see you contemplating ordering a pastry, they may try to persuade you to do otherwise. When they see you, they may specifically ask you how the dietary change is going, and praise you if it's going well, or give you encouragement to give it another try if you tell them you're struggling to stick with it. You may feel highly uncomfortable at the prospect of ordering a pastry in their company, and you may even feel uncomfortable ordering one when you are by yourself, because doing so is inconsistent with your stated intentions to change. On the other hand, if you keep your intended dietary change to yourself, support from your friends will be absent, and they may even inadvertently encourage you to alter your intended course by offering you all the goodies you are trying to avoid. Furthermore, the social pressure to keep to your stated intentions will be absent. In short, through a variety of inter- and intrapersonal mechanisms, making your planned change in diet known to others can make it more likely that you will accomplish your goal.

Giving JICs the homework assignment of telling important people in their lives about the changes they plan to make in their substance use can be similar to the pastry scenario described above: It can make this behavioral goal more tangible, provide a greater sense of accountability for achieving it, and allow them to obtain support from the people who matter most to them. Moreover, this homework assignment need not be restricted to JICs who need to make *major* changes in their substance use. You can encourage JICs who plan on making relatively minor changes in their alcohol or drug use to make it known to important people in their life, and to solicit support from others.

This is not an easy assignment, however. JICs may be uncertain of what to say, or may find the prospect of telling close friends or family members about this step to be embarrassing. They may also fear that it will lead to uncomfortable questions. For these reasons, we recommend practicing this assignment in session before having a JIC carry it out as homework. Be adventurous and role-play a potential situation of self-disclosure that may occur. Form 12.4, together with Script 12.2 (both provided at the end of the chapter), can be used to structure the assignment for the first time.

In Step 1, have the JIC identify one or two people who are likely to be supportive of the change. Discuss the suitability of the identified person(s). You are looking for an "easy case" for the first trial. An easy case is a friend or family member with whom the JIC has regular contact, and who will probably readily support the planned change. In Step 2, provide Form 12.4 to help the JIC develop a script that can be used for telling the other person. The script should not be long; it is best to communicate the planned change briefly, perhaps in four to eight sentences. The script should be structured into four parts. First, it should provide a brief introduction of the topic that tells the other person about the planned change in substance use. Second, the script should explain why the JIC is making this change. The client can list a few reasons that relate to decreasing the chances of criminal justice involvement or improving other life areas. Third, the script should explain that the client is telling people who are important to him or her, in order to make it more likely that the client will be successful in making this change. Last, the script should explain that the JIC is hoping the other person will support him or her. If possible, it should also let the other person know one specific way to be helpful in supporting this change. A completed script for Hank is presented in Figure 12.3.

In Step 3, ask the JIC to read the script out loud to you as a rehearsal. Provide the client with positive feedback by identifying one thing that strikes you as effective about the script. If necessary, provide some constructive feedback about a few things to change, and have the JIC make revisions. Rehearse the new script with the JIC a few times until the client is comfortable delivering it. Establish an approximate date and time when the JIC thinks he or she will be able to carry out the assignment, and let the client know that you will be following up next time to see how it goes.

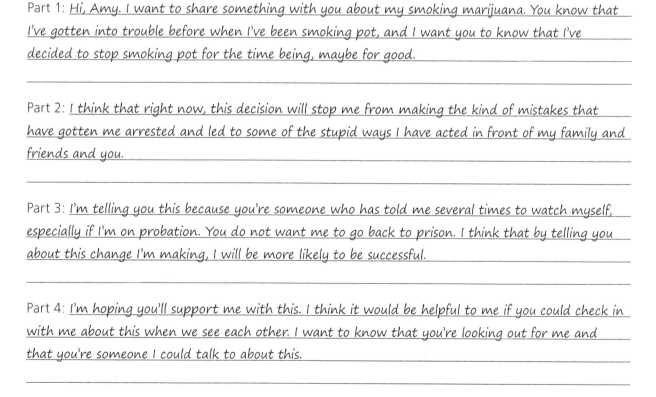

Part 1: *Hi, Amy. I want to share something with you about my smoking marijuana. You know that I've gotten into trouble before when I've been smoking pot, and I want you to know that I've decided to stop smoking pot for the time being, maybe for good.*

Part 2: *I think that right now, this decision will stop me from making the kind of mistakes that have gotten me arrested and led to some of the stupid ways I have acted in front of my family and friends and you.*

Part 3: *I'm telling you this because you're someone who has told me several times to watch myself, especially if I'm on probation. You do not want me to go back to prison. I think that by telling you about this change I'm making, I will be more likely to be successful.*

Part 4: *I'm hoping you'll support me with this. I think it would be helpful to me if you could check in with me about this when we see each other. I want to know that you're looking out for me and that you're someone I could talk to about this.*

FIGURE 12.3. Hank's completed Announcing Change form.

In the subsequent session, explore how the change-announcing episode went. If the JIC has completed the assignment, reinforce the follow-through. If it went well, work to identify another person or two the JIC thinks it would be helpful to tell, and then modify the script if necessary, to fit the new person(s). Over time, it may be possible to have the JIC gradually announce intended changes to his or her larger network of family and friends, as well as to individuals who have traditionally been negative influences, such as friends or family members with whom the JIC has used substances in the past.

If the JIC has not been successful in completing the assignment, do not simply reassign it without first discussing the nature of the difficulty that came up. If the barrier appears to have been one of discomfort, consider having the JIC rehearse the script several more times until it feels more automatic. If the barrier is related to a concern about how the other person will respond, help the JIC identify a more suitable target who will be highly supportive. When you feel confident that barriers have been resolved and the JIC is in a position to succeed, go ahead and set up a new approximate date and time for completing the assignment.

MANAGING ANGER

In working with Hank, Brenda has come to realize that he has a problem with emotion dysregulation (specifically anger), and she considers this an important treatment target. (Like substance use, this domain is not relevant for Jackie.) Most crucial is that Hank's anger appears to be a driver for the sorts of physically aggressive behaviors that have been a major source of his criminal justice problems. Hank's anger also interferes with his ability to maintain romantic relationships, which is one of his values. Providing Hank with anger management skills will reduce his risk and improve his overall interpersonal functioning.

For some cases, a higher level of treatment or care may be required to address excessive emotional dysregulation, and this is certainly true of out-of-control anger. Depending on the setting where you work and on your training and expertise, you may be equipped to provide such in-depth treatment. In this section, we describe some basic steps for providing JICs with a foundation of anger management skills. See Appendix B for additional resources for addressing anger problems.

Conceptualizing Pathological Anger

Most JICs do not voluntarily attend treatment for anger problems, any more than they voluntarily attend substance abuse treatment. They typically participate in treatment at the insistence of friends, family members, employers, or the criminal justice system, and are ambivalent about whether anger is a problem they want to work on. To make matters worse, several common beliefs can interfere with responsiveness to anger treatment.

The prevailing mindset of most people experiencing anger is to see themselves as having been transgressed upon or otherwise treated unfairly, and to believe that other people *should* have acted differently (Fernandez, 2010; McCullough, Kurzban, & Tabak, 2013; Wranik & Scherer, 2010). In addition, it is typical for people to view their own actions as justified when they are recalling the circumstances surrounding their anger reactions.

Another thinking pattern likely to interfere with the success of anger treatment is the idea that it is healthy to express anger. Venting anger sometimes feels right and may provide the temporary illusion of relief (in the same way that avoiding talking to new people feels right for those with social anxiety). Few would argue that avoidance cures anxiety or that venting makes people less angry. The notion that anger must be expressed or it will build up and lead to physical illness or increased aggression has been largely debunked, with most experts agreeing that venting (e.g., catharsis) as an intervention actually makes people worse (Bushman, 2002; Lohr, Olatunji, Baumeister, & Bushman, 2007).

Another common view is that anger is completely controlled by outside forces. You will regularly hear JICs say that "He [she, they, or it] made me angry." People who see the cause of their anger as wholly externally controlled will be unlikely to want to change it. Other beliefs that can interfere with anger treatment are related to the functionality of anger episodes: "My anger protects me," and "Anger gets me what I want."

In work on the anger domain with JICs, you will have to begin with acknowledging perceived transgressions at the hands of others. Over time however, these conversations must shift away from the "bad," "immoral," or "unfair" behavior of others to exploring whether JICs' reactions really help them face their problems effectively, negotiate outcomes they want, or live according to what they value most. Also, a lack of skills (e.g., social, cognitive, and problem-solving skills) can contribute to the idea that anger is an automatic and uncontrollable reaction to adversity. Exploring the outcomes of anger episodes and developing new skills for responding to life's challenges provide the foundation for treatment.

Hallmarks of Disturbed Anger

Because anger is a normal and common human experience, and there is no agreed-upon formal diagnostic criteria set for an anger disorder, it is sometimes difficult to determine whether anger is a worthwhile treatment target. There are four hallmarks of disturbed anger that will serve as useful guides (Tafrate & Kassinove, 2018). First is *frequency:* How often is the JIC feeling angry? Normal adults feel anger about once or twice a week; incidents of anger beyond these normal frequencies indicate a potential problem. Second is anger *intensity:* How strong is the anger experience? Most well-adjusted adolescents and adults can modulate their anger, more or less, depending upon the triggering stimulus. JICs who seem to have "all-or-nothing" responses to negative life events will have intense anger experiences that can be associated with verbal conflict and aggression. Third is *duration:* How long does the anger last? Most anger episodes last from a few minutes to a few hours. Anger that is connected to ongoing rumination about the triggering event, and that festers for weeks or even years, is beyond the normal experience. The final hallmark of disturbed anger is the *extent to which anger is connected to negative life outcomes:* What are the problematic consequences of anger reactions? There are both benefits and costs to anger. When anger episodes result in vocational or school disruption, serious conflicts, criminal justice involvement, significant damage to relationships, road rage, aggressive behaviors, and/or substance use, these are markers that treatment is necessary.

The Anger Episode Model

It is generally not productive to talk with JICs about anger in generalities or abstract terms; focusing on recent and specific anger episodes from JICs' lives will be more effective. Anger occurs as part of a chain of events, and all anger episodes follow a predictable pattern. The *anger episode model* (Figure 12.4) provides a structure for understanding the five basic components of anger as they naturally occur for a particular JIC (Kassinove & Tafrate, 2002; Tafrate & Kassinove, 2018).

Anger begins with a *triggering event,* which usually involves an unwanted and aversive action by another person or persons. Triggers are most commonly verbal (e.g., insults, criticisms, or being the target of wrong accusations, disrespect, or gossip), but they can also be physical (e.g., being pushed, shoved, or hit). For Hank's most recent offense, the trigger was being pressured by a female acquaintance to lend his car to her.

The second component is *thinking,* or belief patterns related to the trigger. These patterns most commonly include *demandingness* (the view that others *must* do what the JIC wants, or the idea because the JIC expects something to happen, it must happen). Other anger-specific thinking patterns are *awfulizing* (blowing things out of proportion when in fact they are manageable), *low frustration tolerance* (underestimating one's ability to handle adversity), *global negative ratings of others* (e.g., viewing a transgressor in extreme terms), and *negative assumptions* (misinterpreting and attributing malevolent intentions to the relatively neutral actions of others, or assuming the worst). Hank's thinking in the incident that led to his arrest was demanding ("She should respect my decision and stop nagging me about this") and also reflected a low tolerance for frustration ("I can't deal with her bullshit").

The third component is the JIC's *personal experience* of anger. This component includes internal elements, such as the intensity of anger (usually as rated on a 0–10 scale), physical sensations (e.g., muscle tension, rapid heart rate, headaches, and gastrointestinal symptoms), and how long the episode lasts (i.e., duration). For Hank, his anger quickly escalated in this situation (i.e., he

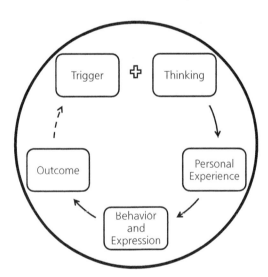

FIGURE 12.4. The anger episode model. Adapted with permission from Impact Publishers, Inc. Copyright © 2009 Raymond Chip Tafrate and Howard Kassinove.

reports that at the time of the altercation it was about a 9 out of 10), and he noticed muscle tension in his back and shoulders. The episode continued for about 30 minutes until the argument worsened and the police arrived.

The fourth component consists of the *behavior and expressive patterns* associated with the specific episode of anger. The most common anger-related behaviors tend to be verbal (e.g., yelling, accusing, threatening, sarcasm, and arguing). Other behaviors include physical expressions (e.g., glaring, provocative gestures, hitting, shoving, and destruction of property), avoidance (e.g., withdrawal and distraction), indirect expression (e.g., gossiping, spreading rumors, not following rules, not responding, and not performing at expected levels), holding anger in (e.g., rumination and holding grudges), and alcohol and drug use. It is also important to recognize that anger is not always bad, and that many anger episodes will include behaviors aimed at fixing or resolving problems. Hank's expressive patterns during the episode in question included swearing and shoving (he harshly pushed the woman to the ground, where she hit her head on the concrete).

The final and most important anger component is *outcome*. Every anger episode results in some type of outcome, which may be negative, neutral, or positive. Short-term outcomes are those that appear immediately (e.g., others' negative reactions or their compliance with angry demands). Some outcomes will be longer-term and require more exploration to raise JICs' awareness of the actual costs of anger (e.g., damage to relationships, loss of respect from others, loss of employment, ongoing legal difficulties, and health problems). The short-term outcome for Hank included getting arrested, while the longer-term outcomes involved ongoing criminal justice problems (a new criminal offense), mandated treatment, loss of his friendship with the woman, and loss of respect from certain friends (the responses of friends varied; some reinforced Hank's aggressive reaction, while others did not).

Often, when anger episodes end negatively, they set the stage for new anger episodes (see the dashed arrow in Figure 12.4). For example, consider a JIC whose anger episode is triggered by an argument with a customer at work. The incident ends with the JIC's insulting the customer and hanging up the phone. The customer then complains to a supervisor, who later confronts the JIC on his or her unprofessional behavior. Unfortunately, this leads directly into a new anger episode—a disagreement with the supervisor. For some JICs, one anger episode cycles into another and still another, creating ongoing drama and chaos.

There are several advantages to analyzing specific episodes of anger. Many JICs are oblivious to the short- and long-term costs associated with their anger, and this type of analysis enhances their awareness, thus setting the stage for treatment. Awareness that anger is having a negative impact on functioning is a prerequisite for taking active steps to change it. This approach also provides details about the specific components of a JIC's anger, allowing you to tailor treatment accordingly. For example, certain triggers can be avoided, thinking patterns can be changed, and new behavioral skills can replace anger responses that lead to bad outcomes. Script 12.3 (provided at the end of the chapter) includes specific questions for analyzing the five components of anger episodes.

Monitoring Anger Episodes

The anger episode model has been translated into a self-monitoring record (see Form 12.5 at the end of the chapter) as a simple way to understand anger patterns. It can be applied in several ways, depending on the level of a JIC's motivation. We recommend that the first Anger Episode Record be completed in session with the JIC, so that you can troubleshoot any problems and address questions. One way to use the record is to have the JIC complete it for the most significant anger episode that has occurred since the last appointment. Reviewing the most significant anger episode can be repeated at the beginning of subsequent sessions and will provide a good snapshot of what anger looks like in the person's day-to-day life. For a JIC who is more motivated to work on anger, the record can be used as an ongoing self-monitoring tool. Provide multiple copies of the record, and ask the JIC to complete a copy for each significant episode of anger experienced. A completed Anger Episode Record for Hank is provided in Figure 12.5.

Interventions

The specific aim of treatment is to reduce a JIC's anger reactivity to commonly experienced triggers, with the overarching goal of reducing future criminal justice involvement. Depending on the nature of the information obtained from the analysis of anger episodes, and on the JIC's awareness of negative anger outcomes and desire to reduce anger, several CBT interventions may be used. Below is a menu of skills-building strategies to consider. Keep in mind that changing entrenched patterns will take time, and that these interventions require active practice and repetition.

Relaxation

The goal of developing relaxation skills is to help a JIC slow down and take stock of a situation, increase awareness of physical activation, and become less immediately reactive to anger triggers. Learning to pause and remain calm in the face of disappointments, setbacks, and provocations interrupts the anger sequence. There are many ways to practice relaxation, such as simple deep breathing (taking calming breaths), repeating calming words, yoga, exercise, mindfulness meditation, and progressive muscle relaxation (a technique that involves tensing and releasing specific muscle groups). A vast array of relaxation videos and instructions can be found on the internet. When deciding on a method, ask the JIC to pick the one that seems most acceptable and that can be practiced most readily as part of his or her daily routine.

Problem Solving

An impulsive and careless problem-solving style is characteristic of how many JICs face life's difficulties. The goals of problem-solving training are to help a JIC invoke a calm and objective perspective when facing challenges; to enable the JIC to search for reasonable (but often not perfect) solutions; and to foster personal growth through the process of finding better solutions to life's problems. JICs often get caught up in their anger and do not ask a very basic question: "Is what I'm doing working?" Reacting constructively to difficult people and situations requires a willingness to slow down the decision-making process and explore new behaviors. The steps for problem solving are (1) identifying an ongoing problem, (2) generating potential solutions or multiple responses, (3) assessing the probable outcomes of each response, (4) putting the best alternative into practice, and (5) evaluating the outcome. Descriptions of problem-solving training can be found in Chang, D'Zurilla, and Sanna (2004) and Tafrate and Kassinove (2018).

Trigger

Describe the event that led to your anger:
A female friend was nagging me about borrowing my car.

Approximate date and time of your anger episode:
Tuesday afternoon about 4:00 P.M.

Where it occurred: ✔ Home ___ Work ___ School
___ Other (describe):

The target (person or object) of my anger was:
Female friend

The situation surrounding my anger was:
Became an argument
Other people were around

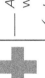

Thinking

(Look at the examples. Then place a check next to each thought that you had.)

✔ *Demandingness* ("I thought the other person should have acted differently.")

___ *Awfulizing* ("At the time, I thought this was one of the worst things that could be happening.")

✔ *Low frustration tolerance* ("I thought I could not handle or deal with this situation.")

___ *Global negative rating of others* ("I thought the other person was bad/worthless/a real #@*%&, etc.")

___ *Negative assumptions* ("I assumed the worst intentions of others without evidence.")

Personal Experience

How intense was your anger in this situation?

0 — None ——— Mild ——— Moderate ——— Strong ——✔— Extreme 10

What physical sensations did you experience? (Place a check next to each physical sensation you experienced.)

✔ Muscle tension	___ Fluttering in stomach	___ Sweating
___ Rapid heart rate	___ Nausea	___ Indigestion
___ Headache	___ Rapid breathing	___ Dizziness
___ Upset stomach	___ Tingling sensations	___ Positive energy

___ Flushing ___ Feelings of unreality
___ Fatigue
___ Trembling

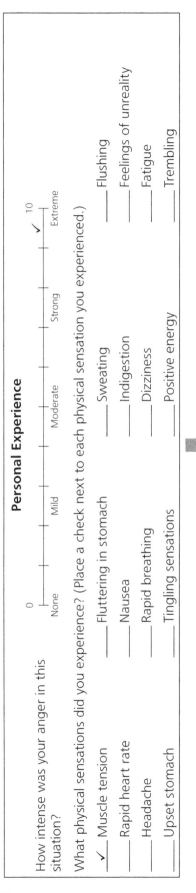

(continued)

FIGURE 12.5. Hank's completed Anger Episode Record. Adapted with permission from Impact Publishers, Inc. Copyright © 2009 Raymond Chip Tafrate and Howard Kassinove.

231

Behaviors and Expressive Patterns

(Place a check next to each behavior you engaged in during this anger episode.)

___ Held anger in (kept things in; boiled inside; held grudges and didn't tell anyone)

___ Indirectly expressed anger (did something secretly harmful to the person; spread rumors or gossip; deliberately didn't follow rules)

✓ Outward expression—verbal (yelled; screamed; argued; threatened; made sarcastic, nasty, or abusive remarks)

✓ Outward expression—physical (fought, hit, kicked, or shoved someone; broke, threw, slammed, or destroyed an object)

___ Outward expression—bodily gestures (rolled eyes; crossed arms; glared; frowned; gave a stern look)

___ Avoidance (escaped or withdrew from the situation; distracted myself by reading, watching TV, or listening to music)

___ Substance use (drank alcohol; took medications such as aspirin, Valium, etc.; took other drugs such as marijuana, cocaine, etc.)

___ Tried to resolve the situation (compromised, discussed, or came to some agreement with the person)

___ Other: _____

List the positive short-term outcomes of this anger episode:
I got her to stop nagging me.

List the negative short-term outcomes of this anger episode:
I got arrested after I pushed her down and she hit her head.

List the positive long-term outcomes of this anger episode:
Some of my friends know that I'm not the kind of guy that takes crap from anyone. They respect it.

List the negative long-term outcomes of this anger episode:
A new charge, maybe probation, I have to come here. Ruined my friendship with her. Some of my friends think what I did was not cool.

FIGURE 12.5. (*continued*)

232

Assertiveness

On the surface, it may seem that JICs with problematic anger reactions have little difficulty expressing themselves. The truth is that many have poor skills for negotiating life's inevitable conflicts. The goal of assertiveness is to teach JICs to approach people and situations through using words and behaviors that are likely to reduce conflict and lead to mutually beneficial solutions to problems (Alberti & Emmons, 2017). Assertiveness often includes a range of social skills, such as (1) reflective listening, (2) expressing desires and preferences, (3) making requests for desired outcomes, (4) accepting compliments, (5) giving compliments, (6) agreeing with others, and (7) disagreeing with others. The specific skills to focus on depend on the situations that are most challenging in JICs' lives. As always, practice, repetition, and follow-up of assertiveness skills are required to make these new behaviors more automatic.

Cognitive Restructuring

As noted above, a range of belief targets go along with anger. The anger episode analysis will allow you to determine which thinking patterns are most relevant for a particular JIC. Cognitive restructuring involves the following steps: (1) identifying the types of thoughts that go through JICs' minds when they are angry; (2) replacing anger-engendering thoughts with more flexible, reasonable, and accurate thinking; and (3) practicing new thinking in day-to-day life. It will take multiple conversations to create major cognitive shifts: Replacing distorted and exaggerated thinking with more realistic perceptions, creating a more flexible and less demanding philosophy, and developing a view of life's challenges as unpleasant but manageable. Table 12.1 provides examples of restructuring specific anger-related thoughts.

Acceptance

Another approach to anger is to teach JICs to become aware of their angry thoughts and feelings, but not to act on or give in to them. People can have impulses, thoughts, and urges, without following through with the behaviors in question (e.g., substance use, sexual behavior, and confrontation). In this approach, JICs deliberately disengage from automatic angry behavior and pursue actions that are more consistent with their values and life priorities (as discussed in Chapter 4; see also Gardner & Moore, 2014a; 2014b). With repetition, internal anger symptoms (e.g., thoughts, sensations, and intensity) diminish over time as JICs practice replacing typical angry behaviors with ones likely to produce better outcomes.

Perspective Taking, Empathy, and Compassion

JICs, especially when angered, have difficulty seeing things from others' perspectives. Perspective taking can aid in the development of empathy and enhance overall anger reduction. In this approach, after listening to a JIC explain the anger-provoking behavior of another, you would ask the JIC to describe the incident from the perspective of the other person. The ability to see things from the other person's perspective can be developed as a skill—one that, like other skills, becomes easier with practice. A higher level of this intervention involves fostering compassion. At

TABLE 12.1. Examples of Cognitive Restructuring for Anger

Anger-related thoughts	Alternative thoughts
Demandingness: "My parole officer should treat me with more respect."	"It would be nice if my parole officer treated me with more respect. However, he seems to have his own style, and he is not likely to change."
Awfulizing: "It is awful that Gina broke up with me."	"Even though I hoped we would stay together, I am capable of moving on with my life and meeting new people."
Low frustration tolerance: "I can't stand having a probation officer."	"I can tolerate my probation officer. It's only for 6 months, and then he will be out of my life."
Global negative rating of others: "My boss is a complete asshole."	"My boss seems to be under a lot of pressure, and he doesn't always talk to me the way I want. In the past, he has treated me well by giving me a chance."
Negative assumptions: "Adam didn't respond to my text. He's blowing me off."	"I don't know what's happening with Adam. I'll reach out again in a few days and see if he responds."

a very basic level, all people are trying to be happy and avoid suffering, at least from their own perspectives. This means that even when people do things that are perceived as inconsiderate, unfair, or harmful, they are often doing those things to avoid pain and enhance their own happiness (Kolts, 2012). Learning to see things from another's point of view is often an antidote to anger.

Getting Started

Once a shared understanding of the impact that anger is having on a JIC's life is established, you and the client can discuss steps to change automatic angry thoughts and behaviors. Form 12.6 (provided at the end of the chapter) can be introduced after several anger episodes have been analyzed and is a good starting point for introducing the interventions described above. As with the other Questions to Ask Myself . . . forms, allow the JIC time in session to complete the form and discuss what next steps might be taken before the next meeting.

KEY POINTS

- Substance misuse and problematic anger reactions will often occur together and can become habitual and destructive patterns in the lives of JICs.

- A large percentage of JICs, both in prison and in the community, will have substance use patterns that put them at risk of further justice involvement and create problems in other life areas.

- A first step in enhancing awareness and motivation to change substance misuse is to have a JIC keep a log to record daily use of alcohol and other drugs.

- Facilitating changes in substance misuse involves identifying specific alternative activities to replace substance use patterns, soliciting support from others, and identifying supportive individuals who will reinforce abstinence or meaningful reductions in the use of substances.

- Anger dysregulation can be a driver for physically aggressive behaviors, disrupt healthy relationships (e.g., romantic, family, and peers), and lead to vocational maladjustment.

- Effective anger treatment begins with analyzing recent and specific episodes of anger, using a five-part anger episode model (triggers, thoughts, experiences, expressive patterns, and outcomes).

- The analysis of anger episodes forms the groundwork for building motivation for change, as well as collaboratively identifying tangible treatment targets.

- The goal of treatment is to reduce a JIC's anger reactivity to frequently experienced triggers. Common interventions include building skills (e.g., relaxation, problem solving, and assertiveness); cognitive restructuring (e.g., fostering more accurate and flexible thinking), and developing acceptance, compassion, and perspective taking.

SCRIPT 12.1. Assigning the Log of Weekly Substance Use

Step 1: Introduce the purpose of the log and the *Description* column.

"We have talked about some of the areas that can cause trouble for you. One of them is your substance use. This log will help us get a picture of your alcohol and drug use during the course of the week, and will show how it changes or stays the same. [Show Form 12.2.] I'd like you to record your substance use on here at the end of each day. If you didn't use any alcohol or drugs during the day, just put a line through the box. On days when you did use, I want you to write down the time you used, the substance or substances you used, the amount of each, and then a phrase or two about the situation, such as 'I was in a bar with my friend,' or 'I was at a party')."

"You may feel a bit uneasy about recording your substance use on this form. This is natural for most people, even those who aren't involved with the criminal justice system. I want you to know that you and I are the only people to see this form, unless you show it to someone else. As I mentioned, the main point of all this is to get a sense of the times and circumstances you may be drinking or using drugs, and the ways we can change them so you don't have problems with the law."

Step 2: Explain the enjoyment and risk ratings.

"Then in these boxes, I want you to rate every episode of use on two characteristics.

"First, rate your level of enjoyment. Put an E in the box if, overall, you found the use to be *enjoyable*. Put a U in the box if, overall, you found the use to be *unpleasant*—maybe you didn't feel well during or afterward, or maybe you just didn't enjoy what happened. Put an OK in the box if, overall, you found the use to be somewhere between enjoyable and unpleasant.

"Second, rate how risky you thought each episode of use was. Put an R in the box if the use strikes you as *risky*. For example, maybe the use could have created a problem with the criminal justice system, such as a dirty urine, or it could have resulted in a fight, a DUI, an arrest, or a problem at work or with your family. Put an N if the use strikes you as *neutral* or safe."

Step 3: Explain how to handle multiple episodes of substance use in a single day.

"If you had more than one episode of use in a day, list and rate each episode separately. For example, if you used alcohol or drugs in the afternoon and then again in the evening, list and rate the afternoon one, and then list and rate the evening one below it. There should be enough space in the box. Include all substance use, even if it seems minor, like a single beer."

Step 4: Ask the client if he or she has questions.

"Does all this make sense, and do you understand it? Does any part of this seem unclear?"

Step 5: Give closing instructions.

"So, at the end of each day, I'd like completing this log to become part of your routine. Please bring it in next time. Remember, it's not going to be used to get you in more trouble. It's a tool to help us work on this area and keep you out of trouble."

SCRIPT 12.2. Steps for Announcing Change

Step 1: Reinforce the JIC's decision to change, and introduce the purpose of the assignment.

"Your decision to work on your substance use is excellent, and I want to do everything I can to help you succeed. One of the steps that often helps people follow through with changes they are going to make is to tell other people about those plans. When you tell other people, you're more likely to follow through with your change plans. So one of the things we're going to do today is figure out one or two people who you can tell about this change and discuss how you will you tell them. Then we'll practice what it would sound like. Lastly, between now and the next time we meet, I'm going to ask you to follow through and do it in real life."

Step 2: Identify and discuss a person to whom the JIC can announce the plan to change.

"Who is one person you are close with that you could tell, and who would support the change you are making?"

"Why did you choose [name of person]?"

"How do you think [person's name] would respond if you told him [her]?"

"In what ways could [person's name] be helpful to you in making this change?"

Step 3: Have the client draft a script of what they will say

"It sounds like you have a good person to talk to about this. Now we're going to come up with a sort of script for what specifically you will say. This is helpful, because having these kinds of talks with someone can be hard. You want to go into it knowing what you will say. So, on this sheet [show the JIC Form 12.4], I want you to write down what you might tell [person's name]. It shouldn't be too long; you can probably say what you need to say in a minute or two. But I want you to cover four things, and each one only needs a sentence or two.

"First, tell [person's name] that you're going to be changing your substance use from what it is now to [the JIC's goal]. Second, tell [person's name] why you are making this change, what you hope to get out of it. Third, tell [person's name] you are letting a few people who are close to you know about this, because it will help you be successful in making this change. Fourth, tell [person's name] that you are hoping he [she] will support you, and try to come up with one specific thing [person's name] could do to help."

(continued)

Step 4: Ask the JIC to read the script out loud, reinforce the client's work, offer feedback, and have the client revise the script as necessary.

> "I'd like us to practice what you've written a little bit. The more you practice saying it, the more comfortable you will feel when you actually do it. So I'd like you to tell me what you've written. Say it to me out loud."

> "Good job. One thing I think works well is . . . [provide one piece of positive feedback about a specific aspect of the script]."

> "Is there anything on the script you want to change? One thing I noticed was . . . [provide a suggestion if necessary for improving the script]."

Step 5: Run through the script until the JIC feels comfortable and no further changes need to be made.

Step 6: Identify when the JIC will carry out the assignment.

Step 7: Give closing instructions.

> "So you'll try this out for real on [day and time identified in Step 6] with [person's name]. You can use the sheet while you do it, or you can try to memorize it. I'll check in with you next time we meet about how it went, and then we may work together to identify some other people to tell as well."

SCRIPT 12.3. Steps for Analyzing Anger Episodes

Step 1: Identify the triggering event.

"[JIC's name], everyone feels anger at times. Anger can be difficult to understand, because it is made up of different parts. In order for me to understand you better, I would like to explore the specific parts that make up your anger. Give me an example of an anger episode you have experienced in the past month. Tell me about what triggered it." [Keep asking questions until you have an understanding of the trigger.]

Step 2: Search for the thinking that emerged immediately prior to the anger episode.

"When you think about your anger in this situation, what was going through your mind when you started to get angry?" [Continue asking questions as necessary.]

Step 3: Assess the personal experience of the anger.

"How angry did you get during this anger episode? That is, how strongly did you feel anger on a scale of 0 to 10, where 0 is not at all angry and 10 is the most anger you have ever experienced?"

"What physical sensations did your notice in your body?"

"How long did this episode last?"

Step 4: Explore the behavior and expressive patterns associated with the anger.

"Now let's look at how you acted in the moment. What did you do when you were angry in this situation?" [Was the reaction verbal, physically aggressive, passive–aggressive, relationally aggressive, or avoidant?]

Step 5: Explore the long- and short-term outcomes of the anger episode.

"What good came out of your anger in this situation?"

"What was not so good about your anger in this situation?"

"How did you feel about this anger episode after the feeling had passed?"

FORM 12.1. Looking at My Substance Use

To get a deeper understanding of how your substance use is influencing your life, complete the information below about the substances you have used in the past year. In the column labeled Substance, list the name of each substance you have used in the past year, including alcohol. In the column labeled Criminal Justice, check the box if use of the substance led to an arrest or could lead to an arrest or technical violation of supervision. In the column labeled Interpersonal Conflict, check the box if use of the substance led to a conflict (a disagreement or fight) with a friend, family member, significant other, or stranger. In the column labeled Work/School, check the box if use of the substance led to a problem with a job or getting a job, or a problem with attending or doing well in school. In the column labeled Emotional, check the box if use of the substance led to depression, anxiety, anger, or other emotional difficulties. In the column labeled Behavioral, check the box if use of the substance led to a loss of control over your behavior (e.g., blackout, injury, attempt at self-harm).

Substance	Problem Areas				
	Criminal Justice	Interpersonal Conflict	Work/School	Emotional	Behavioral
1.					
2.					
3.					
4.					
5.					
6.					
7.					

FORM 12.2. Log of Weekly Substance Use

Over the next week, record your substance use at the end of each day. Record the time, type of substance, amount, and a brief phrase about the situation in which it occurred. Then rate your level of enjoyment by writing an E if you found the substance use *enjoyable,* a U if you found the use *unpleasant,* or an OK if it was somewhere in between. In the last column, rate the riskiness of the use by writing an R next to incidents of use that were *risky* (could have potentially resulted in criminal justice problems), and an N next to episodes of use that you thought were *neutral* in terms of likely legal problems.

Day	Description of Use (time of day, type of substance, amount of use, situation)	Rating of Enjoyment (E, U, OK)	Rating of Risk (R, N)
Monday			
Tuesday			
Wednesday			
Thursday			
Friday			
Saturday			
Sunday			

FORM 12.3. Questions, Answers, and Next Steps for My Substance Use

Write your answer to each question below with a short sentence or two. Be prepared to discuss them afterward.

Question: In what situations is my use most likely to lead to trouble?
Answer: _____

_____

Next Step: One step I can take right away to avoid those situations is _____

_____

Question: Who are some people I know who might hold me back in changing my pattern of use?
Answer: _____

_____

Next Step: One step I can take right away to avoid those people is _____

_____

Question: Who are some people I know who will probably encourage me in changing my pattern of use?
Answer: _____

_____

Next Step: One step I can take right away to spend more time with them is _____

_____

Question: What are some *new* activities that I could try out when I would otherwise be using?
Answer: _____

_____

Next Step: One step I can take right away to try these new activities is _____

_____

Question: What are some *old* activities that I used to enjoy (but haven't been doing lately), and that I can try again?
Answer: _____

_____

Next Step: One step I can take right away to do these activities is _____

_____

FORM 12.4. Announcing Change

In the space below, come up with a script that you can follow when you tell other people about the change you are going to make in your substance use. The script doesn't have to be long. It should be able to be delivered in a minute or two.

Organize your script into four parts. In Part 1, let the person(s) know you have something important to say, and tell them specifically what you are changing about your substance use. In Part 2, briefly let the person(s) know why you are making this change: You can include how it will help you with the criminal justice system and how you think it will help in any other life areas. In Part 3, let them know why you are sharing this with them—why you think they would be good person(s) to tell about this change. In Part 4, let the person(s) know you are hoping they will support you, and try to come up with one specific way you think they could help you with this change.

Part 1: _____
_____
_____
_____
_____
_____

Part 2: _____
_____
_____
_____
_____
_____

Part 3: _____
_____
_____
_____
_____
_____

Part 4: _____
_____
_____
_____
_____
_____

FORM 12.5. Anger Episode Record

Fill out a record for a recent episode of anger that you experienced. Provide information in each box.

Trigger

Describe the event that led to your anger:

Approximate date and time of your anger episode:

Where it occurred: ___ Home ___ Work ___ School
___ Other (describe):

The target (person or object) of my anger was:

The situation surrounding my anger was:

Thinking

(Look at the examples. Then place a check next to each thought that you had.)

___ *Demandingness* ("I thought the other person should have acted differently.")

___ *Awfulizing* ("At the time, I thought this was one of the worst things that could be happening.")

___ *Low frustration tolerance* ("I thought I could not handle or deal with this situation.")

___ *Global negative rating of others* ("I thought the other person was bad/worthless/a real #@*%&, etc.")

___ *Negative assumptions* ("I assumed the worst intentions of others without evidence.")

Personal Experience

How intense was your anger in this situation?

```
0        Mild      Moderate      Strong     10
None                                      Extreme
```

What physical sensations did you experience? (Place a check next to each physical sensation you experienced.)

✓ Muscle tension ___ Fluttering in stomach ___ Sweating ___ Flushing
___ Rapid heart rate ___ Nausea ___ Indigestion ___ Feelings of unreality
___ Headache ___ Rapid breathing ___ Dizziness ___ Fatigue
___ Upset stomach ___ Tingling sensations ___ Positive energy ___ Trembling

(continued)

FORM 12.5. Anger Episode Record (page 2 of 2)

Behaviors and Expressive Patterns

(Place a check next to each behavior you engaged in during this anger episode.)

____ Held anger in (kept things in; boiled inside; held grudges and didn't tell anyone)

____ Indirectly expressed anger (did something secretly harmful to the person; spread rumors or gossip; deliberately didn't follow rules)

____ Outward expression—verbal (yelled; screamed; argued; threatened; made sarcastic, nasty, or abusive remarks)

____ Outward expression—physical (fought, hit, kicked, or shoved someone; broke, threw, slammed, or destroyed an object)

____ Outward expression—bodily gestures (rolled eyes; crossed arms; glared; frowned; gave a stern look)

____ Avoidance (escaped or withdrew from the situation; distracted myself by reading, watching TV, or listening to music)

____ Substance use (drank alcohol; took medications such as aspirin, Valium, etc.; took other drugs such as marijuana, cocaine, etc.)

____ Tried to resolve the situation (compromised, discussed, or came to some agreement with the person)

____ Other: _____

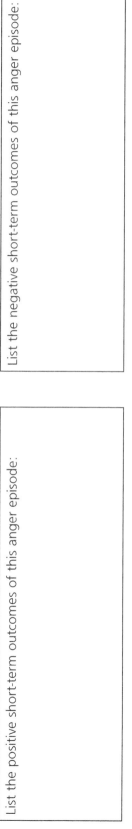

List the negative short-term outcomes of this anger episode:

List the negative long-term outcomes of this anger episode:

List the positive short-term outcomes of this anger episode:

List the positive long-term outcomes of this anger episode:

FORM 12.6. Questions to Ask Myself about My Anger

Write your answer to each question below with a short sentence or two. Be prepared to discuss potential solutions or next steps that you might come up with.

Questions to Ask Myself	Answers, Solutions, and Next Steps
What types of problems is my anger creating in my life?	
What do I stand to lose if I do not address my anger?	
What steps can I take to slow myself down and not react so quickly when I'm angry?	
What steps can I take to make better decisions when I'm angry?	
How can I deal with disagreements with others in a way that leads to better outcomes for everyone?	
How can I be more flexible in my thinking when others do things I don't like?	
What are some things I could do not to act on my angry thoughts and feelings—things that would be more consistent with my values?	

PART VI

PRACTICE MANAGEMENT

CHAPTER 13

Documentation and Report Writing

In many settings, it is a professional requirement to maintain records of clinical interactions with JICs, and written documentation thus becomes an important aspect of the treatment process. Styles and formats can range from rudimentary clinical notes to comprehensive assessment evaluation reports, but an underlying purpose of all clinical record keeping is to provide a thoughtful analysis and description of JICs. Although documentation may be a tedious aspect of clinical work, it nonetheless offers benefits to practitioners, the JICs themselves, and third-party stakeholders.

Apart from documentation being a professional necessity, there are several underappreciated advantages to the process. In working with JICs, you have two essential tasks: to provide treatment guidance (i.e., support increases in awareness and motivation for change; create a structure for cognitive and behavioral steps for self-improvement), and to show enthusiasm (positive reinforcement) for meaningful achievements. As discussed throughout this treatment planner, both of these tasks are facilitated when you understand JICs' functioning across relevant criminal risk domains, recognize their realistic potential for change, and interact with them in a positive and encouraging style.

The combination of a specified treatment plan (whether formal or informal) with regular written monitoring of treatment progress is an excellent method for providing feedback in general, and for expressing enthusiasm about JICs' achievements in particular. It is often easy to notice and provide encouragement for noteworthy successes; unfortunately, not all JICs respond to treatment according to expectations. In fact, it is common among any caseload of JICs for there to be more than a few cases with minimal or no clinical improvements, despite your best efforts. In such situations, it can be easy to overlook small treatment gains. The practice of preparing written documentation at relevant junctures of the treatment process can help you attend to less noticeable fluctuations in thinking and behavior, which can be helpful for maintaining a positive attitude toward these JICs, keeping them motivated for treatment, and directing the nature and course of treatment.

From JICs' perspectives, making documentation available to them whenever it is possible and practical to do so can serve as a rich source of feedback. The essence of self-improvement is a combination of understanding what must be changed to achieve cognitive and behavioral outcomes within relevant criminal risk domains, and having a commitment to change (i.e., motivation). Feedback is a vital component in both increasing understanding and maintaining motivation throughout the treatment process. During sessions, you may offer informal feedback such as verbal statements related to certain clinical issues, but your message may not always be memorable or may not resonate to a sufficient degree to promote change. Written documentation that encapsulates germane issues in JICs' lives, however, can have a strong and enduring influence.

The third benefit of documentation relates directly to the interests of third-party stakeholders. The vast majority of JICs have third parties involved in their cases, primarily representatives of the legal system (officers of the court, probation and parole personnel, legal counsel, etc.). These third-party entities have interests in making decisions about JICs—decisions that can be influenced by practitioners' professional opinions as expressed through documentation. For example, the frequency of probation or parole contacts in community supervision contexts is often based on estimates of JICs' functioning. Greater frequency of contacts is likely to occur when JICs are nonadherent with expectations; less supervision is likely to occur when JICs are functioning well. These types of supervision decisions are often aided by documentation provided by those working directly with the JICs. Documentation may also be necessary for collaborating effectively with professionals in other disciplines who provide auxiliary resources or services (e.g., practitioners whose focus is medical, educational, or occupational).

In summary, there is no escaping that documentation is a necessary part of working with JICs. It is possible to reduce the strain and time demands of record keeping by following a general framework. The remainder of this chapter offers templates for different types of documentation that can be helpful in diverse treatment settings. Three specific types are described: (1) an assessment and treatment plan report, (2) a method for monitoring and documenting clinical progress across sessions, and (3) a treatment summary report.

TIPS FOR WRITING AN EFFECTIVE ASSESSMENT AND TREATMENT PLAN REPORT

An assessment and treatment plan report is essentially a formal written narrative about a JIC. Although there is no consensus about what constitutes a proper report of this type, we wish to emphasize a few features of effective reports. A useful assessment and treatment plan report provides a clear and credible description of the methods used and the conclusions reached. There should also be a logical connection between the assessment information and the ultimate recommendations offered.

Most importantly, the report should add value by contributing distinct information about the JIC to third-party stakeholders. Authors of formal assessment and treatment plan reports are typically regarded as "experts" (i.e., they often have advanced education, specialized training, and experience), which means that they can offer a unique perspective on JICs to end users of the reports. For such a report to be maximally beneficial, however, it is critical that any documentation provided is easily understood by third parties. These parties are most likely to include community supervision officers, correctional counselors, or judges, depending upon the nature and circumstances of each referral. Unfortunately, practitioners are notorious for using excessive professional jargon and detailed explanations of clinical events in their documentation. The guiding principles of parsimony and simplicity, discussed earlier as hallmarks of effective case formulation (see Chapter 6), are also essential in all types of documentation and report writing. Technical material is best described in a user-friendly manner that is logically connected to the conclusions.

In forensic practice, one of the most fundamental assessment issues is JICs' potential risk for reoffending. For this reason, *risk assessment* often becomes a logical starting point for an assessment and treatment plan report; that is, it sets the stage for the development of a plan that targets relevant criminal risk domains. The purpose of this treatment planner is to provide step-by-step guidance on how to conduct CBT interventions with JICs; therefore, a full description of risk assessment procedures and instruments is beyond the scope of this book. Nonetheless, as noted in earlier chapters, it is well established that the most effective and accurate method of determining a JIC's criminal risk potential is the use of a validated risk assessment instrument (see Appendix A for recommendations). The failure to incorporate an instrument that is designed specifically to measure criminal risk potential suggests that questions about future criminality may be inadequately assessed.

It is important to note that the strength of the conclusions in a report is dependent upon a convergence of relevant clinical information, much of which is derived from traditional sources (interview information, file review, psychometric test results, etc.). No one piece of information is flawless. Persuasive clinical recommendations emerge when there is a logical connection among, and a convergence of, clinical, historical, and testing data. At times there may be a divergence between different sources of information, which requires thoughtful explanation. The final result should be a reasonably coherent presentation of complementary information that builds the case for the eventual recommendations.

A TEMPLATE FOR AN ASSESSMENT AND TREATMENT PLAN REPORT

We now describe a template for an assessment and treatment plan report. The format and style are based on considerable experience in conducting psychological assessments with JICs. The basic structure and design of the report are similar to those commonly found in the assessment literature. However, this template provides a uniform format that can assist you in conducting assessments of JICs with many different characteristics (e.g., gender, age, race, offense type). The advantage of templates is that they assist in standardizing the evaluation process, can help reduce errors or omissions of clinical information, can decrease the overall time spent completing an evaluation report, and can improve the quality of evaluation products.

It is important to note that this template reflects a psychological evaluation and is geared toward psychologists and other mental health professionals legally qualified for, and capable of, conducting this style of evaluation. However, discussion of this template has value to non-psychological third-party end users as well, because a better understanding of the inner workings of assessment reports should lead to better utilization and integration of the information into the overall decision-making and treatment processes.

The completed Assessment and Treatment Plan Report provided at the end of this section (see Figure 13.1) is consistent with the completed Criminal Event Analysis and Case Formulation Worksheet provided in Chapter 6 for the case of Hank (see Figures 6.1 and 6.5, respectively). Figure 13.1 focuses on his current criminal situation and explores linkages to historical patterns of criminal and prosocial behavior. Two central goals of this process are to identify Hank's potential for antisocial conduct and to determine his abilities for positive life functioning. This is accomplished by identifying clinical markers of relevant issues, offering a brief exemplar of each marker, and commenting about the importance of any single marker or combination of markers.

Our Assessment and Treatment Plan Report Template is provided in Form 13.1 (at the end of this chapter). As can be seen, it has seven main sections, with subcategories within each section. The template is flexible, in that sections may be added or removed as deemed necessary by the practitioner.

Template Structure

The first section of the template (without a label of its own) is for basic identifying information, including the JIC's name and date of birth, as well as the author of the evaluation report and the completion date. Additional information (such as office location or case number) can be provided as necessary.

The second section is labeled Purpose and Outline of Assessment. This section describes the reason for the evaluation and the methods used to gather the information. It can be helpful to provide a very brief statement about the JIC's circumstances and the context of the evaluation. In regard to any assessment instruments that may have been administered, the content area measured is mentioned, followed by the specific test used to measure the content area.

The third section, Overview of Current Offenses and Legal History, describes the JIC's current involvement with the legal system, past involvements, and custody experiences (subcategories exist for Current Offenses, Legal History, and Custody Behavior, respectively). The description of the current legal involvement should be taken from official sources; it should provide a brief synopsis of events and capture the essence of the JIC's actions. It is important to augment the official accounts with a brief comment giving the JIC's version of events. A comment about the degree of correspondence between the official documentation and the JIC's account is relevant, because it can reflect the JIC's personality style and the overall honesty of his or her self-report information. The Legal History subcategory relates to the JIC's history of involvement with the justice system. This reflects the frequency and severity of any conflict between the JIC and the law in the past, both of which provide clinical information related to risk for future offending. The age of first contact with the law (arrest, prosecution, etc.), number of convictions, types of offenses, dispositions (fine, community supervision, custody), and responses to disposition (compliance vs. noncompliance, time span between offenses, etc.) should also be noted. The Custody Behavior subcategory relates to the JIC's history of custody. Brief notations should be made about the age of first custody, the length of custody, the security level, and the JICs response to custody (complying vs. incurring institutional infractions).

The fourth section, Background Information, includes several subcategories of sociodemographic information related to criminality. Descriptions of social history may be the most tempting areas in which to be overly comprehensive and/or to allow the injection of personal bias, either of which can lead to faulty conclusions or recommendations about the JIC. It is important that information presented in this section be brief and focused on clinical markers that support or refute the JIC's criminality potential. The Developmental History subcategory describes the JIC's early family circumstances, such as geographic location of birth and/or upbringing, family composition (number and ordering of siblings, relations between family members, etc.), parental characteristics, and child-rearing practices. Also included in this subcategory is information about features of the JIC's early years and any notable strengths or difficulties.

The Connections to School/Work subcategory reflects the JIC's educational and vocational experiences and achievements. Comments should be included about the JIC's school and work interests and ethics. The Physical Health Concerns/Psychopathology subcategory relates to any notable medical or mental health considerations that may influence the JIC's behavior in either positive or negative ways (particularly any limitations related to employment, treatment success, or compliance with correctional supervision). Specific comments should be made about emotion regulation (e.g., anger control) and any aggressive tendencies or events. The Substance Abuse/Misuse subcategory relates to the JIC's historical and current use of substances. Comments should include the type, frequency, severity, and consequences of alcohol and other drug use, with particular reference to any criminality that is a direct result of using substances or associating with substance users.

The Family/Romantic Relationships/Companions subcategory reflects the full range of the JIC's relationships, as well as social skills, abilities, and potential deficiencies. Comments related to the characteristics of the JIC's social companions (e.g., prosocial vs. antisocial) and to the proportion of time spent with each are also important. The Self-Improvement Experiences subcategory relates to attempts the JIC has made to improve his or her lifestyle or functioning. This includes participation in both self-help (e.g., weight reduction, smoking cessation, educational upgrading) and structured treatment initiatives. The final subcategory is Professional Assessment History, which relates to any past formal legal, mental health, or substance abuse evaluations in which the JIC has participated (either voluntarily or involuntarily). Comments about the nature of past evaluations, their outcome, and the consistency between these evaluations and the current assessment are important.

The fifth section is labeled Interview(s) and Test Results. This area reflects the central clinical aspects of the present evaluation and includes three subcategories. The first one, Clinical Presentation, is for a general description of the JIC and any notable features or characteristics, as well as the reliability and accuracy of the client's self-report style. In addition, comments are provided about any indicators of violence toward self or others, as well as general mental status, which is generally assessed by way of a mental status examination. The second subcategory, Test Results, is for recording the results of any standardized tests administered. It is important to describe the JIC's style of interacting with the administration of the tests (i.e., was the client cooperative, alert, and attentive to the task, or uncooperative, or inattentive/indifferent?), as this may offer information related to the accuracy of the results. A brief notation about the name of each test, the domain(s) it assesses, and the JIC's score(s)/performance on the test is required. For tests with multiple subtests, it is important to present a synthesis of the test data rather than a pedantic subtest-by-subtest description. Parsimony of presentation is critical; otherwise, the manner in which standardized tests provide insightful information may be underappreciated by end users. The final subcategory, Case Formulation of Interview and Test Data, is for an integration of all clinical information into an opinion about the JIC. This opinion offers an explanation of the JIC's criminal behavior, both past and current, and projections of his or her criminality potential. Again, it is imperative that the entry in this subcategory be kept brief and straightforward.

The sixth section is labeled Summary and Recommendations. This section not only represents a concise integration and summary of all clinical information and data, but expresses a clinical opinion. Generally, this opinion relates to the JIC's criminal risk potential, the factors that give rise to this potential, and prognostications about the potential for future antisocial acts. General comments about the correctional disposition/actions are also made.

The final section, Treatment Plan Recommendations, describes the treatment steps that should be pursued. It is important to describe the areas in need of modification and the dosage of intervention that may optimally benefit the JIC. In some cases, a target for intervention may be identified, but a method to address that issue may not be immediately available. For example, the JIC may require a cognitive treatment that targets criminal thinking, but the agency responsible does not offer such a program, or a practitioner is currently unavailable for various reasons (e.g., all available practitioners have waiting lists). It is important to identify what is required for the JIC, and whether such intervention is readily available or not. Treatment targets will also tend to match up with those identified in case formulation (see Chapter 6, Form 6.3). The completed Assessment and Treatment Plan Report for Hank appears in Figure 13.1.

PROVIDING FEEDBACK TO JICs ON THEIR CLINICAL DATA

The discussion of the assessment and treatment plan report thus far has concerned tailoring the document to third-party end users. We now turn our attention to the task of providing JICs with feedback on the report. Practitioners may use a thoughtful assessment and case formulation approach, and offer a range of intervention options, only to be met with confusion, defensiveness, or indifference by JICs if such information is not presented in a manner they can understand. It can be common for a practitioner to describe assessment- and treatment-relevant topics to a JIC, only to have him or her respond with "I hear you, but what does it all mean?" One way to avoid this type of situation is to present germane information to the JIC via a graphic representation of the clinical data. In other words, a chart of relevant test data will often resonate with a JIC. In Form 13.2 (at the end of this chapter), we provide an Assessment Profile Template as a method of presenting report information and test data to a JIC.

The X-axis of Form 13.2 represents different assessment domains or areas of functioning. We recommend that the number of domains presented be limited to the main criminal risk domains and any relevant secondary domains that may have been assessed. Form 13.2 has spaces for six columns: one reflecting primary criminal risk factors assessed by way of a validated risk assessment instrument (Risk/Need), and five specialized domains that include Imprecision (i.e., response bias), Criminogenic Thinking, Emotion (i.e., dysregulated anger), Substances, and Readiness to Change. The specialized or secondary domains are measured by way of specialized assessment instruments and are likely to vary depending on several factors, such as a JIC's characteristics, a practitioner's level of expertise and comfort with specific instruments, and the assessment tools generally available to the practitioner in his or her work setting. A chart such as Form 13.2 should be designed to be flexible to accommodate the addition or removal of different instruments, based on the type of information desired for any particular JIC.

(text resumes on page 261)

Client's name: Parker, Hank

Assessor's name: Wilson, Brenda

D.O.B.: April 1, 1992

Date report completed: June 20, 2017

PURPOSE AND OUTLINE OF ASSESSMENT

Mr. Parker is currently on probation for assaulting a female acquaintance. A psychological assessment was requested by the Court to evaluate his current emotional state, factors that may have been responsible for his criminal behavior, and his potential for future criminal conduct. Recommendations for any treatment considerations will also be offered. The assessment was based on a review of the relevant file information, a clinical assessment interview of approximately 2 hours, and psychological testing. Psychological testing included measures of intelligence (Shipley Institute of Living Scale), response bias (Paulhus Deception Scales), anger (Anger Disorders Scale), criminal attitudes (Criminal Sentiments Scale—Modified), substance use (Substance Use Behavior Survey), amenability for lifestyle change (Self-Improvement Orientation Scheme—Self Report), and a broad-based criminal risk instrument (Level of Service Inventory—Revised).

At the beginning of the interview, Mr. Parker was advised of the purpose and methodology (i.e., review of file material, clinical interview, administration of psychological tests) used in the evaluation, including the benefits and costs of participating. He was also advised of the limits of confidentiality and the distribution of the report. Mr. Parker indicated that he understood all issues, allowed unconditional access to all potential sources of information, and consented freely to participate.

OVERVIEW OF CURRENT OFFENSES AND LEGAL HISTORY

Current Offenses

Mr. Parker is a 25-year-old male who was involved in an aggressive incident involving a female acquaintance. According to file information, Mr. Parker and the victim are connected by way of mutual friends. On the day of the offense, Mr. Parker was socializing with a group of friends, and the victim was present. At some point, a disagreement occurred among various people, and Mr. Parker pushed the victim in an aggressive manner. Although the victim hit her head on the concrete, she did not sustain any notable physical injuries. Mr. Parker was arrested by police without incident shortly after this event.

During the present interview, Mr. Parker described a version of his offense that was consistent with official documentation. Although he tended to downplay the extent of his actions, he also showed some insight into the circumstances surrounding the event, which reflected modest remorse and a desire to change his lifestyle.

Legal History

Mr. Parker's contact with the criminal justice system began when he was approximately 18 years old. He has been convicted of three prior offenses: possession and sale of narcotics, larceny, and DUI. He was briefly jailed and sentenced to terms of

(continued)

FIGURE 13.1. Assessment and Treatment Plan Report for Hank.

probation for these offenses. He has been generally compliant with all correctional supervision.

Custody Behavior

Mr. Parker was briefly detained in jail upon his arrest for his current offense. He also has been detained in jail on a previous offense. Mr. Parker was cooperative with the routine and expectations, and displayed no outbursts of noncompliant behavior during these occasions.

BACKGROUND INFORMATION

Developmental History

Mr. Parker reported that he was born and raised in a small town in Florida. He is the younger of two children (he has an older brother) reared by his biological parents. According to Mr. Parker, he was reared in a disadvantaged neighborhood (social housing, high crime, etc.) and a chaotic family environment characterized by social dysfunction (e.g., poor finances, lax house routine and rules, and parental substance abuse). However, Mr. Parker had generally positive relationships with family members while growing up, and he maintains approximately monthly contact with his brother and parents at the present time.

Mr. Parker reported relatively normal early child development and behavior patterns in spite of his family situation. This changed, however, when he was approximately 15 years old, when he developed behavioral problems both within and outside the family. He became more impulsive and oppositional toward authority figures (e.g., parents and teachers). There were no significant efforts for treatment or intervention presented to Mr. Parker at the time.

Connections to School/Work

Mr. Parker has an uninspired vocational history. With respect to school, he had a reasonably positive attitude toward school, but was academically "average." Although he had no grade failures or chronic school or behavior problems, he described his academic career as "borderline" problematic. He reported being suspended for fighting on at least one occasion, which seems to have been related to anger control problems.

Mr. Parker left school after completing the 11th grade but he completed a GED; his employment history appears disjointed, much as his school career was. He has been involved in "a few" manual-labor-type jobs, but has a poor attitude toward working and puts in minimal effort. He has been fired on one occasion for poor performance. Mr. Parker described the intention to be involved in "truck driving," but has not sought out information that would make him eligible for such work. He was unemployed at the time of his current offense.

Physical Health Concerns/Psychopathology

Mr. Parker is in adequate physical condition for his age and has no health issues that would interfere with his ability for positive life functioning or compliance with any criminal justice supervision or treatment.

(continued)

FIGURE 13.1. *(continued)*

Mr. Parker reported that he has no history of psychiatric or mental health problems. He also denied any history of self-harm.

Substance Abuse/Misuse

Mr. Parker drinks to intoxication a few times a month when he is with his friends. He also smokes marijuana. He began using these substances in his mid-teenage years and has been involved with them ever since. The frequency of his marijuana use tends to be relatively sporadic (i.e., whenever he has sufficient money, or if he is in the company of friends who provide substances to him). Moreover, his use of substances is routinely related to behavior problems, and virtually all his criminal incidents are related to the use of these substances. To Mr. Parker's credit, he has had periods of abstinence and is mindful of the need to pay attention to his use of substances, although he has never attended substance use treatment.

Family/Romantic Relationships/Companions

Mr. Parker is a person with adequate social skills and has the capability for positive social relationships. Unfortunately, he tends to be somewhat of a follower, and the majority of his social relationships are with individuals who have conflict with the law.

With respect to romantic relationships, Mr. Parker indicated that he is heterosexual in orientation and has had "a few" romantic relationships, although none that have lasted for any significant period of time. His description of his relationships indicates that he tends to become involved with volatile women who are impulsive/aggressive and abuse alcohol. Mr. Parker is currently single, but would like to be a relationship with someone who is "stable."

Self-Improvement Experiences

Self-improvement relates to a person's interest/attempt to alter undesirable aspects of his or her life. Change requires skills, aptitudes, and motivation to be successful, and a history of self-improvement can be reflective of a person's current potential for success. Mr. Parker has a limited history of self-improvement. Although he has never attended a formal substance use treatment program, he has quit cigarette smoking and attempted to reduce his use of substances.

Professional Assessment History

Mr. Parker has no history of participating in previous mental health or criminal risk assessments.

INTERVIEW(S) AND TEST RESULTS

Clinical Presentation

Mr. Parker attended a clinical interview in the morning of March 28, 2017, which lasted 2 hours. He presented as a white male of average height and normal weight, and he appeared to be his stated age. He was casually dressed but unshaven. During the interview, Mr. Parker was somewhat hesitant in his responses to questions, but

(continued)

FIGURE 13.1. *(continued)*

his answers seemed to be genuine. There was no evidence that he was deceptive in his responses.

A mental status examination conducted during the interview found that Mr. Parker had normal mood and no evidence of hallucinations, flight of ideas, or loose associations that would indicate the presence of a major mental illness. He did, however, present as a person with emotion dysregulation difficulties (namely, anger control problems). Aside from this, Mr. Parker has normal psychological and psychiatric functioning at the present time.

Test Results

Mr. Parker completed a series of self-report psychological questionnaires. He showed good concentration and completed the measures in a conscientious manner within expected time limits.

The Shipley Institute of Living Scale is a general screening measure of intellectual performance. Mr. Parker's scores on this measure placed him in the average range compared to standardized norms. These findings are consistent with clinical impressions; they suggest that he has sufficient intellectual abilities for effective life management and decision making, and for any vocational aspirations or rehabilitation initiatives he may wish to pursue.

The Paulhus Deception Scale (PDS) is an assessment inventory that measures the degree to which a test taker provides socially desirable responses on self-report questionnaires. This can be considered as an index of imprecision and is used to assess the honesty of respondents, which serves as a gauge for the validity of other self-report questionnaires. Mr. Parker's profile of scores on the PDS was in the low range, at the 23rd percentile relative to offender normative data. These findings suggest that his scores on other self-report measures are accurate reflections of his current personal orientation.

Research shows that excessive emotion dysregulation in the form of anger is linked to a behavioral disposition that may trigger criminal conduct, including violence. The Anger Disorders Scale (ADS) is a self-report instrument designed to measure a person's propensity toward anger problems. Higher scores on the instrument indicate a greater predisposition toward experiencing and expressing anger. Mr. Parker's score on the ADS was in the high range, at the 95th percentile compared to normative data. These results are consistent with his current clinical functioning and with his behavioral history of aggressiveness. On balance, Mr. Parker shows signs of acting in an aggressive manner when sufficiently provoked.

Criminological theory and research indicate that criminal attitudes are linked to antisocial behavior. Mr. Parker completed the Criminal Sentiments Scale—Modified, which is a measure of criminal thinking. Higher scores on this instrument are reflective of greater criminal attitudes/values and an increased risk for antisocial behavior. Mr. Parker's score on this measure placed him in the high range, at the 79th percentile relative to offender norms. These results are consistent with clinical impressions and his behavioral history.

The Substance Use Behavior Survey (SUBS) is a structured professional judgment instrument that examines behavioral indicators of substance use problems. No distinction is made between alcohol and other drugs. It consists of 14 items

(continued)

FIGURE 13.1. *(continued)*

separated into two categories: Part A consists of 11 items that examine substance use, and Part B consists of 3 items related to potential for change. Mr. Parker's scores on the SUBS were in the high range, at the 75th percentile compared to relevant normative data. These results are consistent with clinical impressions and his recent history of substance use.

The Self-Improvement Orientation Scheme—Self Report (SOS-SR) is a clinical measure designed to evaluate a person's amenability to making positive changes in his or her life. It consists of a total score and several subscales that measure different aspects of life change potential. Mr. Parker's scores on the SOS-SR were in the low range (at the 30th percentile relative to normative data), suggesting that he has limited motivation to make positive changes in his life. These findings are consistent with clinical impressions and his behavioral history.

The Level of Service Inventory—Revised (LSI-R) is a broad-based actuarial risk/need instrument used to classify offenders according to their risk for criminal conduct and need for treatment. The instrument is scored by way of a semistructured interview with the client and a review of file information. Empirical and clinical evidence indicates that the instrument predicts criminal conduct criteria (i.e., general and violent reoffending) and is useful as a case management tool. The instrument consists of a Criminal History domain that provides a static (historical) appraisal of risk, and several dynamic domains that provide information on modifications to the static risk estimate. Mr. Parker's scores on the LSI-R placed him in the high risk/need range. Normative data from the publisher of the LSI-R indicates that scores such as these are related to a 68% probability of reoffending. According to the LSI-R scores, Mr. Parker is at risk for future criminal conduct if he is uninvolved in positive vocational activities, associates with antisocial peers, is involved in substance abuse, and/or acts on his criminal thinking.

Case Formulation Based on Interview and Test Data

The overall clinical profile portrays a person who has sufficient intellectual abilities and social skills, and is open and honest in discussing his life functioning issues. Mr. Parker's criminal risk potential based on his lifestyle factors is in the high range and is related to his social connections, use of substances, weak involvement in vocational pursuits, anger difficulties, and a moderate level of criminal thinking. His ability to modify these issues is considered poor at the present time, due to his lack of motivation and readiness for change.

SUMMARY AND RECOMMENDATIONS

Mr. Parker is a young adult male who was recently involved in the assault of a female acquaintance. At the time of his offense, he was leading a dysfunctional lifestyle and was active in antisocial conduct. He was not suffering from any psychiatric or psychological problems at the time of his offenses. Predicting future conduct as it relates to criminality relies on a combination of science and practice. From a scientific perspective, several assessment instruments have been developed to determine the probability of a future criminal event. The practice of risk assessment

(continued)

FIGURE 13.1. *(continued)*

relates to the integration of clinical information into a case formulation of the risk of future criminality, and the likely circumstances under which it will occur. In the case of Mr. Parker, the science and practice of criminality indicate that he is in the high-risk range.

In summary, I am satisfied I have had sufficient clinical contact with Mr. Parker, and am sufficiently confident in the psychological tests administered to him, to form an opinion regarding his psychological status and risk for future criminality. Broadly speaking, a convergence of clinical and psychometric information indicates that Mr. Parker is a psychologically stable person who is unlikely to experience hallucinations, delusions, or manic episodes. From a criminal risk perspective, he is considered to be at high risk for future criminal conduct, with an actuarial estimate of risk for recidivism at minimum being in the 68% range. He has a limited criminal record, but has a history of being surrounded by negative social influences (e.g., his current peer relations and use of substances). He also has weak connections to sustained involvement in prosocial activities, such as employment and leisure pursuits. He also has difficulty managing his anger reactions in challenging situations. These issues must change if Mr. Parker is to lead a prosocial (noncriminal) lifestyle.

TREATMENT PLAN RECOMMENDATIONS

- Readiness for Change: Mr. Parker is weak in this area, which may compromise success in all areas of treatment. It will be necessary to increase his awareness of the costs connected to some of his current patterns (e.g., peers, use of substances, problematic anger reactions). Integrating "motivational enhancements" into intervention sessions is recommended.

- Criminogenic Thinking: Mr. Parker has a long-standing connection to antisocial individuals and has a moderate degree of criminal thinking. Participation in treatment designed to modify criminal thinking is recommended. Addressing the thinking component across problematic life areas (e.g., peers, substance use) is also suggested.

- Emotion Dysregulation: Mr. Parker is assessed as having above-average difficulty with anger dysregulation, which seems to be related to his history of aggressive behaviors. Participation in an anger management rehabilitation initiative of moderate intensity is recommended.

- Substance Abuse/Misuse: Mr. Parker is assessed as having above-average substance use difficulties; his criminal involvements are related to his use of alcohol and marijuana. Participation in a substance abuse treatment of moderate intensity is recommended.

- Connections to School/Work: Mr. Parker has a weak vocational history and a maladaptive attitude toward employment. He presents with some ambition to become a truck driver, and he should be encouraged and supported to pursue this employment direction.

- Psychopathology: Mr. Parker has no mental health history; however, he has skills deficits (e.g., impulsivity, poor decision making) that compromise effective life functioning. These issues should be addressed in intervention programs.

Report author's name and credentials: Brenda Wilson, M.A.

FIGURE 13.1. (*continued*)

The Y-axis of Form 13.2 represents the scaling procedure, or points of reference for displaying findings from the individual assessment domains. The power of an assessment instrument is derived from a comparison of a specific JIC's score on the measurement device to the instrument's normative data. In situations where multiple assessment domains are examined, a common metric is used to determine relative ranking between domains. Several test standardization procedures exist for this purpose (e.g., z-scores, T-scores); however, the percentile rank method may offer a considerable practical advantage. With the percentile rank approach, a given score is precisely compared to normative data. A percentile rank expresses the percentage of scores that are lower than a given score. To give a simple example, a score of 75 on a scale of scores ranging from 0 to 100 is at the 75th percentile, meaning that it is higher than 74% of scores. This approach offers both precision and ease of understanding, which are important in practical applications.

A completed Assessment Profile for Hank appears in Figure 13.2. The information shown in this figure comes from the original Case Formulation Worksheet for Hank (Figure 6.5) and the Assessment and Treatment Plan Report for him (Figure 13.1). Hank's percentile rankings on the domains listed are as follows: Risk/Need, 68th percentile; Imprecision (based on the faking measure), 23rd percentile; Criminogenic Thinking, 79th percentile; Emotion, 95th percentile; Substances, 75th percentile; and Readiness to Change, 30th percentile.

Although a chart of test data can be illuminating to a JIC on its own, it is important to discuss the findings with the JIC in a way that fosters understanding and allows for opportunities to answer any questions. A sample script for reviewing an Assessment Profile is presented in Script 13.1 (provided at the end of this chapter); Hank's data are used for ease of presentation, but of course each JIC's own data should be substituted for these. A similar script for providing feedback on standardized test results appears in Chapter 7 (Script 7.5).

Name: *Hank Parker*   Date: *June 20, 2017*

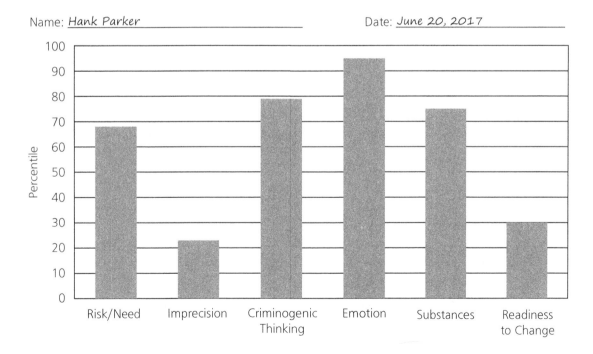

FIGURE 13.2. Assessment Profile for Hank.

MONITORING AND DOCUMENTING CLINICAL PROGRESS
WITHIN SESSIONS

Practitioners providing treatment to JICs are exposed to and must process a large amount of clinical information. Documenting relevant elements of this information not only is a professional requirement, but can enhance the effects of treatment for JICs, as noted at the start of this chapter. Research has shown that documenting clinical progress enhances the decision making of both practitioners and clients (Meier, 2008), which in turn improves therapeutic outcomes (Lambert, Hansen, & Finch, 2001). At the same time, however, many practitioners perceive recording information about treatment progress as a burden (Hatfield & Ogles, 2004). This quandary can be partially resolved by employing a simple but informative method for recording treatment progress. The Session Record Template in Form 13.3 (provided at the end of the chapter) is our recommended solution. The essence of this documentation approach is merging clinical narrative information with quantitative ratings of treatment performance (a fuller discussion of this approach is available in Simourd, 2014).

The Session Record Template has three components. The top portion of the document is reserved for basic information, such as the JIC's name, the date and duration of the session, and the location. The middle portion provides a system for rating the JIC in four treatment progress areas: (1) Participation (the JIC's degree of activity–inactivity in the session); (2) Understanding (the degree to which the JIC seemed to understand the topics discussed); (3) Self-Application (the degree to which the JIC seemed to see the session material as being applicable to his or her life); and (4) Overall (an omnibus rating of the JIC's session performance).

Each of these areas is rated on a typical Likert-type scale, which ranges from 1 (Far below Expectation) to 5 (Far above Expectation). The rating approach in the Session Record Template, however, differs from what most practitioners may be used to: It is an intraindividual approach in which the JIC is rated against him- or herself, as opposed to an interindividual approach in which comparisons are made to some external normative standard. In completing the ratings for each category in the Session Record, you will pose this question: "How did [JIC's name] do in this session, relative to what I would expect of him [her]?" Although the intraindividual nature of the ratings may be unfamiliar to most of our readers, our experience has been that the benefits of this method far outweigh the initial discomfort. As with anything new, it may take practice and repetition for you to become accustomed to this approach—but you will probably become reasonably proficient in it within a short period of time.

The (large) bottom portion of the Session Record Template is simply labeled Notes. This is the area in which to make narrative notations about the JIC. This approach is consistent with traditional clinical note taking, in which a variety of pertinent information is typically recorded. For example, it is common to include comments related to mental status or mood issues (e.g., "The client seemed quite forgetful this session," "The client was in a negative mood this session and was inclined to argue"), topics discussed (e.g., "Today we discussed companions"), other relevant issues (e.g., "Today the client mentioned applying for a job"), and a comment about what is to occur next session (e.g., "We will meet next week and discuss companions again").

The space allotted to the Notes section in Form 13.3 comprises approximately two-thirds of a page. This is intended to encourage efficiency in the documentation practices. A strong clinical note is one in which there is a balance between comprehensiveness and parsimony; in other words, pertinent information is included, but in an efficient manner. Too often, practitioners become overly verbose or detailed in their descriptions of clinical progress, which ultimately diminishes the richness of their comments about JICs. Having a limited amount of recording space provides a natural incentive to be parsimonious.

Only a modest amount of time is required to complete the Session Record Template. Moreover, the time requirement is either on a par with those for traditional methods of recording session progress or even slightly less, due to the structured format. With respect to completion frequency, the maximum benefit of this approach is achieved when the Session Record Template is completed for each interaction with a JIC, which we routinely do in our own treatment activities. However, we recognize that some users may have competing time demands and may be unable to complete a record for each session. In such cases, it is recommended that the document be completed "as often as practical" —although it should be kept in mind that the greater the frequency, the greater the clinical clarity regarding the assessment of participation and progress. Two examples of a completed Session Record are presented for Hank in Figures 13.3 and 13.4: One for his initial session, and one for his 10th session. The focus of these sessions was on his emotion dysregulation, and a specific anger management intervention was pursued.

A TEMPLATE FOR A TREATMENT SUMMARY REPORT

A treatment summary report is a document that summarizes overall progress. It provides a synopsis of the clinical activities that occurred over the course of treatment, offers comments about a JIC's performance in those activities, and describes any benefits for the JIC's life functioning. Like other types of clinical documentation, the treatment summary report is a professional necessity and can be useful to both practitioner and JIC. And like other forms of documentation, it is often considered by practitioners to be a time-consuming burden.

A template of our recommended approach for a treatment summary report is provided in Form 13.4. As can be seen, there are five main sections. The (unlabeled) initial section provides case-specific information, such as the JIC's name and identifying information (date of birth in this case, but other information, such as the client's ID number, can be added); the name of the practitioner who provided the treatment and/or who wrote the treatment summary report; the date the report was completed; and the name or type of intervention or program. The second section, Client Background, is reserved for information about the JIC. This should contain a brief account of the circumstances of how the client came to be referred to the intervention, as well as any supporting clinical information (test data, behavioral markers, etc.).

The third section, Intervention, should contain a brief description of the treatment activities. This may include a description of the intervention(s) employed (e.g., commercial product or program, number of sessions or modules, group vs. individual). The fourth section, Client Performance, is reserved for information related to the JIC's overall progress in the intervention(s). This includes comments about attendance, participation, completion of any intervention requirements (e.g., role plays, homework assignments), and any pre- to posttreatment test data. The Session

(text resumes on page 266)

| Name: | Parker, Hank | Date: | July 5, 2017 |
| Time: | 1:00–2:00 P.M. | Location: | Office |

	Far below Expectation	Below Expectation	Meets Expectation	Above Expectation	Far above Expectation
Participation		×			
Understanding		×			
Self-Application	×				
Overall		×			

NOTES

- Mr. Parker attended his initial individual session.
- He arrived 10 min. late for his scheduled appointment and seemed in a poor mood.
- Mr. P. is a 25-year-old male of average height/weight, with no distinguishing features.
- He was soft-spoken but had an aloof style of conversation; it seemed as though he didn't want to be at the session.
- Mr. P. has recently been convicted of an assault against a female acquaintance. He has a modest history of convictions that began in his late teens.
- He has a poor social history (raised in a chaotic and dysfunctional family setting). He has poor connections to school/work, uses substances that cause problems, and has emotional dysregulation.
- Mr. P. was initially referred for anger management treatment. His pretreatment assessment indicated a high level of problems in emotion dysregulation. In addition, his readiness for change was deemed to be weak.
- Mr. P. was suspicious and resentful about being referred for anger management treatment. He disagreed with the idea that he had anger problems. He is also mandated to undergo drug testing, which he resented.
- Future treatment considerations were explained to Mr. P. These included specific issues addressed and the aim of treatment (e.g., to reduce the frequency, intensity, and duration of his verbal and physical anger expressions). The benefits of success were also highlighted.
- He grudgingly agreed to attend other sessions.
- Next appointment: July 19, 2017, 1:00 P.M.
  - Continue with rapport building.
  - Introduce first steps of anger management.

FIGURE 13.3. Session Record: Initial session with Hank.

Name:	Parker, Hank	Date:	October 20, 2017
Time:	1:00–2:00 P.M.	Location:	Office

	Far below Expectation	Below Expectation	Meets Expectation	Above Expectation	Far above Expectation
Participation				X	
Understanding				X	
Self-Application				X	
Overall				X	

NOTES

- Mr. P. attended his 10th individual session to address emotion dysregulation issues.
- He arrived on time, was in a positive mood, and was talkative. This is typical of his presentation during the past several sessions.
- At the outset, Mr. P. reported he had taken steps to gain employment as a truck driver.
- He recognizes the need for positive work experiences and obtaining a source of income.
- As for treatment targets, Mr. P completed five thought records of his anger experiences since the last session. He provided considerable detail and related the thought records to personal changes he has had in the past few sessions. His effort and amount of self-application were excellent.
- This session focused on specific anger situations related to his friends.
- Mr. P's friends are of an antisocial nature and have a negative influence on him. He has been making efforts to distance himself from them, but finds that this creates conflict and anger; he rates the anger as 8/10 (1 being no anger and 10 being extreme).
- We reviewed the A-B-C model and applied it to the situations with his friends.
- Mr. P. agreed to work on this for our next session.
- He continues to show steady and gradual improvements in his anger management. He used to have anger episodes of high frequency and strong intensity, but both frequency and intensity have decreased considerably.
- Next appointment: November 3, 2017, 1:00 P.M.
  - Review A-B-C model of anger with friends.
  - Introduce relapse prevention and begin planning for treatment termination.

FIGURE 13.4. Session Record: 10th session with Hank.

Record approach described above can be particularly useful in completing this section, because the narrative and quantitative records kept across intervention sessions can be easily integrated into the treatment summary report. The final section, Summary, is for a synopsis of the JIC's overall response to the intervention.

To offer a practical example, Figure 13.5 presents the Treatment Summary Report for Hank's anger management treatment. Keep in mind that Hank's course of treatment addresses several criminal risk domains. This sample report is specific to the anger intervention.

In conclusion, clinical documentation is a necessary and important part of the treatment process with JICs. It can be perceived as a burden, but this does not have to be the case if a focused, parsimonious, and relevant approach is undertaken. This chapter has offered a practical framework for the smooth but informative completion of documentation that is vital to all stakeholders in the management of JICs.

KEY POINTS

- Documentation is an importation aspect of clinical work with JICs and can be helpful to practitioners, the clients, and third-party stakeholders.

- An effective assessment and treatment plan report provides a clear and credible description of the assessment methods used and the conclusions reached. There should also be a clear and logical connection between the assessment information and the ultimate recommendations offered.

- All clinical documentation should be clear and concise. The use of professional jargon should be kept to a minimum.

- We recommend providing JICs with feedback on assessment results in a manner they can understand and appreciate.

- Treatment performance information can be efficiently documented by using session-by-session ratings and notations.

- A treatment summary report provides valuable information about treatment activities and highlights JICs participation and overall progress.

Client's name: Parker, Hank   **D.O.B.:** April 1, 1992
Practitioner's name: Wilson, Brenda   **Date report completed:** December 7, 2017
Name or type of intervention: Anger management

CLIENT BACKGROUND

Mr. Parker is a 25-year-old male who was recently convicted of an assault against a female acquaintance. He was referred to anger management treatment by his probation officer due to this event, and also because he has a history of anger dysregulation difficulties that have caused problems in his life.

   Mr. Parker participated in a personal evaluation as part of his court proceedings, which are described in the Assessment and Treatment Plan Report. This report indicated that Mr. Parker had elevations in his anger, as measured by the Anger Disorders Scale, which is a standardized measure of anger difficulties. The overall conclusion was that anger treatment (given his high need) would be beneficial to Mr. Parker.

INTERVENTION

Mr. Parker was offered the Anger Reduction Program (ARP), which is a standardized intervention designed to improve emotion regulation related to anger. The ARP consists of 15 separate modules, with each module lasting 1.5 hours. It has a cognitive-behavioral focus with a relapse prevention context. The ARP incorporates pre- to posttreatment test data, session-by-session ratings of participant performance, and rated homework into its method of evaluating participant progress. The ARP is typically a group-operated intervention; however, it was delivered to Mr. Parker on an individual basis, because no group class was available at the time of his admission.

CLIENT PERFORMANCE

Mr. Parker attended 13 of 15 sessions of the ARP. He was ill for one session and had a conflict related to pursuing employment for the other session. The information he missed during the missed sessions was integrated into other sessions, and as such, he was deemed to have met all the requirements of the ARP.

   Clinically, Mr. Parker was reasonably well engaged with the ARP, and a positive therapeutic rapport was established. He was somewhat hesitant at the outset of the program to reveal personal information about his anger

(continued)

FIGURE 13.5. Treatment Summary Report for Hank's anger management intervention.

that could serve as a basis for discussion. However, he became more relaxed after a few sessions and was genuine and open in his self-disclosures. He commented several times about how the ARP brought to light for him the fact that his anger problems have existed for some time and have caused problems in his life. He was thus motivated to improve his anger control, both reducing the frequency and intensity of his reactions.

Mr. Parker's performance in each session was rated by a practitioner rating method. This included four areas: Participation (his degree of activity–inactivity in the session), Understanding (the degree to which he understood intervention information), Self-Application (the degree to which he applied intervention information in his life functioning), and Overall (a summary comment about his progress in session). These criteria were rated on a 5-point scale ranging from "Far below Expectation" to "Far above Expectation." Mr. Parker had ratings in the 2–3 range across the four criteria at the beginning of the ARP, but by the fifth intervention session, his session ratings were regularly in the 4–5 range.

In addition to the session ratings, Mr. Parker completed standardized tests at pretreatment, and these were readministered at posttreatment. The tests included measures of anger, response bias, and readiness for change. Mr. Parker had positive change scores on these tests that reflected improvement in his anger problems. Specifically, his pretreatment anger score was in the high range, and this was reduced to the low–moderate range at the end of the intervention. Moreover, the measures of response bias and readiness for change also improved at the end of intervention, reflecting greater honesty and a greater interest in improving his life.

SUMMARY

Mr. Parker is a relatively young man who has a history of emotion dysregulation that has caused both life functioning problems and criminal involvement. He was referred to the ARP by his probation officer, with the hope of reducing the frequency, duration, and intensity of his anger episodes and the resulting negative consequences. Mr. Parker was actively engaged in the ARP and had a positive response. This was evident from both his in-session performance and the results of standardized tests. Also, Mr. Parker was a pleasure to work with in the ARP. Although he has made gains, Mr. Parker is encouraged to continue to utilize the techniques he has learned, so that he does not return to old patterns.

Practitioner's name   Brenda Wilson, M.A.

FIGURE 13.5. *(continued)*

SCRIPT 13.1. Describing an Assessment Profile: The Example of Hank

"Hello, Hank. I want to review with you the results of the questionnaires you completed as part of the assessment phase. As a reminder, the purpose of doing the assessment and completing the questionnaires was to gain an understanding of some of the reasons why you have had trouble with the law. I have a chart that shows some of the questionnaire results, and I want to show them to you.

"I'll begin by describing the chart. First, there are six separate categories for different areas that were measured. As you can see, these categories are shown along the bottom row of this chart. The height of the column for each category relates to how high or low you scored in that area, compared to other people who have taken the same tests. Most of the scores are presented so that the higher the score, the more it is a concern.

"Let me start with the first column, Risk/Need. This shows the results of the big-picture test of your overall lifestyle as it relates to getting into trouble with the law. Your score is almost at the 70th percentile, which is in an elevated range. Based on this, I would say that your chances of getting into trouble with the law in the future are somewhat high unless you make some changes in your life.

"Now let's look at the second column, called Imprecision. This relates to the mindset you had toward completing the self-report questionnaires, particularly whether the answers included some untruths (either intentionally or unintentionally). This influences the accuracy of the test results; the more untruthful you are, the less accurate the results. Your score is a little over the 20% level, which is in the low range. This means that you were more or less honest in your answers, which tells me that the results of the other self-report tests are most likely accurate reflections of your opinions. In this case, lower scores are better.

"The third column is called Criminogenic Thinking. This column relates to thoughts and attitudes that may lead to trouble with the law. The more of these a person has, the more likely it is that this person will get in trouble in the future when a risky situation presents itself. Your score in this area is in the high range, at the 79th percentile. This means your thinking is such that you are at risk for making destructive decisions and possibly having further conflict with the law.

"The fourth column is called Emotion. This column relates to how much of a problem anger is for you. Your score here is at the 95th percentile, which is in the high range. This means your anger can be a serious problem that interferes with your relationships and puts you at risk for getting into conflicts with people.

"The fifth column is called Substances, which measures your substance use. You are at the 75th percentile level here, which is in the high range. This tells me that your use of substances is causing notable amounts of difficulty in your life and could increase your chances of getting into trouble in the future.

"The last column is called Readiness to Change; it measures your overall interest in improving your life or making changes. Your score in this area is at the 30th percentile, which is in the low area. This tells me that you have some problems getting yourself interested and motivated to make changes in your life.

"Overall, what the chart shows is that you have a high likelihood of getting into trouble with the law in the future, and that your thinking, anger, and use of substances are areas related to your risk of future legal problems. Also, at the moment you don't seem overly interested in making changes to your lifestyle, which is a bit concerning to me.

"I want you to know that all these scores can change over time, but your energy and participation will be necessary to make that happen.

"Does this information make sense? And do you have any questions?"

(continued)

[Use some of the following questions to elicit change talk.]

"What do you think about all this information I've shown you?"

"Can you tell me in your own words what the basic message from all these tests is?"

"How does this fit with the way you see your life and criminal risk potential?"

"How could your life be different if you didn't have these criminal risk factors?"

"Tell me about any downsides of your current lifestyle." [Search for complications related to relationships, personal happiness, finances, and personal freedoms.]

"Give me a sense of what your life will be like if you deal with your criminal risk factors."

"Thanks. Your ability to talk about these things is helpful to both of us."

FORM 13.1. Assessment and Treatment Plan Report Template

Client's name: D.O.B.:

Assessor's name: Date report completed:

PURPOSE AND OUTLINE OF ASSESSMENT

OVERVIEW OF CURRENT OFFENSES AND LEGAL HISTORY

Current Offenses

(continued)

Legal History

Custody Behavior

BACKGROUND INFORMATION

Developmental History

Connections to School/Work

(continued)

Physical Health Concerns/Psychopathology

Substance Abuse/Misuse

Family/Romantic Relationships/Companions

Self-Improvement Experiences

Professional Assessment History

(continued)

INTERVIEW(S) AND TEST RESULTS

Clinical Presentation

Test Results

(continued)

Case Formulation Based on Interview and Test Data

SUMMARY AND RECOMMENDATIONS

(continued)

TREATMENT PLAN RECOMMENDATIONS

- Treatment Target 1 (Brief comment and method of achievement)

- Treatment Target 2 (Brief comment and method of achievement)

- Treatment Target 3 (Brief comment and method of achievement)

- Treatment Target 4 (Brief comment and method of achievement)

- Treatment Target 5 (Brief comment and method of achievement)

- Treatment Target 6 (Brief comment and method of achievement)

Report author's name and credentials:

FORM 13.2. Assessment Profile Template

Name: _____   Date: _____

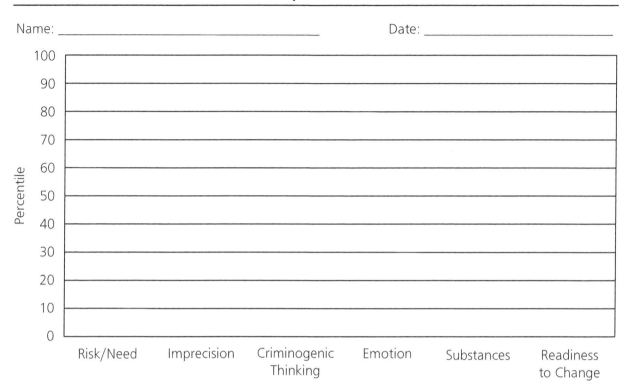

FORM 13.3. Session Record Template

Name:		Date:	
Time:		Location:	

	Far below Expectation	Below Expectation	Meets Expectation	Above Expectation	Far above Expectation
Participation					
Understanding					
Self-Application					
Overall					

NOTES

FORM 13.4. Treatment Summary Report Template

Client's name: **D.O.B.:**

Practitioner's name: **Date report completed:**

Name or type of intervention:

CLIENT BACKGROUND

INTERVENTION

(continued)

CLIENT PERFORMANCE

SUMMARY

Practitioner's name

Postscript

"How shall I lose the sin, yet keep the sense,
And love th' offender, yet detest th' offence?"
—ALEXANDER POPE, *Eloisa to Abelard* (1717)

To borrow the *tool* metaphor common to clinical training workshops, throughout this book we have endeavored to share our clinical tools with you so that you can add them to your toolbox. We hope you have found the scripts, forms, strategies/techniques, and other tools to be useful additions to your toolkit. To carry the metaphor a little further, if we were to construct the very toolbox itself, the materials we would make it out of would include a focus on criminal risk domains (rather than mental health symptoms) and the development of *approach* as well as *avoidance* goals centered around those risk domains. MI would serve as the glue holding the box together—enhancing motivation for change in clients who are commonly coerced into the office, and providing a communication style that is practical and compassionate. From our perspective, mental health symptoms are not unimportant, but their reduction will not necessarily reduce future criminal behavior. Addressing criminal risk domains that drive repeated involvement with the criminal justice system is the most empirically supported approach to curbing recidivism and improving the lives of JICs.

We hope that reading this book is not the end of your learning and clinical work with JICs. There are many excellent books devoted to in-depth coverage of one or more of the concepts covered in this treatment planner, and we have listed a sampling of them in Appendix B. A list of professional associations that provide training, networking, and education in forensic treatment is also provided in Appendix B. We hope that you will take advantage of these resources and continue your professional development in this complex, but worthwhile, area of clinical practice.

The cost of incarceration, the wasted potential of incarcerated members of society, and—most importantly—the suffering of victims and their families all make forensic treatment an important area of practice. There is a considerable need for competent CBT practitioners to make an impact on such a large and significant social problem. Just as a single offense can create a ripple effect and have far-reaching negative consequences on a large network of individuals, desistance from a pattern of offending can prevent a potentially enormous amount of human suffering.

We thank you, our readers, for spending time with this treatment planner, and we hope it has provided you with the necessary foundation of knowledge for working effectively with JICs.

Standardized Test Recommendations

There has been exponential growth over the years in the development of assessment instruments suitable for JICs, so that practitioners now have a number of options from which to choose. One unintended consequence of this growth is that the wide availability of instruments can create indecision about which specific instrument to use. It is good clinical practice to administer assessment instruments in a judicious and balanced manner—in other words, to administer those that accomplish clinical goals but are not burdensome to JICs. This means that practitioners must decide which instruments to include in a test battery and which to exclude. Decisions in this regard are often dependent on practitioners' preferences and may be related to any number of considerations, such as forensic experience, degree of commitment to the scientist-practitioner model, availability of assessment resources, familiarity with certain instruments, and theoretical orientation. Bonta (2002) has offered a set of guidelines to consider in selecting standardized assessment instruments. With these in mind, we recommend choosing instruments that are (1) predominantly dynamic (i.e., they assess risk domains on which clients can change) rather than predominantly static; (2) are simple and fluid to administer (i.e., they have limited complexity of administration and scoring/interpretation); and (3) have some level of psychometric evidence/relevant normative data consistent with the characteristic features of the JICs with whom you work.

Tables A.1–A.6 present suggestions for instruments with which we have some clinical familiarity, along with references or information for further reading and exploration. The instruments listed are those that adhere to the selection issues noted above. Some instruments are commercial test products and copyrighted, while others are in the public domain. We recognize that practitioners have many options and may opt for different instruments, or may work in a setting that dictates what instruments are used.

We recommend utilizing broad-based risk tools *in addition to* an interview, rather than *in place of* an interview. For the assessment of criminal risk domains, several broad-based criminal risk/need assessment instruments have been developed (see Table A.1), such as the Level of Service tools (which include the Level of Service/Case Management Inventory (LS/CMI) for use with adults, and the Youth Level of Service/Case Management Inventory [YLS/CMI] for youth) and the Offender Screening Tool (OST). All of these tools rely on a semistructured interview that classifies JICs in terms of risk level (e.g., low, medium, high) for supervision purposes, and that identifies specific criminal risk domains in need of change. Their advantage in terms of treatment planning is that they examine multiple criminal risk domains and have empirical support in predicting recidivism. Their limitation is that the depth of information they are designed to obtain in any given risk area is somewhat less than what may be desired for treatment planning. For example, both criminal thinking and emotional dysregulation related to anger are important criminogenic factors, but they are inadequately measured for treatment-planning purposes by most broad-based instruments.

Additional testing is therefore needed and can be accomplished by way of specialized test instruments. We recommend that supplemental testing occur in areas of interest that are sub-optimally assessed by the broad-based tools. These may include, but is not limited to the areas of substance abuse, response bias, anger, and readiness to change. Some recommendations for specialized tools can be found in Tables A.2–A.6.

TABLE A.1. Selected Instruments for Assessing Broad–Based Criminal Risk Domains

Instrument	Features	Further information about instrument
Level of Service tools: Level of Service/Case Management Inventory (LS/CMI); Youth Level of Service/Case Management Inventory (YLS/CMI)	LSI-R (adults): 54 items, 10 subscales YLS/CMI (youth): 42 items, 8 subscales	• Olver, M. E., Stockdale, K. C., & Wormith, J. S. (2014). Thirty years of research on the Level of Service scales: A meta-analytic examination of predictive accuracy and sources of variability. *Psychological Assessment, 26*, 156–176. • *www.mhs.com*
Offender Screening Tool (OST)	44 items, 10 subscales	• Casey, P. M., Elek, J. K., Warren, R. K., Cheesman, F., Kleiman, M., & Ostrom, B. (2014). *Offender risk and needs assessment instruments: A primer for the courts.* Williamsburg, VA: National Center for State Courts. • *www.acesink.com*

TABLE A.2. Specialized Tests for Assessing Criminogenic Thinking

Instrument	Features	Further information about instrument
Psychological Inventory of Criminal Thinking Styles (PICTS)	80 items, 8 subscales	• Walters, G. D. (2012). *Crime in a psychological context: From career criminals to criminal careers.* Thousand Oaks, CA: SAGE.
Criminal Sentiments Scale—Modified (CSS-M)	41 items, 5 subscales	• Simourd, D. J. (1997). The Criminal Sentiments Scale—Modified and Pride in Delinquency Scale: Psychometric properties and construct validity of two measures of criminal attitudes. *Criminal Justice and Behavior, 24*, 52–70.
Criminogenic Thinking Profile (CTP)	65 items, 8 subscales	• Mitchell, D., & Tafrate, R. C. (2012). Conceptualization and measurement of criminal thinking: Initial validation of the Criminogenic Thinking Profile. *International Journal of Offender Therapy and Comparative Criminology, 56*, 1080–1102.

TABLE A.3. Specialized Tests for Assessing Substance Use

Instrument	Features	Further information about instrument
Adult Substance Use Scale—Revised (ASUS-R)	96 items, 18 subscales	• Wanberg, K. W., & Milkman, H. B. (2008). *Criminal conduct and substance abuse treatment: Strategies of self-improvement and change—Pathways to responsible living. Provider guide.* Thousand Oaks, CA: SAGE. • *http://aodassess.com*
Texas Christian University Drug Screen (TCUDS II)	31 items, total score	• Simpson, D. D., Joe, G. W., Knight, K., Rowan-Szal, G. A., & Gray, J. S. (2012). Texas Christian University (TCU) short forms for assessing client needs and functioning in addiction treatment. *Journal of Offender Rehabilitation, 51,* 34–56. • *http://ibr.tcu.edu*

TABLE A.4. Specialized Tests for Assessing Dysfunctional Anger

Instrument	Features	Further information about instrument
Anger Disorders Scale (ADS) [adults]	74 items, 22 scores/ subscales	• DiGiuseppe, R., & Tafrate, R. (2004). *Anger Disorders Scale.* North Tonawanda, NY: Multi-Health Systems. • *www.mhs.com*
Anger Regulation and Expression Scale (ARES) [youth]	75 items, 25 scores/ subscales	• DiGiuseppe, R., & Tafrate, R. (2011). *Anger Regulation and Expression Scale (ARES).* North Tonawanda, NY: Multi-Health Systems. • *www.mhs.com*
Novaco Anger Scale and Provocation Inventory (NAS-PI)	81 items, 6 scores/ subscales	• Novaco, R. (2003). *Novaco Anger Scale and Provocation Inventory (NAS-PI).* Torrance, CA: Western Psychological Services. • *www.wpspublish.com*

TABLE A.5. Specialized Tests for Assessing Response Bias

Instrument	Features	Further information about instrument
Paulhus Deception Scales (PDS)	40 items, 2 subscales	• Paulhus, D. L. (1998). *Paulhus Deception Scales.* North Tonawanda, NY: Multi-Health Systems. • *www.mhs.com*
Marlowe–Crowne Social Desirability Scale (MCSDS)	33 items, total score	• Tatman, A. W., & Schouten, C. (2008). Measuring social desirability in adult male probation and parole clients. *Perspectives: The Journal of the American Probation and Parole Association, 32,* 49–53.

TABLE A.6. Specialized Tests for Assessing Readiness to Change

Instrument	Features	Further information about instrument
University of Rhode Island Change Scale (URICA)	32 items, 4 subscales	• Polaschek, D. L. L., Anstiss, B., & Wilson, M. (2010). The assessment of offending-related stage of change in offenders: Psychometric validation of the URICA with male prisoners. *Psychology, Crime and Law, 16,* 305–325. • *http://habitslab.umbc.edu*
Self-Improvement Orientation Scheme—Self Report (SOS-SR)	72 items, 13 subscales	• Simourd, D. J., & Olver, M. E. (2011). Use of the Self-Improvement Orientation Scheme—Self Report (SOS-SR) among incarcerated offenders. *Psychological Services, 8,* 200–211. • *www.acesink.com*

Resources for Practitioners

BOOKS

Bishop, F. M. (2001). *Managing addictions: Cognitive, emotive, and behavioral techniques.* Northvale, NJ: Aronson.

Bonta, J., & Andrews, D. A. (2017). *The psychology of criminal conduct* (6th ed.). New York: Routledge.

Marlatt, G. A., & Donovan, D. M. (Eds.). (2005). *Relapse prevention: Maintenance strategies in the treatment of addictive behaviors* (2nd ed.). New York: Guilford Press.

Miller, W. R., & Rollnick, S. (2013). *Motivational interviewing: Helping people change* (3rd ed.). New York: Guilford Press.

Mills, J. F., Kroner, D. G., & Morgan, R. D. (2011). *Clinician's guide to violence risk assessment.* New York: Guilford Press.

Najavits, L. M. (2002). *Seeking safety: A treatment manual for PTSD and substance abuse.* New York: Guilford Press.

Polaschek, D., Day, A., & Hollin, C. (Eds.). (2018). *Wiley handbook of correctional psychology.* Chichester, UK: Wiley.

Singh, J. P., Kroner, D. G., Wormith, J. S., Desmarais, S. L., & Hamilton, Z. (2018). *Handbook of recidivism risk/needs assessment tools.* Chichester, UK: Wiley.

Tafrate, R. C., & Kassinove, H. (2018). *Anger management for everyone* (2nd ed.): *Ten proven strategies to help you control anger and live a happier life.* Oakland, CA: New Harbinger.

Tafrate, R. C., & Mitchell, D. (Eds.). (2014). *Forensic CBT: A handbook for clinical practice.* Chichester, UK: Wiley.

Walters, G. D. (2012). *Crime in a psychological context: From career criminals to criminal careers.* Thousand Oaks, CA: Sage.

Wanberg, K. W., & Milkman, H. B. (2008). *Criminal conduct and substance abuse treatment: Strategies for self-improvement and change—Pathways to responsible living. Provider guide.* Thousand Oaks, CA: Sage.

PROFESSIONAL ORGANIZATIONS

Many of the large professional organizations in psychology have forensic specialty subsections. There are also several professional organizations that are solely forensically oriented. Both types provide conferences, continuing education, and networking opportunities. A sample of relevant organizations is provided below.

Organization: Association for Behavioral and Cognitive Therapies (ABCT)
Specialty subsection: Forensic and Externalizing Behaviors Special Interest Group
Website: *www.abct.org/Members/?m=mMembers&fa=SIG_LinkToAll#forensic*

Organization: American Psychological Association (APA)
Specialty subsection: Division 41, American Psychology–Law Society
Website: *www.apa.org/about/division/div41.aspx*

Organization: Australian Psychological Society
Specialty subsection: College of Forensic Psychologists
Website: *https://groups.psychology.org.au/cfp*

Organization: British Psychological Society (BPS)
Specialty subsection: Division of Forensic Psychology
Website: *www.bps.org.uk/networks-and-communities/member-microsite/division-forensic-psychology*

Organization: Canadian Psychological Association (CPA)
Specialty subsection: Criminal Justice Psychology Section
Website: *www.cpa.ca/aboutcpa/cpasections/criminaljusticepsychology*

Organization: European Association for Behavioural and Cognitive Therapies (EABCT)
Specialty subsection: Forensic CBT Special Interest Group
Website: *http://eabct.eu/portfolio-item/forensic-cbt*

Organization: International Association for Correctional and Forensic Psychology (IACFP)
Website: *www.aa4cfp.org*

Organization: International Community Corrections Association (ICCA)
Website: *http://iccalive.org/icca*

Organization: Motivational Interviewing Network of Trainers (MINT)
Website: *www.motivationalinterviewing.orgv*

References

Alberti, R. E., & Emmons, M. L. (2017). *Your perfect right: Assertiveness and equality in your life and relationships* (10th ed.). Oakland, CA: New Harbinger.

American Psychiatric Association. (2013). *Diagnostic and statistical manual of mental disorders* (5th ed.). Arlington, VA: Author.

Amrod, J., & Hayes, S. C. (2014). ACT for the incarcerated. In R. C. Tafrate & D. Mitchell (Eds.), *Forensic CBT: A handbook for clinical practice* (pp. 43–65). Chichester, UK: Wiley.

Andía, J. F., Deren, S., Robles, R. R., Kang, S. Y., Colón, H. M., Oliver-Velez, D., & Finlinson, A. (2005). Factors associated with injection and non-injection drug use during incarceration among Puerto Rican drug injectors in New York and Puerto Rico. *The Prison Journal, 85,* 329–342.

Andrews, D. A., & Bonta, J. (2010a). Rehabilitating criminal justice policy and practice. *Psychology, Public Policy, and the Law, 16,* 39–55.

Andrews, D. A., & Bonta, J. (2010b). *The psychology of criminal conduct* (5th ed.). New Providence, NJ: LexisNexis Matthew Bender.

Andrews, D. A., Bonta, J., & Hoge, R. D. (1990). Classification for effective rehabilitation: Rediscovering psychology. *Criminal Justice and Behavior, 17,* 19–52.

Andrews, D. A., Bonta, J., & Wormith, J. S. (2006). The recent past and near future of risk and/or need assessment. *Crime and Delinquency, 52,* 7–27.

Andrews, D. A., Zinger, I., Hoge, R. D., Bonta, J., Gendreau, P., & Cullen, F. T. (1990). Does correctional treatment work?: A psychologically informed meta-analysis. *Criminology, 28*(3), 419–429.

Australian Bureau of Statistics. (2015). Corrective services, Australia, December quarter 2015. Retrieved from *www.abs.gov.au/ausstats/abs@.nsf/mf/4512.0.*

Babcock, J. C., Green, C. E., & Robie, C. (2004). Does batterers' treatment work?: A meta-analytic review of domestic violence treatment. *Clinical Psychology Review, 23,* 1023–1053.

Babor, T. F., & Higgins-Biddle, J. C. (2001). *Brief intervention for hazardous and harmful drinking: A manual for use in primary care.* Geneva, Switzerland: World Health Organization.

Barrick, K., Lattimore, P. K., & Visher, C. A. (2014). Reentering women: The impact of social ties and long-term recidivism. *The Prison Journal, 94,* 279–304.

Beck, A. T. (1963). Thinking and depression: I. Idiosyncratic content and cognitive distortions. *Archives of General Psychiatry, 9,* 324–444.

Beck, A. T. (1967). *Depression: Causes and treatment.* Philadelphia: University of Pennsylvania Press.

Beck, A. T., Davis, D. D., & Freeman, A. (Eds.). (2015). *Cognitive therapy of personality disorders* (3rd ed.). New York: Guilford Press.

Beck, J. S. (2011). *Cognitive behavior therapy: Basics and beyond* (2nd ed.). New York: Guilford Press.

Berg-Smith, S. M. (2010). *Guiding the learning of motivational interviewing: A resource for trainers* [DVD]. Larkspur, CA: AIM for Change. Available from *www.berg-smithtraining.com/dvd.html.*

Bishop, F. M. (2001). *Managing addictions: Cognitive, emotive, and behavioral techniques.* Northvale, NJ: Jason Aronson.

Bishop, F. M. (2014). An integrated REBT-based approach to the treatment of addicted offenders. In R. C. Tafrate & D. Mitchell (Eds.), *Forensic CBT: A handbook for clinical practice* (pp. 233–251). Chichester, UK: Wiley.

Bonczar, T. P., & Mumola, C. J. (1998). *Substance abuse and treatment of adults on probation, 1995.* Washington, DC: Bureau of Justice Statistics.

Bonta, J. (2002). Offender risk assessment: Guidelines for selection and use. *Criminal Justice and Behavior, 29,* 355–379.

Bonta, J., & Andrews, D. A. (2007). *Risk–need–responsivity model of offender assessment and rehabilitation 2007–06.* Ottawa: Public Safety Canada.

Bonta, J., & Andrews, D. A. (2017). *The psychology of criminal conduct* (6th ed.). New York: Routledge.

Bonta, J., Blais, J., & Wilson, H. A. (2014). A theoretically informed meta-analysis of the risk for general and violent recidivism for mentally disordered offenders. *Aggression and Violent Behavior, 19,* 278–287.

Bonta, J., Bourgon, G., Rugge, T., Scott, T.-L., Yessine, A., Gutierrez, L., & Li, J. (2011). An experimental demonstration of training probation officers in evidence-based community supervision. *Criminal Justice and Behavior, 38*(11), 1127–1148.

Bonta, J., Law, M., & Hanson, R. K. (1998). The prediction of criminal and violent recidivism among mentally disordered offenders: A meta-analysis. *Psychological Bulletin, 123,* 123–142.

Bushman, B. J. (2002). Does venting anger feed or extinguish the flame?: Catharsis, rumination, distraction, anger, and aggressive responding. *Journal of Personality and Social Psychology, 28,* 724–731.

Carson, E. A. (2015, September). Prisoners in 2014. Retrieved from *www.bjs.gov/content/pub/pdf/p14.pdf.*

Centers for Disease Control and Prevention. (2015, August 10). Heart disease behavior. Retrieved from *www.cdc.gov/heartdisease/behavior.htm.*

Chang, E. C., D'Zurilla, T. J., & Sanna, L. J. (2004). *Social problem solving: Theory, research, and training.* Washington, DC: American Psychological Association.

Correctional Services Program, Statistics Canada. (2015). Adult correctional statistics in Canada, 2013/2014. Retrieved from *www.statcan.gc.ca/pub/85-002-x/2015001/article/14163-eng.htm.*

Cottle, C., C., Lee, R., J., & Heilbrun, K. (2001). The prediction of criminal recidivism in juveniles: A meta-analysis. *Criminal Justice and Behavior, 28,* 367–394.

Cox, S. M., Bantley, K., & Roscoe, T. (2005). *Evaluation of the Court Support Services Division's Probation Transition Program and Technical Violation Unit.* Wethersfield, CT: Court Support Services Division.

Dowden, C., & Andrews, D. A. (1999a). What works for female offenders: A meta-analytic review. *Crime and Delinquency, 45,* 438–452.

Dowden, C., & Andrews, D. A. (1999b). What works in young offender treatment: A meta-analysis. *Forum on Corrections Research, 11,* 21–24.

Dumas, L. L., & Ward, T. (2016). The good lives model of offender rehabilitation. *The Behavior Therapist, 39,* 175–177.

Ellis, A. (1957). Rational psychotherapy and individual psychology. *Journal of Individual Psychology, 13,* 38–44.

Ellis, A. (1962). *Reason and emotion in psychotherapy.* New York: Lyle Stuart.

Fazel, S., Bains, P., & Doll, H. (2006). Substance abuse and dependence in prisoners: A systematic review. *Addiction, 101,* 181–191.

Fernandez, E. (2010). Toward an integrative psychotherapy for maladaptive anger. In M. Potegal, G. Stemmler, & C. Spielberger (Eds.), *International handbook of anger: Constituent and concomitant biological, psychological, and social processes* (pp. 499–513). New York: Springer.

Fortune, C. A., & Ward, T. (2014). Integrating strength-based practice with forensic CBT: The good lives model of offender rehabilitation. In R. C. Tafrate & D. Mitchell (Eds.), *Forensic CBT: A handbook for clinical practice* (pp. 436–455). Chichester, UK: Wiley.

Garb, H. N. (1998). *Studying the clinician: Judgment research and psychological assessment.* Washington, DC: American Psychological Association.

Garcia, C. A. (2015). Community-based sanctions and juveniles: What works, what does not, and what looks promising. In M. D. Krohn & J. Lane (Eds.), *The handbook of juvenile delinquency and juvenile justice* (pp. 459–494). Chichester, UK: Wiley-Blackwell.

Gardner, F. L., & Moore, Z. E. (2014a). Contextual anger regulation therapy (CART): An acceptance-based treatment for domestic and non-domestic violent offenders. In R. C. Tafrate & D. Mitchell (Eds.), *Forensic CBT: A handbook for clinical practice* (pp. 161–183). Chichester, UK: Wiley.

Gardner, F., & Moore, Z. (2014b). *Contextual anger regulation therapy.* New York: Routledge.

Gendreau, P., Goggin, C., & Paparozzi, M. (1996). Principles of effective assessment for community corrections. *Federal Probation, 60,* 64–70.

Gendreau, P., & Smith, P. (2007). Influencing the 'people who count': Some perspectives on the reporting of meta-analytic results for prediction and treatment outcomes with offenders. *Criminal Justice and Behavior, 34,* 1536–1559.

Glynn, L. H., & Moyers, T. B. (2010). Chasing change talk: The clinician's role in evoking client language about change. *Journal of Substance Abuse Treatment, 39,* 65–70.

Hanson, R. K., Bourgon, G., Helmus, L., & Hodgson, S. (2009). The principles of effective correctional treatment also apply to sexual offenders: A meta-analysis. *Criminal Justice and Behavior, 36,* 865–892.

Hanson, R. K., & Bussiere, M. T. (1998). Predicting relapse: A meta-analysis of sexual offender recidivism studies. *Journal of Consulting and Clinical Psychology, 66,* 348–362.

Hare, R. D. (1996). Psychopathy: A clinical construct whose time has come. *Criminal Justice and Behavior, 23,* 25–54.

Hare, R. D. (2003). *The Hare Psychopathy Checklist—Revised manual* (2nd ed.). Toronto: Multi-Health Systems.

Hare, R. D., & Neumann, C. S. (2008). Psychopathy as a clinical and empirical construct. *Annual Review of Clinical Psychology, 4,* 217–246.

Hatfield, D. R., & Ogles, B. M. (2004). The use of outcome measures by psychologists in clinical practice. *Professional Psychology: Research and Practice, 35,* 485–491.

Hoffman, S. G., Asnaani, A., Vonk, I. J. J., Sawyer, A. T., & Fang, A. (2012). The efficacy of cognitive behavioral therapy: A review of meta-analyses. *Cognitive Therapy and Research, 36,* 437–440.

Kaeble, D., Maruschak, L. M., & Bonczar, T. P. (2015, November). Probation and parole in the United States, 2014. Retrieved from *www.bjs.gov/content/pub/pdf/ppus14.pdf.*

Karberg, J. C., & Mumola, C. J. (2006). *Drug use and dependence, state and federal prisoners, 2004.* Washington, DC: Bureau of Justice Statistics.

Kassinove, H., & Tafrate, R. C. (2002). *Anger management: The complete treatment guidebook for practitioners.* Atascadero, CA: Impact.

Kassinove, H., & Tafrate, R. C. (2014). *Anger management in counseling and psychotherapy* [DVD]. Mill Valley, CA: Psychotherapy.net.

Keulen-de Vos, M., Bernstein, D. P., & Arntz, A. (2014). Schema therapy for aggressive offenders with personality disorders. In R. C. Tafrate & D. Mitchell (Eds.), *Forensic CBT: A handbook for clinical practice* (pp. 66–83). Chichester, UK: Wiley.

Knight, K., Garner, B. R., Simpson, D. D., Morey, J. T., & Flynn, P. M. (2006). An assessment for criminal thinking. *Crime and Delinquency, 52,* 159–177.

Kolts, R. (2012). *The compassionate mind guide to managing your anger: Using compassion-focused therapy to calm your rage and heal your relationships.* Oakland, CA: New Harbinger.

Kolts, R., & Chodron, T. (2013). *Living with an open heart: How to cultivate compassion in everyday life.* London: Constable & Robinson.

Kroner, D. G., & Morgan, R. D. (2014). An overview of strategies for the assessment and treatment of criminal thinking. In R. C. Tafrate & D. Mitchell (Eds.), *Forensic CBT: A handbook for clinical practice* (pp. 87–103). Chichester, UK: Wiley.

Lambert, M. J., Hansen, N. B., & Finch, A. E. (2001). Patient focused research: Using patient outcome data to enhance treatment effects. *Journal of Consulting and Clinical Psychology, 69,* 159–172.

Landenberger, N. A., & Lipsey, M. W. (2005). The positive effects of cognitive behavioral programs for offenders: A meta-analysis of factors associated with effective treatment. *Journal of Experimental Criminology, 1*(4), 451–476.

Leahy, R. L., Holland, S. J., & McGinn, L. K. (2012). *Treatment plans and interventions for depression and anxiety disorders* (2nd ed.). New York: Guilford Press.

Lipsey, M. W., Chapman, G. L., & Landenberger, N. A. (2001). Cognitive-behavioral programs for offenders. *Annals of the American Academy of Political and Social Science, 578*, 144–147.

Lipsey, M. W., & Cullen, F. T. (2007). The effectiveness of correctional rehabilitation: A review of systematic reviews. *Annual Review of Law and Social Science, 3*, 297–320.

Lipsey, M. W., Landenberger, N. A., & Wilson, S. J. (2007). Effects of cognitive-behavioral programs for criminal offenders. *Campbell Systematic Reviews, 6*, 1–27. Retrieved from *www.campbellcollaboration. org/media/k2/attachments/1028_R.pdf.*

Lohr, J. M., Olatunji, B. O., Baumeister, R. F., & Bushman, B. J. (2007). The psychology of anger venting and empirically supported alternatives that do no harm. *Scientific Review of Mental Health Practice, 5*, 53–64.

Mandracchia, J. T., Morgan, R. D., Garos, S., & Garland, J. T. (2007). Inmate thinking patterns: An empirical investigation. *Criminal Justice and Behavior, 34*, 1029–1043.

Marlatt, G. A., & Donovan, D. M. (Eds.). (2005). *Relapse prevention: Maintenance strategies in the treatment of addictive behaviors* (2nd ed.). New York: Guilford Press.

Martin, M. S., Dorken, S. K., Wamboldt, A. D., & Wooten, S. E. (2012). Stopping the revolving door: A meta-analysis on the effectiveness of interventions for criminally involved individuals with major mental disorders. *Law and Human Behavior, 36*, 1–12.

Martinez, D. J., & Abrams, L. S. (2013). Informal social support among returning young offenders: A meta-synthesis of the literature. *International Journal of Offender Therapy and Comparative Criminology, 57*, 169–190.

Martinson, R. (1974). What works?: Questions and answers about prison reform. *The Public Interest, 35*, 22–54.

McCullough, M. E., Kurzban, R., & Tabak, B. A. (2013). Cognitive systems for revenge and forgiveness. *Behavioral and Brain Sciences, 36*, 1–15.

Meier, S. T. (2008). *Measuring change in counseling and psychotherapy.* New York: Guilford Press.

Miller, W. R., Moyers, T. B., Ernst, D., & Amrhein, P. (2008, January 8). *Manual for the Motivational Interviewing Skill Code version 2.1.* Retrieved from *http://casaa.unm.edu/download/misc.pdf.*

Miller, W. R., Moyers, T. B., & Rollnick, S. (2013). *Motivational interviewing professional training* [DVD series]. Carson City, NV: The Change Companies.

Miller, W. R., & Rollnick, S. (2013). *Motivational interviewing: Helping people change* (3rd ed.). New York: Guilford Press.

Miller, W. R., Rollnick, S., & Moyers, T. B. (1998). *Motivational interviewing professional training* [VHS/ DVD series]. Albuquerque: University of New Mexico Center on Alcoholism, Substance Abuse, and Addictions (UNM/CASAA).

Mills, J. F., Kroner, D. G., & Forth, A. E. (2002). Measures of Criminal Attitudes and Associates (MCAA): Development, factor structure, reliability, and validity. *Assessment, 9*, 240–253.

Mitchell, D., & Tafrate, R. C. (2012). Conceptualization and measurement of criminal thinking: Initial validation of the Criminogenic Thinking Profile. *International Journal of Offender Therapy and Comparative Criminology, 56*, 1080–1102.

Mitchell, D., Tafrate, R. C., & Freeman, A. (2015). Antisocial personality disorder. In A. T. Beck, D. D. Davis, & A. Freeman (Eds.), *Cognitive therapy of personality disorders* (3rd ed., pp. 346–365). New York: Guilford Press.

Morani, N. M., Wikoff, N., Linhorst, D. M., & Bratton, S. (2011). A description of the self-identified needs, service expenditures, and social outcomes of participants of a prisoner re-entry program. *The Prison Journal, 91*, 347–365.

Morgan, R. D., Flora, D. B., Kroner, D. G., Mills, J. F., Varghese, F. P., & Steffan, J. S. (2012). Treating offenders with mental illness: A research synthesis. *Law and Human Behavior, 36*, 37–50.

Morrison, J. (2014). *The first interview* (4th ed.). New York: Guilford Press.

Moyers, T. B., Martin, T., Houck, J. M., Christopher, P. J., & Tonigan, J. S. (2009). From in-session behaviors to drinking outcomes: A causal chain for motivational interviewing. *Journal of Consulting and Clinical Psychology, 77*, 1113–1124.

Moyers, T., Martin, T., Manuel, J., Miller, W., & Ernst, D. (2010, January 22). *Motivational Interviewing Treatment Integrity Instrument 3.1.1.* Retrieved from *http://casaa.unm.edu/download/MITI3_1.pdf.*

National Institute of Corrections (NIC) & Crime and Justice Institute (CJI). (2004). *Implementing evidence-based practice in community corrections: The principles of effective intervention.* Retrieved from *http://nicic.gov/Library/019342.*

National Institute of Mental Health. (n.d.). *What is prevalence?* Retrieved November 2014 from *www.nimh.nih.gov/health/statistics/prevalence/index.shtml.*

Novaco, R. W. (1994). Anger as a risk factor for violence among the mentally disordered. In J. Monahan & H. J. Steadman (Eds.), *Violence and mental disorder: Developments in risk assessment* (pp. 21–59). Chicago: University of Chicago Press.

Novaco, R. W. (2011a). Anger dysregulation: Driver of violent offending. *Journal of Forensic Psychiatry and Psychology, 22*, 650–668.

Novaco, R. W. (2011b). Perspectives on anger treatment: Discussion and commentary. *Cognitive and Behavioral Practice, 18*, 251–255.

Ogloff, J. R. P. (2006). Psychopathy/antisocial personality disorder continuum. *Australian and New Zealand Journal of Psychiatry, 40*, 519–528.

Parhar, K. K., Wormith, J. S., Derkzen, D. M., & Beauregard, A. M. (2008). Offender coercion in treatment: A meta-analysis of effectiveness. *Criminal Justice and Behavior, 35*, 1109–1135.

Persons, J. B. (2008). *The case formulation approach to cognitive-behavior therapy.* New York: Guilford Press.

Peterson, J. K., Skeem, J., Kennealy, P., Bray, B., & Zvonkovic, A. (2014). How often and how consistently do symptoms directly precede criminal behavior among offenders with mental illness? *Law and Human Behavior, 38*, 439–449.

Quinsey, V. L., Harris, G. T., Rice, M. E., & Cormier, C. A. (1998). *Violent offenders: Appraising and managing risk.* Washington, DC: American Psychological Association.

Rhodes, W., Dyouus, C., Kling, R., Hunt, D., & Luallen, J. (2013). *Recidivism of offenders on federal community supervision.* Washington, DC: Bureau of Justice Statistics.

Rosengren, D. B. (2018). *Building motivational interviewing skills: A practitioner workbook.* New York: Guilford Press.

Rosengren, D. B., Baer, J. S., Hartzler, B., Dunn, C. W., Wells, E. A., & Ogle, R. (2009, April). *Video Assessment of Simulated Encounters (VASE-R): Administration and scoring manual.* Retrieved from *http://adai.washington.edu/instruments/PDF/VASERScoringManual_145.pdf.*

Rowell, T. L., Wu, E. Hart, C. L., Haile, R., & El-Bassel, N. (2012). Predictors of drug use in prison among incarcerated black men. *American Journal of Drug and Alcohol Abuse, 38*, 593–597.

Rugge, T., & Bonta, J. (2014). Training community corrections officers on cognitive-behavioral intervention strategies. In R. C. Tafrate & D. Mitchell (Eds.), *Forensic CBT: A handbook for clinical practice* (pp. 122–136). Chichester, UK: Wiley.

Salisbury, E. J., & Van Voorhis, P. (2009). Gendered pathways: A quantitative investigation of women probationers' paths to incarceration. *Criminal Justice and Behavior, 36*, 541–566.

Scott, W. (2008). *Effective clinical practices in treating clients in the criminal justice system* (Accession No. 023362). Washington, DC: U.S. Department of Justice.

Seeler, L., Freeman, A., DiGuiseppe, R., & Mitchell, D. (2014). Traditional cognitive-behavioral therapy models for antisocial patterns. In R. C. Tafrate & D. Mitchell (Eds.), *Forensic CBT: A handbook for clinical practice* (pp. 15–42). Chichester, UK: Wiley.

Simourd, D. J. (1997). The Criminal Sentiments Scale—Modified and Pride in Delinquency Scale: Psychometric properties and construct validity of two measures of criminal attitudes. *Criminal Justice and Behavior, 24*, 52–70.

Simourd, D. J. (2014). Session-by-session assessment of client participation and progress. In R. C. Tafrate

& D. Mitchell (Eds.), *Forensic CBT: A handbook for clinical practice* (pp. 393–410). Chichester, UK: Wiley.

Skeem, J., Kennealy, P., Monahan, J., Peterson, J. K., & Appelbaum, P. (2016). Psychosis uncommonly and inconsistently precedes violence among high-risk individuals. *Clinical Psychological Science, 4*, 40–49.

Skeem, J. L., Schubert, C., Odgers, C., Mulvey, E. P., Gardner, W., & Lidz, C. (2006). Psychiatric symptoms and community violence among high risk patients: A test of the relationship at the weekly level. *Journal of Consulting and Clinical Psychology, 74*, 967–979.

Skeem J. L., Steadman, H. J., & Manchak, S. M. (2015). Applicability of the risk–need–responsivity model to persons with mental illness involved in the criminal justice system. *Psychiatric Services, 66*, 916–922.

Smith, P., Goggin, C., & Gendreau, P. (2002). *Effects of prison sentences and intermediate sanctions of recidivism: General effects and individual differences* (Accession No. CJA0370040004098s). Ottawa: Solicitor General of Canada,

Staton-Tindall, M., Havens, J., R., Oser, C. B., & Burnett, M. C. (2011). Substance use prevalence in criminal justice settings. In C. Leukefeld, T. P. Gullota, & J. Gregich (Eds.), *Handbook of evidence-based substance abuse treatment in criminal justice settings* (pp. 81–101). New York: Springer Science + Business Media.

Steadman, H. J., Osher, F. C., Robbins, P. C., Case, B., & Samuels, S. (2009). Prevalence of serious mental illness among jail inmates. *Psychiatric Services, 60*, 761–765.

Substance Abuse and Mental Health Services Administration. (2011, March 3). The TEDS report: Characteristics of probation and parole admissions aged 18 or older. Retrieved from *http://archive.samhsa.gov/data/2k10/231Parole2k11Web/231Parole2k11.htm*.

Sun, K. (2014). Treating depression and PTSD behind bars: An interaction schemas approach. In R. C. Tafrate & D. Mitchell (Eds.), *Forensic CBT: A handbook for clinical practice* (pp. 456–470). Chichester, UK: Wiley.

Swanston, M. C. (1987). Effects of rational–emotive imagery on self-reported affect and behavioral infractions in prisoners. *Dissertation Abstracts International: Section B. Sciences and Engineering, 49*(1), AAT 8800465.

Sykes, G. M., & Matza, D. (1957). Techniques of neutralization: A theory of delinquency. *American Sociological Review, 22*, 664–673.

Tafrate, R. C., & Kassinove, H. (2018). *Anger management for everyone* (2nd ed.): *Ten proven strategies to help you control anger and live a happier life*. Oakland, CA: New Harbinger.

Tafrate, R. C., & Luther, J. D. (2014). Integrating motivational interviewing with forensic CBT: Promoting treatment engagement and behavior change with justice-involved clients. In R. C. Tafrate & D. Mitchell (Eds.), *Forensic CBT: A handbook for clinical practice* (pp. 411–435). Chichester, UK: Wiley.

Tafrate, R. C., Mitchell, D., & Novaco, R. (2014). Forensic CBT: Five recommendations for clinical practice and five topics in need of more attention. In R. C. Tafrate & D. Mitchell (Eds.), *Forensic CBT: A handbook for clinical practice* (pp. 473–486). Chichester, UK: Wiley.

Tangney, J. P., Steuwig, J., Furukawa, E., Kopelovich, S., Meyer, P. J., & Crosby, B. (2012). Reliability, validity, and predictive utility of the 25-item Criminogenic Cognitions Scale (CCS). *Criminal Justice and Behavior, 39*, 1340–1360.

U.K. Ministry of Justice. (2013, September 19). Transforming rehabilitation: A summary of evidence on reducing reoffending. Retrieved from *www.gov.uk/government/publications/transforming-rehabilitation-a-summary-of-evidence-on-reducing-reoffending*.

U.K. Ministry of Justice. (2017, January 13). Prison population figures: 2016. Retrieved from *www.gov.uk/government/statistics/prison-population-figures-2016*.

U.S. Department of Health and Human Services. (2013). *Results from the 2012 national survey on drug use and health: Summary of national findings*. Retrieved from *www.samhsa.gov/data/sites/default/files/NSDUHresults2012/NSDUHresults2012.pdf*.

Van Dieten, M., & King, E. (2014). Advancing the use of CBT with justice-involved women. In R. C. Tafrate & D. Mitchell (Eds.), *Forensic CBT: A handbook for clinical practice* (pp. 329–353). Chichester, UK: Wiley.

Visher, C. A. (2013). Incarcerated fathers: Pathways from prison to home. *Criminal Justice Policy Review,* *24*, 9–26.

Visher, C., Debus, S., & Yahner, J. (2008). *Employment after prison: A longitudinal study of releases in three states.* Washington, DC: Urban Institute Justice Policy Center.

Visher, C. A., Winterfield, L., & Goggeshall, M. B. (2005). Ex-offender employment programs and recidivism: A meta-analysis. *Journal of Experimental Criminology, 1,* 295–315.

Walmsley, R. (2013). World prison population list (10th ed.). Retrieved from *www.apcca.org/uploads/10th_ Edition_2013.pdf*

Walters, G. D. (1995). The Psychological Inventory of Criminal Thinking Styles: I. Reliability and preliminary validity. *Criminal Justice and Behavior, 22,* 307–325.

Walters, G. D. (2012). *Crime in a psychological context: From career criminals to criminal careers.* Thousand Oaks, CA: SAGE.

Walters, G. D. (2014). Applying CBT to the criminal thought process. In R. C. Tafrate & D. Mitchell (Eds.), *Forensic CBT: A handbook for clinical practice* (pp. 104–121). Chichester, UK: Wiley.

Wanberg, K. W., & Milkman, H. B. (2008). *Criminal conduct and substance abuse treatment: Strategies for self-improvement and change—Pathways to responsible living. Provider guide.* Thousand Oaks, CA: SAGE.

Wanberg, K. W., & Milkman, H. B. (2014). Social and community responsibility therapy (SCRT): A cognitive-behavioral model for the treatment of substance abusing judicial clients. In R. C. Tafrate & D. Mitchell (Eds.), *Forensic CBT: A handbook for clinical practice* (pp. 252–277). Chichester, UK: Wiley.

Ward, T. (2010). The good lives model of offender rehabilitation: Basic assumptions, aetiological commitments, and practice implications. In F. McNeill, P. Raynor, & C. Trotter (Eds.), *Offender supervision: New directions in theory, research and practice* (pp. 41–64). Abingdon, UK: Willan.

White, B. A., Olver, M. E., & Lilienfeld, S. O. (2016). Psychopathy: Its relevance, nature, assessment, and treatment. *the Behavior Therapist, 39,* 154–161.

World Health Organization. (1992). *International classification of diseases and related health problems* (10th rev.). Geneva, Switzerland: Author.

Wranik, T., & Scherer, K. R. (2010). Why do I get angry?: A componential appraisal approach. In M. Potegal, G. Stemmler, & C. Spielberger (Eds.), *International handbook of anger: Constituent and concomitant biological, psychological, and social processes* (pp. 243–266). New York: Springer.

Index

Note. *f* or *t* following a page number indicates a figure or a table.

Ability, change talk and, 117, 118, 119*t*
Abuse, childhood, 16
Academic functioning
   assessment and, 68
   case formulation and, 96*f*–104*f*
   criminogenic thinking and, 137*f*
   forms to use in the case formulation and, 109–114
   overview, 18*t*
   risks–thoughts–decisions (RTD) sequence and, 141, 151
   scripts for, 78–79, 151
   template for report writing and, 253
Acceptance, 233, 235
Acceptance and commitment therapy (ACT), 27–28, 43
Activation, 117, 118, 119*t*
Active involvement in sessions, 11
Activity monitoring
   forms for, 192–195
   job search and, 184–185
   overview, 175–179, 177*f*, 178*f*, 187
   scripts for, 188–189
Advancement, 187
Advice, 218–219
Affirmations. *See also* OARS skills (open questions, affirmations, reflections, summarizations)
   change talk and, 117–118
   coding sheet for, 41
   engagement and, 32–33, 34*t*
   lifestyle changes and, 174
   motivational interviewing (MI), 25
Agenda for sessions, 11, 12*f*
Agenda-setting strategies, 121
Aggression, 235. *See also* Anger dysregulation
Alcohol abuse. *See* Substance abuse/misuse
Anger dysregulation
   assessment and, 70, 87
   case formulation and, 96*f*–104*f*, 109–114

criminogenic thinking and, 137*f*
   forms for, 109–114, 244–246
   managing anger, 226–234, 228*f*, 231*f*–232*f*, 234*t*
   overview, 17, 18*t*, 234–235
   risks–thoughts–decisions (RTD) sequence and, 141, 152
   scripts for, 87, 152, 239
Anger episode model, 228–230, 228*f*, 235
Anger Episode Record (Form 12.5)
   complete, 244–245
   examples of, 231*f*–232*f*
   overview, 229–230
Announcing Change (Form 12.4)
   complete, 243
   examples of, 225*f*
   overview, 224–225
Antisocial behavior, 67, 74–75. *See also* Behavior patterns
Antisocial companions. *See also* Peer factors; Relationships
   assessment and, 68, 71*t*, 81–82
   case formulation and, 96*f*–104*f*, 109–114
   criminogenic thinking and, 137*f*, 138*t*
   forms to use in the case formulation and, 109–114
   overview, 18*t*
   restructuring friendships and, 199–203, 201*f*, 203*f*
   risks–thoughts–decisions (RTD) sequence and, 141, 142–144, 147
   scripts for, 81–82, 147
Antisocial decision making, 145–146. *See also* Decision making
Antisocial label, 9–10
Antisocial orientation
   assessment and, 69–70, 86
   case formulation and, 96*f*–104*f*, 109–114
   forms to use in the case formulation and, 109–114
   overview, 17, 18*t*
   script for assessing, 86
Antisocial personality disorder (ASPD), 9

Anxiety
    assessment and, 66
    cognitions that promote criminality and, 21
Approach goals. *See also* Goals
    overview, 28, 281
    values and, 43
Asking permission, 123
Assertiveness, 233, 235
Assessment. *See also* Case formulation
    criminogenic thinking and, 22–23
    eliciting thinking patterns and, 71t–72t
    engagement and, 39
    focusing and, 121
    overview, viii, 4, 65–66, 70
    providing feedback regarding, 254, 261, 261f
    report writing and, 250–251, 266
    risk domains and, 66–70
    scripts for, 66–70, 73–87, 131, 269–270
    standardized tests and, 124, 125t, 283–284,
        284t–286t
    template for report writing and, 251–254, 255f–260f
Assessment and Treatment Plan Report Template
        (Form 13.1)
    Assessment Profile and, 261
    complete, 271–276
    examples of, 255f–260f
    overview, 251–254
Assessment interview, 66–70
Assessment Profile
    providing feedback regarding, 254, 261, 261f
    scripts for, 269–270
Assessment Profile Template (Form 13.2), 254, 261, 277
Attribution bias
    case formulation and, 105–106
    managing anger and, 226–227
Automatic thoughts, 22, 23–24, 145. *See also* Immediate
        Thinking; Thinking patterns
Avoidance goals, 28, 281. *See also* Goals
Awfulizing, 228, 228f

B

Base rate neglect, 105, 106–108
Behavior and expressive patterns, 228f, 229
Behavior patterns, 136, 173–174, 215–226, 220f, 223f,
        225f. *See also* Lifestyle
Behavioral interventions
    managing anger, 226–234, 228f, 231f–232f, 234t
    overview, 173–174
    restructuring friendships and, 200, 202
    substance use and abuse and, 218, 222–224, 223f
Better Thinking. *See also* Thinking Helpsheet (Form 9.1)
    overview, 163
    restructuring interventions and, 158–163, 159f
    scripts for, 166–169

Bias, 105–108
"Big Four" risk factors, 15. *See also* Risk domains
Blame
    attribution bias and, 106
    working with justice-involved clients and, 4

C

Career planning, 179–187, 181f, 183f
Case formulation. *See also* Assessment
    avoiding bias in, 105–108
    estimates of risk and, 89–91
    focusing and, 121
    forms for, 92–93, 96f–104f, 109–114
    overview, 4, 10–11, 65–66, 70, 88–89, 108
    providing feedback regarding, 254, 261, 261f
    template for report writing and, 253
    treatment plans and, 96f–104f
    treatment targets, 91–93, 92t, 94f–95f, 105
Case Formulation Worksheet (Form 6.3)
    Assessment Profile and, 261
    complete, 111–114
    examples of, 97f–104f
    overview, 93
Case management, 40
CAT (commitment, activation, and taking steps)
        acronym, 117, 118. *See also* Change talk
"Central Eight" risk factors, 15, 16–17. *See also* Risk
        domains
Change. *See also* Change talk
    motivation for, 24–27, 116–121, 118f, 119t
    overview, 281
    scripts for, 237–238
    standardized tests and, 286t
    substance use and abuse and, 219, 224–226, 225f,
        234–235
    values and, 43–44
Change planning, 25, 26
Change talk. *See also* Change
    eliciting, 118, 119t
    lifestyle changes and, 174
    overview, 116–121, 118f, 119t, 126
    recognizing, 117–118, 118f
    strategies for focusing conversations and, 121–124,
        122t, 125t
    substance use and abuse and, 219
Check-ins, 10, 12f
Childhood abuse, 16
Children of the offender, 16
Choices
    discrepancy between values and decisions and,
        50–53
    mental health problems and, 53
    overview, 28
Client-centered focus, 36

Closed questions
    coding sheet for, 41
    engagement and, 32, 33*t*
    minimizing the use of, 39
Coaching, 187
Coding sheets, 37–38
Coercion, 27, 28
Cognitions
    levels of, 22
    risk domains and, 135–136
    that promote criminality, 21–24, 23*t*
Cognitive restructuring, 233, 234*t*, 235
Cognitive schematic processing, 106
Cognitive-behavioral therapy (CBT)
    diagnosis and, 9–10
    effectiveness of, 8–9
    engagement and, 36
    overview, 281
Collaborative goals, 115, 121–124, 122*t*, 125*t*, 126. *See also* Goals
Collecting summary, 34, 35*t*. *See also* Summarizations
Commitment, 117, 118, 119*t*
Communication skills
    employment and, 185
    restructuring friendships and, 202
Community settings for treatment, 6
Compassion
    engagement and, 36
    managing anger and, 233–234, 235
    overview, 13
    working with justice-involved clients and, 4
Confidentiality
    court-mandated services and, 6
    custody settings for treatment and, 7
Confirmatory bias
    attribution bias and, 106
    case formulation and, 105
Conflicts, 186
Confrontation
    coding sheet for, 41
    motivational interviewing (MI) and, 27
Connecting interventions, 136
Contextual domains, 94*f*–95*f*, 136
Continuity, 11
Control
    assessment and, 71*t*
    criminogenic thinking and, 138*t*
Coping strategies
    assessment and, 72*t*
    criminogenic thinking and, 139*t*
Core beliefs (schemas), 22. *See also* Thinking patterns
Correctional treatment settings, 6–7
Court-mandated client. *See* Justice-involved clients (JICs)
Court-mandated services. *See also* Treatment
    community settings for treatment and, 6
    motivation for change and, 24

overview, 13
substance use and abuse and, 219
Criminal behavior
    assessment and, 67
    risk levels and, 89–90
    script for assessing, 74–75
    substance use and abuse and, 216
Criminal Cognitions Scale, 22
Criminal Event Analysis
    case formulation and, 92–93, 108
    complete, 109
    examples of, 94*f*–95*f*
Criminal risk domains. *See* Risk domains
Criminal Risk Domains Quiz, 15, 16*t*
Criminal Risk Domains Worksheet
    complete, 110
    examples of, 96*f*
    overview, 108
Criminal Sentiments Scale—Modified, 22
Criminogenic thinking. *See also* Thinking patterns
    assessment and, 69–70, 71*t*–72*t*, 86
    automatic thoughts and, 23–24
    case formulation and, 96*f*–104*f*, 109–114
    focusing and, 123, 129–130
    forms to use in the case formulation and, 109–114
    levels of, 136–137, 137*f*, 138*t*–139*t*
    monitoring assignments and, 155–158
    overview, 17, 18*t*, 22–23, 23*t*, 28, 135–136, 145–146
    restructuring interventions and, 158–163, 159*f*
    risk domains and, 140–145
    scripts for, 86, 141–144
    standardized tests and, 284*t*
    substance use and abuse and, 218, 221
Criminogenic Thinking Profile, 22
Crisis focus, 10–11
Criticism, 186
Curious stance, 32, 36, 39
Custody settings for treatment, 6–7

D

Daily activities, 173–174. *See also* Leisure time activities; Lifestyle; Routines
DARN (desire, ability, reasons, and need) acronym, 117, 118. *See also* Change talk
Day reporting centers, 6
Decision making
    automatic thoughts and, 23–24
    discrepancy between values and, 50–53, 54, 58–59
    overview, 135–136, 145–146
    risk domains and, 137, 140–145
    scripts for, 141–144
    substance use and abuse and, 219
Decisional balance technique, 120

Defensiveness
  diagnostic labels and, 9–10
  motivational interviewing (MI) and, 27
  substance use and abuse and, 218–219
Demandingness, 228, 228f
Demand for excitement
  assessment and, 71t
  criminogenic thinking and, 139t
Depression
  assessment and, 66
  cognitions that promote criminality and, 21
Desire, 117, 118, 119t
Destructive patterns, 173–174. *See also* Behavior
    patterns
Destructive values, 52–53. *See also* Values
Diagnosis, 9–10, 13. *See also* Mental health factors
Diagnostic and Statistical Manual of Mental Disorders,
    fifth edition (DSM-5), 9
Disability, intellectual
  case formulation and, 92t, 96f–104f
  forms to use in the case formulation and, 109–114
Disagreements, 186, 187
Dispositional characteristics, 90–91, 94f–95f
Disregard for others, 71t, 138t
Dissocial personality disorder, 9
Distancing, 206
Documentation. *See also* Report writing
  of clinical progress, 262–263
  court-mandated services and, 6
  examples of, 255f–260f, 264f–265f
  forms for, 271–280
  overview, 12f, 249–250, 266
  providing feedback regarding, 254, 261, 261f
  template for, 251–254, 255f–260f
  treatment summary report, 263, 266, 267f–268f
Drug testing, 6. *See also* Substance abuse/misuse
Dysfunctional family/romantic relationships
  assessment and, 67–68, 76–77
  case formulation and, 96f–104f, 109–114
  changing family dynamics, 204–208, 205f, 207f
  criminogenic thinking and, 137f
  forms to use in the case formulation and, 109–114
  overview, 18t
  risks–thoughts–decisions (RTD) sequence and, 141,
    149
  scripts for, 76–77, 149
  standardized tests and, 285t
  template for report writing and, 253

E

Education, 179–187, 181f, 183f, 187, 196–197
Education and Employment History Checklist (Form
    10.6), 182, 197
Emotion regulation, 70

Emotional disengagement
  assessment and, 71t
  criminogenic thinking and, 138t
Emotional dysregulation, 226–234, 228f, 231f–232f,
    234t. *See also* Anger dysregulation
Empathy
  engagement and, 36
  managing anger and, 233–234
  working with justice-involved clients and, 4
Employment. *See also* Work, connection to
  forms for, 196–197
  overview, 179–187, 181f, 183f, 187
  scripts for, 190–191
Engagement
  coding sheet for, 41
  motivational interviewing and OARS skills and,
    25–26, 32–35, 33t, 34t, 35t
  overview, 4, 31–32, 39
  in practice, 37–38, 38t
  tips for the initial session, 36–37
Entitlement
  assessment and, 71t
  criminogenic thinking and, 138t
Estimating the likelihood, 161–162, 163
Evoking intrinsic motivation, 25–26, 116–121, 118f,
    119t. *See also* Intrinsic motivation; Motivation
Excitement demands
  assessment and, 71t
  criminogenic thinking and, 139t
Expectations, 12
Exploitation
  assessment and, 72t
  criminogenic thinking and, 139t
Exploratory stance, 32, 39

F

Fact gathering, 39
Family factors
  assessment and, 67–68, 76–77
  case formulation and, 96f–104f, 109–114
  changing family dynamics, 204–208, 205f, 207f
  criminogenic thinking and, 137f
  forms to use in the case formulation and, 109–114
  overview, 18t
  risks–thoughts–decisions (RTD) sequence and, 141, 149
  scripts for, 76–77, 149, 210
  template for report writing and, 253
Feedback
  documentation and, 249–250, 266
  employment and, 186, 187
  regarding the assessment and treatment plan report,
    254, 261, 261f
  scripts for, 124, 131
  standardized tests and, 124, 125t

First impressions
    employment and, 183–184
    overview, 187
    restructuring friendships and, 202
Flexibility, 10–11
Focusing
    lack of agreement on, 125
    motivational interviewing (MI), 25–26
    overview, 121, 126
    scripts for, 123, 124, 127–131
    strategies for, 121–124, 122*t*, 125*t*
Focusing questions, 122, 122*t*, 126
Friendships. *See also* Peer factors; Relationships
    restructuring, 199–203, 201*f*, 203*f*
    scripts for, 209
Frustration tolerance, 228, 228*f*
Functioning, 5, 11. *See also* Goals

G

Gender-related differences, 16
Global negative ratings of others, 228, 228*f*
Goals. *See also* Collaborative goals; Functioning;
    Recidivism; Reductions in criminal behavior
    compared to values, 44–45, 53
    overview, 5, 8–9, 13, 28, 281
    strategies for establishing, 121–124, 122*t*, 125*t*, 126
    values and, 42–43, 48–50
Good lives model (GLM), 27–28, 43
Grandiosity
    assessment and, 71*t*
    criminogenic thinking and, 138*t*

H

Habits, 173–174, 215–226, 220*f*, 223*f*, 225*f*. *See also*
    Substance abuse/misuse
Halfway houses, 6, 217
Health concerns
    case formulation and, 92*t*, 96*f*–104*f*
    forms to use in the case formulation and, 109–114
History of criminal/antisocial behavior
    assessment and, 67, 74–75
    case formulation and, 90–91, 92–93, 96*f*–104*f*,
        109–114
    forms to use in the case formulation and, 109–114
    overview, 18*t*
    script for assessing, 74–75
    template for report writing and, 252–253
Homework
    noncompliance with, 157–158
    overview, 11, 12*f*
    substance use and abuse and, 218, 224–226, 225*f*
    values and, 49–50

Honesty
    employment and, 185–186
    lifestyle changes and, 174
Hostility
    assessment and, 71*t*, 72*t*
    criminogenic thinking and, 138*t*, 139*t*
Housing factors
    case formulation and, 92*t*, 96*f*–104*f*
    forms to use in the case formulation and, 109–114

I

Immediate Thinking. *See also* Automatic thoughts;
    Thinking Helpsheet (Form 9.1)
    overview, 163
    restructuring interventions and, 158–163, 159*f*
    scripts for, 166–169
Imminence, outcome, 90
Impressions, first
    employment and, 183–184
    overview, 187
    restructuring friendships and, 202
Incarceration, 7–8, 8–9
Individual domains, 94*f*–95*f*
Individualized treatment, 19
Initial sessions
    coding sheet for, 37–38, 41
    engagement and, 36–37
    overview, 39
Inmate. *See* Justice-involved clients (JICs)
Insight, 24–25
Integrity, 185–186
Intellectual disability
    case formulation and, 92*t*, 96*f*–104*f*
    forms to use in the case formulation and, 109–114
Intermediate beliefs (attitudes, rules, and assumptions),
    22–23, 23*t*. *See also* Thinking patterns
International Classification of Diseases, 10th revision
    (ICD-10), 9
Interventions. *See also* Treatment
    motivational interviewing (MI), 25–27
    overview, 4
    treatment summary report, 263, 266, 267*f*–268*f*
Interview skills, 183–184, 187. *See also* Employment
Intrinsic motivation, 25, 28. *See also* Evoking intrinsic
    motivation; Motivation
Irrational beliefs, 21–24, 23*t*

J

Job search, 184–185, 187. *See also* Employment
Job skills, 182–183, 187. *See also* Employment
Judgment, 107
Judgmental statements, 41

Justice-involved clients (JICs)
    overview, 3–4, 13
    statistics regarding, 7–8
    terminology, viii–ix
    working with, 4–5
Justifications. *See also* Sustain talk
    assessment and, 72*t*
    criminogenic thinking and, 139*t*
    motivational interviewing (MI) and, 27
    overview, 116
Juvenile delinquent. *See* Justice-involved clients (JICs)

L

Labels, 9–10, 13
Lack of connection to work/school, 18*t*
Least resistance, path of
    assessment and, 72*t*
    criminogenic thinking and, 139*t*
Leisure time activities. *See also* Lifestyle
    assessment and, 68–69, 83
    case formulation and, 96*f*–104*f*, 109–114
    criminogenic thinking and, 137*f*
    forms to use in the case formulation and, 109–114
    overview, 18*t*, 173, 174–179, 177*f*, 178*f*, 187
    risks–thoughts–decisions (RTD) sequence and, 148
    scripts for, 83, 148, 188–189
Levels of cognitions, 22. *See also* Cognitions
Life Areas That Put Me at Risk (Form 7.1), 132
Lifestyle. *See also* Behavior patterns; Daily activities;
        Leisure time activities; Routines
    changing substance use patterns and, 215–226, 220*f*,
        223*f*, 225*f*
    employment and education and, 179–187, 181*f*, 183*f*
    managing anger, 226–234, 228*f*, 231*f*–232*f*, 234*t*
    overview, 19, 173–174, 187
    scripts for, 188–191
Likelihood estimations, 161–162, 163
Listening
    engagement and, 36, 39
    strategies for focusing conversations and, 121–124,
        122*t*, 125*t*
Log of Weekly Substance Use (Form 12.2)
    complete, 241
    overview, 221, 222
    scripts for, 236
Looking at My Close Friends (Form 11.1)
    complete, 211
    examples of, 201*f*
    overview, 200
Looking at My Family and Romantic Relationship
    (Form 11.3)
    complete, 213
    examples of, 205*f*
    overview, 204

Looking at My Substance Use (Form 12.1)
    complete, 240
    examples of, 220*f*
    overview, 219, 221

M

Maladaptive leisure time. *See also* Leisure time
    activities
    assessment and, 68–69, 83
    case formulation and, 96*f*–104*f*
    criminogenic thinking and, 137*f*
    forms to use in the case formulation and, 109–114
    overview, 18*t*
    risks–thoughts–decisions (RTD) sequence and, 148
    scripts for, 83, 148
Mandated treatment, 28
Measure of Offender Thinking Styles, 22
Measures of Criminal Attitudes and Associates, 22
Mental health factors
    case formulation and, 92*t*
    gender-related differences and, 16
    risk domains and, 16–17, 28
    template for report writing and, 253
    treatment and, 137
    values and, 53, 54
Menu of options, 123
Minimization. *See also* Sustain talk
    assessment and, 72*t*
    criminogenic thinking and, 139*t*
    motivational interviewing (MI) and, 27
    overview, 116
    working with justice-involved clients and, 4
Mobilizing change talk, 117. *See also* Change talk
Modeling, 136
"Moderate Four" risk factors, 15. *See also* Risk domains
Monitoring interventions
    anger episode model and, 229–230, 231*f*–232*f*
    overview, 136, 155–158, 163
    scripts for, 164
    substance use and abuse and, 219, 221
Motivation
    enhancing, 24–27
    evoking, 116–121, 118*f*, 119*t*
    overview, 28, 281
    values and, 43–44
    working with justice-involved clients and, 5
Motivational interviewing (MI)
    discrepancy between values and decisions and, 51
    engagement and, 32–35, 33*t*, 34*t*, 35*t*
    overview, 25–27, 116, 281
My Typical Weekday (Form 10.1)
    complete, 192–193
    examples of, 177*f*
    overview, 176

N

Need, 117, 118, 119*t*
Need principle, 19
Negative assumptions, 228, 228*f*
Neutralizations, 21

O

OARS skills (open questions, affirmations, reflections, summarizations)
  coding sheet for, 37–38, 41
  engagement and, 32–35, 33*t*, 34*t*, 35*t*
  motivational interviewing (MI) and, 26
  opening statements and, 36–37
  overview, 25–26, 39
  in practice, 37
Offender. *See* Justice-involved clients (JICs)
Open questions. *See also* OARS skills (open questions, affirmations, reflections, summarizations)
  change talk and, 117–118
  coding sheet for, 41
  engagement and, 32, 33*t*
  focusing and, 122, 122*t*
  motivational interviewing (MI), 25
  responding to sustain talk and, 119–120, 119*t*
Opening statements
  coding sheet for, 37–38, 41
  engagement and, 36–37
  examples of, 40
  overview, 39
  scripts for, 73
Opportunity, 90–91
Optimism, 13
Outcome, 90, 228*f*, 229
Outpatient counseling, 40

P

Parole officer, ix, 6
Parolees, 6. *See also* Justice-involved clients (JICs)
Path of least resistance
  assessment and, 72*t*
  criminogenic thinking and, 139*t*
Patient. *See* Justice-involved clients (JICs)
Peer factors. *See also* Antisocial companions; Friendships; Relationships
  assessment and, 68, 81–82
  case formulation and, 96*f*–104*f*
  criminogenic thinking and, 137*f*
  forms to use in the case formulation and, 109–114
  overview, 18*t*
  restructuring friendships and, 199–203, 201*f*, 203*f*

risks–thoughts–decisions (RTD) sequence and, 141, 142–144, 147
  scripts for, 81–82, 147, 209
Personal experience of anger, 228, 228*f*. *See also* Anger dysregulation
Perspective taking, 233–234, 235
Physical health
  case formulation and, 92*t*, 96*f*–104*f*
  forms to use in the case formulation and, 109–114
Positive psychology movement, 27
Positive reinforcement, 49–50
Power
  assessment and, 71*t*
  criminogenic thinking and, 138*t*
Practitioners, ix
Predicting risk, 89–91. *See also* Risk level; Risk domains
Prediction, 107
Preparatory change talk, 116–117. *See also* Change talk
Present-moment focus, 36
Pretrial defendants, 6, 24. *See also* Justice-involved clients (JICs)
Preventive orientation, 19
Priorities. *See also* Values
  clarifying, 27–28
  overview, 53
  restructuring interventions and, 162, 163
Prison-based services, 40
Prisoner. *See* Justice-involved clients (JICs)
Probation officer, ix, 6
Probationers, 6. *See also* Justice-involved clients (JICs)
Probation/parole services, 40
Problem solving, 230, 235
Productive thinking, 162, 163
Programming. *See* Treatment
Progress
  monitoring and documenting, 262–263, 264*f*–265*f*
  progress review, 179, 203
  treatment summary report, 263, 266, 267*f*–268*f*
Promotions, 187
Prosocial goals, 43
Prosocial thinking, 162, 163
Psychological Inventory of Criminal Thinking Styles, 22
Psychopathic label, 9–10
Psychopathology, 92*t*, 96*f*–104*f*, 109–114. *See also* Mental health factors
Psychopathy Checklist—Revised (PCL-R), 9

Q

Questions, Answers, and Next Steps for My Substance Use (Form 12.3)
  complete, 242
  examples of, 223*f*
  overview, 222

Questions, closed
    coding sheet for, 41
    engagement and, 32, 33t
    minimizing the use of, 39
Questions, open. *See also* OARS skills (open questions,
        affirmations, reflections, summarizations)
    change talk and, 117–118
    coding sheet for, 41
    engagement and, 32, 33t
    focusing and, 122, 122t
    motivational interviewing (MI), 25
    responding to sustain talk and, 119–120, 119t
Questions to Ask Myself about Education and
        Employment (Form 10.5)
    complete, 196
    examples of, 181f
    overview, 181–182
Questions to Ask Myself about How I Spend My Time
        (Form 10.4)
    complete, 195
    examples of, 178f
    overview, 176, 178–179
Questions to Ask Myself about My Anger (Form 12.6),
        234, 246
Questions to Ask Myself about My Close Friends (Form
        11.2)
    complete, 212
    examples of, 203f
    overview, 202
Questions to Ask Myself about My Family and
        Romantic Relationships (Form 11.4), 206, 207f,
        214

R

Rationalizations, 218–219
Readiness to change, 286t. *See also* Change
Reasons, 117, 118, 119t
Recidivism, 5, 8–9, 13, 89–90. *See also* Goals; Risk
        domains
Recognizing Change Talk exercise, 117–118, 118f
Reductions in criminal behavior, 5, 8–9, 13. *See also*
        Goals; Risk domains
Referral mechanisms, 4–5, 13
Reflections. *See also* OARS skills (open questions,
        affirmations, reflections, summarizations)
    change talk and, 117–118
    coding sheet for, 41
    engagement and, 33–34, 35t
    motivational interviewing (MI), 25
Reinforcement
    change talk and, 126
    overview, 115
    strategies for focusing conversations and, 121–124,
        122t, 125t

Relationships. *See also* Peer factors; Restructuring
        relationships; Romantic relationships
    assessment and, 67–68, 71t, 76–77
    case formulation and, 96f–104f, 109–114
    changing family dynamics, 204–208, 205f, 207f
    criminogenic thinking and, 137f
    forms for, 109–114, 211–214
    overview, 18t, 198–199, 208
    risks–thoughts–decisions (RTD) sequence and, 141,
        149
    scripts for, 76–77, 149, 209–210
    template for report writing and, 253
Relaxation skills, 230, 235
Remorse, 4
Reoffending risks. *See* Risk domains
Report writing. *See also* Documentation
    clinical progress and, 262–263
    effective assessment and treatment plan report,
        250–251
    examples of, 255f–260f, 264f–265f
    forms for, 271–280
    overview, 249–250, 266
    providing feedback regarding, 254, 261, 261f
    scripts for, 269–270
    template for, 251–254, 255f–260f
    treatment summary report, 263, 266, 267f–268f
Resistance
    motivational interviewing (MI) and, 27
    substance use and abuse and, 218–219
Respectful stance, 36
Response bias, 285t
Responsibility taking, 4
Responsiveness, 10–11
Responsivity principle, 20–21, 28
Restructuring interventions, 136, 158–163, 159f,
        164–169
Restructuring relationships. *See also* Relationships
    changing family dynamics, 204–208, 205f, 207f
    close friendships and, 199–203, 201f, 203f
    forms for, 211–214
    overview, 198–199, 208
    scripts for, 200, 204, 209–210
Risk assessment, 251
Risk level, 88, 89–91. *See also* Predicting risk; Risk
        domains
Risk principle, 20–21, 28, 89
Risk reduction approach
    implications of, 18–20
    risk domains and, 15–21, 16t, 18t
Risk domains. *See also* Recidivism; Risk level
    assessment and, 66–70, 74–87
    case formulation and, 88, 91, 96f–104f, 108, 109–114
    change talk and, 126
    cognitive component of, 135–136
    criminogenic thinking and decision making and,
        137, 137f, 140–146

focusing and, 123, 125, 128
forms for, 109–114
overview, 11, 12f, 15–21, 16t, 18t, 28, 281
scripts for, 74–87
standardized tests and, 284t
treatment planner focus on, 17–18, 18t
values and, 43
Risk–need–responsivity (RNR) model, 15, 19, 20–21
Risks–thoughts–decisions (RTD) sequence, 141–144, 145–146, 147–152
Role play
    employment and, 186
    restructuring interventions and, 158–161
    scripts for, 166–167
Romantic relationships. *See also* Relationships
    assessment and, 67–68, 76–77
    case formulation and, 96f–104f
    changing family dynamics, 204–208, 205f, 207f
    criminogenic thinking and, 137f
    forms to use in the case formulation and, 109–114
    overview, 18t
    risks–thoughts–decisions (RTD) sequence and, 141, 149
    scripts for, 76–77, 149
    template for report writing and, 253
Routines, 173–179, 177f, 178f, 187. *See also* Lifestyle

S

Schemas. *See* Core beliefs (schemas)
School, connection to
    assessment and, 68, 78–79
    case formulation and, 96f–104f, 109–114
    criminogenic thinking and, 137f
    forms to use in the case formulation and, 109–114
    overview, 18t
    risks–thoughts–decisions (RTD) sequence and, 141, 151
    scripts for, 78–79, 151
    template for report writing and, 253
Scripts
    academic functioning, 78–79, 151
    activity monitoring, 188–189
    anger dysregulation, 87, 152, 239
    assessment, 66–70, 73–87, 131, 269–270
    Better Thinking, 166–169
    change and, 237–238
    criminogenic thinking and decision making and, 86, 141–144
    discrepancy between values and decisions, 51
    employment, 151, 190–191
    family factors, 76–77, 149, 210
    feedback, 124, 131
    focusing, 123, 124, 127–131
    Immediate Thinking, 166–169

leisure time activities, 83, 148, 188–189
lifestyle changes and, 188–191
monitoring assignments, 164
opening statements, 37, 40, 73
overview, vii–viii
peer factors, 81–82, 147, 200, 209
relationships, 76–77, 149, 200, 204, 209–210
report writing and, 269–270
restructuring interventions, 200, 209–210
risk domains, 74–87
risks–thoughts–decisions (RTD) sequence, 147–152
role plays, 166–167
romantic relationships, 76–77, 149
substance use and abuse, 150, 236–238
Thinking Helpsheet (Form 9.1), 164–165
thinking pattern impact (TPI) analysis, 153–154
values, 45, 48, 55–59
Self-efficacy, 50
Self-monitoring, 229–230, 231f–232f
Session Record Template (Form 13.3)
    complete, 278
    examples of, 264f–265f
    overview, 262–263
Sessions
    coding sheet for, 37–38, 41
    engagement and, 36–37
    overview, 10–11, 12t, 39
Severity, outcome, 90
Sexual offenders
    base rate neglect and, 107
    restructuring friendships and, 199–200
Situational reinforcement contingencies, 136
Skills-building orientation, 11
Social domains, 94f–95f
Social skills
    restructuring friendships and, 202
    template for report writing and, 253
Sociopathic label, 9–10
Standardized tests
    focusing and, 124, 125t
    providing feedback regarding, 261, 264f–265f
    recommendations for, 283–284, 284t–286t
    scripts for, 131
Structure of sessions, 11
Substance abuse/misuse
    assessment and, 69, 84–85
    case formulation and, 96f–104f, 109–114
    changing substance use patterns and, 215–226, 220f, 223f, 225f
    criminogenic thinking and, 137f
    forms for, 109–114, 240–243
    overview, 18t, 234–235
    restructuring friendships and, 199–200
    risks–thoughts–decisions (RTD) sequence and, 141, 150
    scripts for, 84–85, 150, 236–238
    standardized tests and, 285t

Summarizations. *See also* OARS skills (open questions, affirmations, reflections, summarizations)
    coding sheet for, 41
    discussing in sessions, 12*f*
    engagement and, 34, 35*t*
    motivational interviewing (MI), 25
Supervision, 12*f*. *See also* Treatment
Support from others, 224–226, 225*f*
Supportive stance, 36
Sustain talk. *See also* Change talk; Justifications; Minimization
    evoking, 120
    overview, 116, 126
    recognizing, 118*f*
    responding to, 119–120
    substance use and abuse and, 219
Sympathy, 4
Synergistic nature of risk domains, 19–20. *See also* Risk domains

T

Taking steps, 117, 118, 119*t*
Termination of care, 7
Texas Christian University Criminal Thinking Scales, 22
Therapeutic relationship. *See also* Working alliance
    engagement and, 31–32
    overview, 173–174
    working with justice-involved clients and, 4
Thinking Helpsheet (Form 9.1)
    complete, 170
    monitoring assignments and, 155–157
    noncompliance with homework and, 157–158
    overview, 163
    restructuring interventions and, 158–163, 159*f*
    scripts for assigning and introducing, 164–165
Thinking pattern impact (TPI) analysis, 144 145, 153–154
Thinking patterns. *See also* Criminogenic thinking
    anger and, 226–234, 228, 228*f*, 231*f*–232*f*, 234*t*
    assessment and, 71*t*–72*t*, 86
    criminogenic thinking and decision making and, 140–146
    focusing and, 123, 129–130
    levels of, 136–137, 137*f*, 138*t*–139*t*
    monitoring assignments and, 155–158
    overview, 145–146
    restructuring interventions and, 158–163, 159*f*
    script for assessing, 86
    substance use and abuse and, 218
    that promote criminality, 21–24, 23*t*
Time management, 184–185, 187
Transitional housing programs, 6
Transitional summary, 34, 35*t*. *See also* Summarizations
Transitions, 187

Treatment. *See also* Interventions
    diagnosis and, 9–10
    effectiveness of, 8–9
    expectations of, 12
    motivation for change and, 24–27
    overview, viii, ix, 13
    overview of sessions in general, 10–11, 12*t*
    settings for, 5–7
    treatment summary report, 263, 266, 267*f*–268*f*
Treatment goals. *See also* Collaborative goals; Functioning; Recidivism; Reductions in criminal behavior
    compared to values, 44–45, 53
    overview, 5, 8–9, 13, 28, 281
    strategies for establishing, 121–124, 122*t*, 125*t*, 126
    values and, 42–43, 48–50
Treatment plans and planning
    assessment and, 65–66
    case formulation and, 88, 96*f*–104*f*
    documentation and, 249–250
    overview, 10, 10*t*, 173–174
    providing feedback regarding, 254, 261, 261*f*
    report writing and, 250–251, 266
    template for report writing and, 251–254, 255*f*–260*f*
    values and, 43
Treatment Summary Report Template (Form 13.4)
    complete, 279–280
    examples of, 267*f*–268*f*
    overview, 263, 266
Treatment targets, 91–93, 92*t*, 94*f*–95*f*, 105
Triggering event, 228, 228*f*, 235
Two Voices role play, 158–161, 159*f*, 163, 166–167

U

Underestimating
    assessment and, 72*t*
    criminogenic thinking and, 139*t*

V

Values
    clarifying, 27–28
    compared to goals, 44–45
    discrepancy between decisions and, 50–53, 54, 58–59
    forms for, 46*f* 47*f*, 60 61
    identifying and discussing, 45–50, 46*f*–47*f*
    overview, 53–54
    reasons to work on with JICs, 42–44
    restructuring interventions and, 162, 163
    scripts for, 55–59
    substance use and abuse and, 218
Values Helpsheet (Form 4.1)
    complete, 60–61
    discrepancy between values and decisions and, 50–51

examples of, 46f–47f
introducing, 55–56
overview, 45, 50

W

Work, connection to. *See also* Employment
  assessment and, 68, 78–79
  case formulation and, 96f–104f, 109–114

criminogenic thinking and, 137f
forms to use in the case formulation and, 109–114
overview, 18t
risks–thoughts–decisions (RTD) sequence and, 141, 151
scripts for, 78–79, 151
template for report writing and, 253
Work Opportunity Tax Credit (WOTC), 180
Working alliance. *See also* Therapeutic relationship
  engagement and, 31–32
  working with justice-involved clients and, 4–5